RN Maternal Newborn Nursing
REVIEW MODULE EDITION 10.0

Contributors

Norma Jean E. Henry, MSN/Ed, RN

Mendy McMichael, DNP, MSN

Janean Johnson, MSN, RN, CNE

Agnes DiStasi, DNP, RN, CNE

Pamela Roland, MSN, RN

Kellie L. Wilford, MSN, RN

Marsha S. Barlow, MSN, RN

Consultants

Jenni L. Hoffman, DNP, FNP-C, CLNC

Jessica Johnson, MSN, RN

Christi Blair, MSN, RN

Director of content review: Kristen Lawler

Director of development: Derek Prater

Project management: Janet Hines, Nicole Burke

Coordination of content review: Norma Jean E. Henry, Mendy McMichael

Copy editing: Kelly Von Lunen, Derek Prater

Layout: Spring Lenox, Randi Hardy

Illustrations: Randi Hardy

Online media: Morgan Smith, Ron Hanson, Nicole Lobdell, Brant Stacy

Cover design: Jason Buck

Interior book design: Spring Lenox

IMPORTANT NOTICE TO THE READER

User's Guide

Welcome to the Assessment Technologies Institute® RN Maternal Newborn Nursing Review Module Edition 10.0. The mission of ATI's Content Mastery Series® Review Modules is to provide user-friendly compendiums of nursing knowledge that will:
- Help you locate important information quickly.
- Assist in your learning efforts.
- Provide exercises for applying your nursing knowledge.
- Facilitate your entry into the nursing profession as a newly licensed nurse.

This newest edition of the Review Modules has been redesigned to optimize your learning experience. We've fit more content into less space and have done so in a way that will make it even easier for you to find and understand the information you need.

ORGANIZATION

This Review Module is organized into units covering antepartum, intrapartum, postpartum, and newborn nursing care. Chapters within these units conform to one of three organizing principles for presenting the content.
- Nursing concepts
- Procedures
- Complications of pregnancy

Nursing concepts chapters begin with an overview describing the central concept and its relevance to nursing. Subordinate themes are covered in outline form to demonstrate relationships and present the information in a clear, succinct manner.

Procedures chapters include an overview describing the procedure(s) covered in the chapter. These chapters provide nursing knowledge relevant to each procedure, including indications, nursing considerations, and complications.

Complications of pregnancy chapters include an overview describing the complication; assessment, including risk factors and expected findings; and patient-centered care, including nursing care, medications, and client education.

ACTIVE LEARNING SCENARIOS AND APPLICATION EXERCISES

Each chapter includes opportunities for you to test your knowledge and to practice applying that knowledge. Active Learning Scenario exercises pose a nursing scenario and then direct you to use an ATI Active Learning Template (included at the back of this book) to record the important knowledge a nurse should apply to the scenario. An example is then provided to which you can compare your completed Active Learning Template. The Application Exercises include NCLEX-style questions, such as multiple-choice and multiple-select items, providing you with opportunities to practice answering the kinds of questions you might expect to see on ATI assessments or the NCLEX. After the Application Exercises, an answer key is provided, along with rationales.

NCLEX® CONNECTIONS

To prepare for the NCLEX-RN, it is important to understand how the content in this Review Module is connected to the NCLEX-RN test plan. You can find information on the detailed test plan at the National Council of State Boards of Nursing's website, www.ncsbn.org. When reviewing content in this Review Module, regularly ask yourself, "How does this content fit into the test plan, and what types of questions related to this content should I expect?"

To help you in this process, we've included NCLEX Connections at the beginning of each unit and with each question in the Application Exercises Answer Keys. The NCLEX Connections at the beginning of each unit point out areas of the detailed test plan that relate to the content within that unit. The NCLEX Connections attached to the Application Exercises Answer Keys demonstrate how each exercise fits within the detailed content outline. These NCLEX Connections will help you understand how the detailed content outline is organized, starting with major client needs categories and subcategories and followed by related content areas and tasks. The major client needs categories are:
- Safe and Effective Care Environment
  - Management of Care
  - Safety and Infection Control
- Health Promotion and Maintenance
- Psychosocial Integrity
- Physiological Integrity
  - Basic Care and Comfort
  - Pharmacological and Parenteral Therapies
  - Reduction of Risk Potential
  - Physiological Adaptation

An NCLEX Connection might, for example, alert you that content within a unit is related to:
- Health Promotion and Maintenance
  - Ante/Intra/Postpartum and Newborn Care
    - Assess client psychosocial response to pregnancy.

QSEN COMPETENCIES

As you use the Review Modules, you will note the integration of the Quality and Safety Education for Nurses (QSEN) competencies throughout the chapters. These competencies are integral components of the curriculum of many nursing programs in the United States and prepare you to provide safe, high-quality care as a newly licensed nurse. Icons appear to draw your attention to the six QSEN competencies.

Safety: The minimization of risk factors that could cause injury or harm while promoting quality care and maintaining a secure environment for clients, self, and others.

Patient-Centered Care: The provision of caring and compassionate, culturally sensitive care that addresses clients' physiological, psychological, sociological, spiritual, and cultural needs, preferences, and values.

Evidence-Based Practice: The use of current knowledge from research and other credible sources, on which to base clinical judgment and client care.

Informatics: The use of information technology as a communication and information-gathering tool that supports clinical decision-making and scientifically based nursing practice.

Quality Improvement: Care related and organizational processes that involve the development and implementation of a plan to improve health care services and better meet clients' needs.

Teamwork and Collaboration: The delivery of client care in partnership with multidisciplinary members of the health care team to achieve continuity of care and positive client outcomes.

ICONS

Icons are used throughout the Review Module to draw your attention to particular areas. Keep an eye out for these icons.

(N) This icon is used for NCLEX Connections.

(G) This icon indicates gerontological considerations, or knowledge specific to the care of older adult clients.

Qs This icon is used for content related to safety and is a QSEN competency. When you see this icon, take note of safety concerns or steps that nurses can take to ensure client safety and a safe environment.

Qpcc This icon is a QSEN competency that indicates the importance of a holistic approach to providing care.

Qebp This icon, a QSEN competency, points out the integration of research into clinical practice.

Qi This icon is a QSEN competency and highlights the use of information technology to support nursing practice.

Qqi This icon is used to focus on the QSEN competency of integrating planning processes to meet clients' needs.

Qtc This icon highlights the QSEN competency of care delivery using an interprofessional approach.

M This icon appears at the top-right of pages and indicates availability of an online media supplement, such as a graphic, animation, or video. If you have an electronic copy of the Review Module, this icon will appear alongside clickable links to media supplements. If you have a hard copy version of the Review Module, visit www.atitesting.com for details on how to access these features.

FEEDBACK

ATI welcomes feedback regarding this Review Module. Please provide comments to comments@atitesting.com.

Table of Contents

UNIT 2   *Intrapartum Nursing Care*

SECTION: *Labor and Delivery*

UNIT 4

Newborn Nursing Care

SECTION: *Low-Risk Newborn*

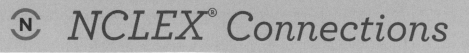

When reviewing the following chapters, keep in mind the relevant topics and tasks of the NCLEX outline, in particular:

Client Needs: Health Promotion and Maintenance

ANTE/INTRA/POSTPARTUM AND NEWBORN CARE: Provide prenatal care and education.

DEVELOPMENTAL STAGES AND TRANSITIONS: Identify expected body image changes associated with the client's developmental age.

LIFESTYLE CHOICES: Assess client's need/desire for contraception.

Client Needs: Physiological Adaptation

ALTERATIONS IN BODY SYSTEMS: Identify signs of potential prenatal complications.

Client Needs: Reduction of Risk Potential

DIAGNOSTIC TESTS: Monitor results of maternal and fetal diagnostic tests.

POTENTIAL FOR COMPLICATIONS OF DIAGNOSTIC TESTS/ TREATMENTS/PROCEDURES: Monitor the client for signs of bleeding.

SYSTEM SPECIFIC ASSESSMENTS: Perform focused assessment.

Client Needs: Basic Care and Comfort

NON-PHARMACOLOGICAL COMFORT INTERVENTIONS: Assess the client's need for alternative and/or complementary therapy.

CHAPTER 1 *Contraception*

Contraception refers to strategies or devices used to reduce the risk of fertilization or implantation in an attempt to prevent pregnancy. The human ovum can be fertilized no later than 12 to 24 hr after ovulation. Motile sperm have been recovered from the uterus and oviducts as long as 60 hr after coitus, but their ability to fertilize the ovum probably lasts no longer than 24 to 48 hr.

A nurse should assess clients' need, desire, and preferences for contraception. A thorough discussion of benefits, risks, and alternatives of each method should be discussed. Qᴘᴄᴄ

Sexual partners often make a joint decision regarding a desired preference (vasectomy or tubal ligation). Postpartum discharge instructions should include the discussion of future contraceptive plans.

Expected outcomes for family planning methods consist of preventing pregnancy until a desired time. Nurses should support clients in making the decision that is best for their individual situations.

Methods of contraception include natural family planning; barrier, hormonal, and intrauterine methods; and surgical procedures.

NATURAL FAMILY PLANNING (FERTILITY AWARENESS-BASED METHODS)

Abstinence

Abstaining from having sexual intercourse eliminates the possibility of sperm entering the vagina.

CLIENT EDUCATION: Refrain from sexual intercourse. This method can be associated with saying "no," but it also can incorporate saying "yes" to other gratifying sexual activities, such as affectionate touching, communication, holding hands, kissing, massage, and oral and manual stimulation.

ADVANTAGES
- Most effective method of birth control.
- Abstinence during fertile periods (rhythm method) can be used, but it requires an understanding of the menstrual cycle and fertility awareness.
- Can eliminate the risk of sexually transmitted infections (STIs) if there is no genitalia contact.

DISADVANTAGES: Requires self-control

RISKS: If complete abstinence is maintained, there are no risks.

Coitus interruptus (withdrawal)

Withdrawal of penis from vagina prior to ejaculation.

CLIENT EDUCATION: Be aware of fluids leaking from the penis.

ADVANTAGES: Possible choice for monogamous couples who do not have another contraceptives available.

DISADVANTAGES
- One of the least effective methods of contraception.
- No protection against STIs.

RISKS
- Influenced by male partner's control.
- Leakage of fluid that contains spermatozoa prior to ejaculation can be deposited in vagina.
- Risk of pregnancy.

Calendar method

A woman records her menstrual cycle by calculating her fertile period based on the assumption that ovulation occurs about 14 days before the onset of her next menstrual cycle, and avoids intercourse during that period. Also taken into account is the timing of intercourse with this method because sperm are viable for 48 to 120 hr, and the ovum is viable for about 24 hr.

CLIENT EDUCATION
- Accurately record the number of days in each cycle counting from the first day of menses for a period of at least six cycles.
- The start of the fertile period is figured by subtracting 18 days from the number of days in the woman's shortest cycle.
- The end of the fertile period is established by subtracting 11 days from the number of days of the longest cycle.

> For example:
> Shortest cycle, 26 - 18 = 8th day
> Longest cycle, 30 - 11 = 19th day
> Fertile period is days 8 through 19.
> Refrain from intercourse during these
> days to avoid conception.

ADVANTAGES
- Most useful when combined with basal body temperature or cervical mucus method.
- Inexpensive

DISADVANTAGES
- Not a very reliable technique.
- Does not protect against STIs
- Requires accurate record-keeping.
- Requires compliance regarding abstinence during fertile periods.

RISKS
- Various factors can affect and change the time of ovulation and cause unpredictable menstrual cycles.
- Risk of pregnancy.

Basal body temperature

Temperature can drop slightly at the time of ovulation. This can be used to facilitate conception, or be used as a natural contraceptive.

CLIENT EDUCATION: Measure oral temperature prior to getting out of bed each morning to monitor ovulation.

ADVANTAGES: Inexpensive, convenient, and no adverse effects

DISADVANTAGES
- Reliability can be influenced by many variables that can cause inaccurate interpretation of temperature changes, such as stress, fatigue, illness, alcohol, and warmth of sleeping environment.
- Does not protect against STIs.

RISKS: Risk of pregnancy

Symptom-based method (cervical mucus)

Fertility awareness method based on ovulation. Ovulation occurs approximately 14 days prior to the next menstrual cycle, which is when a woman is fertile. Following ovulation, the cervical mucus becomes thin and flexible under the influence of estrogen and progesterone to allow for sperm viability and motility. The ability for the mucus to stretch between the fingers is greatest during ovulation. This is referred to as spinnbarkeit sign.

CLIENT EDUCATION
- Engage in good hand hygiene prior to and following assessment.
- Begin examining mucus from the last day of the menstrual cycle.
- Mucus is obtained from the vaginal introitus. It is not necessary to reach into the vagina to the cervix.
- Do not douche prior to assessment.

ADVANTAGES
- A woman can become knowledgeable in recognizing her own mucus characteristics at ovulation, and self-evaluation can be very accurate.
- Self-evaluation of cervical mucus can be diagnostically helpful in determining the start of ovulation while breastfeeding, noting the commencement of menopause, and planning a desired pregnancy.

DISADVANTAGES
- Some women are uncomfortable with touching their genitals and mucus, and therefore find this method objectionable.
- Does not protect against STIs.

RISKS/POSSIBLE COMPLICATIONS
- Assessment of cervical mucus characteristics can be inaccurate if mucus is mixed with semen, blood, contraceptive foams, or discharge from infections.
- Risk of pregnancy.

BARRIER METHODS

Male condom

A thin rubber sheath a man wears on his penis during sexual intercourse as a contraceptive or as protection against infection. Male condoms can be made of latex rubber, polyurethane, or natural membrane.

CLIENT EDUCATION
- Place a condom on the erect penis, leaving an empty space at the tip for a sperm reservoir.
- Following ejaculation, withdraw the penis from the vagina while holding the rim of the condom to prevent any semen spillage to the vulva or vaginal area.
- Can be used in conjunction with spermicidal gel or cream to increase effectiveness.

ADVANTAGES
- Protects against STIs and involves the male in the birth control method.
- No adverse effects.
- Readily accessible.

DISADVANTAGES

- High rate of noncompliance.
- Can reduce spontaneity of intercourse.
- The penis must be erect to apply a condom.
- Withdrawing the penis while still erect, can interfere with sexual intercourse.

RISKS/POSSIBLE COMPLICATIONS/CONTRAINDICATIONS

- Condoms can rupture or leak, potentially resulting in pregnancy.
- Condoms have a one-time usage, which creates a replacement cost.
- Condoms made of latex should not be worn by those who are sensitive or allergic to latex.
- Only water-soluble lubricants should be used with latex condoms to avoid condom breakage.

Female condom

Vaginal sheath made of nitrile, a nonlatex synthetic rubber with flexible rings on both ends

CLIENT EDUCATION: The closed end of the pouch is inserted into the vagina by the client prior to intercourse and anchored around the cervix. The open ring covers the labia. The condom is removed and thrown away after intercourse.

ADVANTAGES: Offers protection against pregnancy and STIs

Diaphragm and spermicide

A dome-shaped cup with a flexible rim made of silicone that fits snugly over the cervix with spermicidal cream or gel placed into the dome and around the rim. Diaphragms are available in different sizes.

CLIENT EDUCATION

- A client should be properly fitted with a diaphragm by a provider.
- Replaced every 2 years and refitted for a 20% weight fluctuation, after abdominal or pelvic surgery, and after every pregnancy.
- Requires proper insertion and removal. Prior to coitus, the diaphragm is inserted vaginally over the cervix with spermicidal jelly or cream that is applied to the cervical side of the dome and around the rim. The diaphragm can be inserted up to 6 hr before intercourse and must stay in place 6 hr after intercourse but for no more than 24 hr.
- Spermicide must be reapplied with each act of coitus.
- A client should empty her bladder prior to insertion of the diaphragm.
- Diaphragm should be washed with mild soap and warm water after each use

ADVANTAGES: Gives a woman more control over contraception

DISADVANTAGES

- Diaphragms are inconvenient, interfere with spontaneity, and require reapplication with spermicidal gel, cream, or foam with each act of coitus to be effective.
- Requires a prescription and a visit to a provider.
- Must be inserted correctly to be effective.
- Does not protect against STIs.

RISKS/POSSIBLE COMPLICATIONS/CONTRAINDICATIONS

- Not recommended for clients who have a history of toxic shock syndrome (TSS), or frequent, recurrent urinary tract infections.
- Increased risk of acquiring TSS, which is caused by a bacterial infection. Clinical findings include high fever, a faint feeling, drop in blood pressure, watery diarrhea, headache, and muscle aches.
- Proper hand hygiene aids in prevention of TSS, as well as removing diaphragm promptly at 6 hr following coitus.
- Risk of allergic reaction

Cervical cap and spermicide

Silicone rubber cap that fits snugly around the base of the cervix. Cervical caps come in three sizes.

CLIENT EDUCATION

- Can be inserted up to 6 hr before intercourse and needs to be left in place at least 6 hr after intercourse but for no more than 48 hr at a time.
- Replaced every 2 years and refitted after any gynecological surgery, birth, or any major weight fluctuation.
- Cervical cap should be washed with mild soap and warm water after each use

DISADVANTAGES

- Possible risk of acquiring TSS
- Risk of allergic reaction
- Does not protect against STIs

RISKS/POSSIBLE COMPLICATIONS/CONTRAINDICATIONS: Not for women who have abnormal Pap test results or those who have a history of TSS

Contraceptive sponge

Small, round, polyurethane sponge containing spermicide

CLIENT EDUCATION

- It is designed to fit over the cervix, and is one size fits all.
- Should be left in place for 6 hr after intercourse and provides protection for up to 24 hr.

DISADVANTAGES: Does not protect against STIs

HORMONAL METHODS

Combined oral contraceptives

Hormonal contraception containing estrogen and progestin, which acts by suppressing ovulation, thickening the cervical mucus to block semen, and altering the uterine decidua to prevent implantation

CLIENT EDUCATION
- Medication requires a prescription and follow-up appointments with the provider.
- Medication requires consistent and proper use to be effective.
- Instruct the client to observe for adverse effects and danger signs of medication. Signs include chest pain, shortness of breath, leg pain from a possible clot, headache, eye problems from a stroke, and hypertension.
- In the event of a client missing a dose, instruct the client that if one pill is missed, take one as soon as possible; if two or three pills are missed, follow the manufacturer's instructions. Instruct the client on the use of alternative forms of contraception or abstinence to prevent pregnancy until regular dosing is resumed.

ADVANTAGES
- Highly effective if taken correctly and consistently.
- Noncontraceptive benefits of combined hormonal contraception containing low-dose estrogen (less than 35 mcg) include decreased menstrual blood loss, decreased iron deficiency anemia, regulation of menorrhagia and irregular cycles, and reduced incidence of dysmenorrhea and premenstrual symptoms. Oral contraception also offers protection against endometrial, ovarian, and colon cancer, reduces the incidence of benign breast disease, improves acne, and protects against the development of functional ovarian cysts.

DISADVANTAGES
- Do not protect against STIs.
- Can increase the risk of thromboembolism, stroke, heart attack, hypertension, gallbladder disease, liver tumor.
- Exacerbates conditions affected by fluid retention, such as migraine, epilepsy, asthma, kidney, or heart disease.
- Adverse effects include headache, nausea, breast tenderness, and breakthrough bleeding. (Common adverse effects of estrogen component include nausea, breast tenderness, fluid retention. Common adverse effects of progestin component include increased appetite, tiredness, depression, breast tenderness, oily skin and scalp, and hirsutism.)

RISKS/POSSIBLE COMPLICATIONS/CONTRAINDICATIONS
- Women who have a history of thromboembolic disorders, stroke, heart attack, coronary artery disease, gallbladder disease, cirrhosis or liver tumor, headache with focal neurological symptoms, uncontrolled hypertension, diabetes mellitus with vascular involvement, breast or estrogen-related cancers, pregnancy, lactating, less than 6 weeks postpartum, or smoking (if over 35 years of age) are advised not to take oral contraceptive medications.
- Oral contraceptive effectiveness decreases when taking medications that affect liver enzymes, such as anticonvulsants and some antibiotics.

Progestin-only pills (Minipill)

Oral progestins that provide the same action as combined oral contraceptives

CLIENT EDUCATION
- Take the pill at the same time daily to ensure effectiveness secondary to a low dose of progestin.
- The client cannot miss a pill.
- The client can need another form of birth control during the first month of use to prevent pregnancy.

ADVANTAGES
- Fewer adverse effects when compared with a combined oral contraceptive.
- Considered safe to take while breastfeeding.

DISADVANTAGES
- Less effective in suppressing ovulation than combined oral contraceptives.
- Increased occurrence of ovarian cysts.
- No protection against STIs.
- Adverse effects include breakthrough, irregular, vaginal bleeding (frequently reported/most common); headache; nausea; and breast tenderness.

RISKS/POSSIBLE COMPLICATIONS/CONTRAINDICATIONS
- Oral contraceptive effectiveness decreases when taking medications that affect liver enzymes, such as anticonvulsants and some antibiotics.
- Contraindications include: bariatric surgery, lupus, severe cirrhosis, liver tumors, current or past breast cancer

Emergency oral contraceptive

Morning-after pill that prevents fertilization from taking place

CLIENT EDUCATION
- Pill is taken within 72 hr after unprotected coitus.
- A provider will recommend an over-the-counter antiemetic to be taken 1 hr prior to each dose to counteract the adverse effects of nausea that can occur with high doses of estrogen and progestin.
- Advise a client to be evaluated for pregnancy if menstruation does not begin within 21 days.
- Provide client with counseling about contraception and modification of sexual behaviors that are risky.
- Considered a form of "emergency birth control."

ADVANTAGES
- Not taken on a regular basis.
- Anyone, regardless of age or gender, is allowed to purchase emergency oral contraceptive at a pharmacy.

DISADVANTAGES
- Nausea, heavier than normal menstrual bleeding, lower abdominal pain, fatigue, and headache.
- Does not provide long-term contraception.
- Does not terminate an established pregnancy.
- Does not protect against STIs.

RISKS/POSSIBLE COMPLICATIONS/CONTRAINDICATIONS
- Contraindicated if a client is pregnant or has undiagnosed abnormal vaginal bleeding.
- If menstruation does not start within 1 week of expected date, a client might be pregnant.

Transdermal contraceptive patch

Contains norelgestromin (progesterone) and ethinyl estradiol, which is delivered at continuous levels through the skin into subcutaneous tissue

CLIENT EDUCATION
- Apply the patch to dry skin overlying subcutaneous tissue of the buttock, abdomen, upper arm, or torso, excluding breast area.
- Requires patch replacement once a week.
- Apply the patch the same day of the week for 3 weeks with no application on the fourth week.

ADVANTAGES
- Maintains consistent blood levels of hormone.
- Avoids liver metabolism of medication because it is not absorbed in the gastrointestinal tract.
- Decreases risk of forgetting daily pill.

DISADVANTAGES
- Does not protect against STIs.
- Same adverse effects as oral contraceptives. Risk of deep-vein thrombosis and venous thromboembolism can be slightly higher in women using the patch because the hormones get into the bloodstream and are processed by the body differently than hormones from OCPs.
- Skin reaction can occur from patch application.

RISKS/POSSIBLE COMPLICATIONS/CONTRAINDICATIONS
- Same as those of oral contraceptives
- Avoid applying of patch to skin rashes or lesions.
- Less effective in women greater than 198 lb.

Injectable progestins

Medroxyprogesterone is an intramuscular or subcutaneous injection given to a female client every 11 to 13 weeks

CLIENT EDUCATION
- Start of injections should be during the first 5 days of a client's menstrual cycle and every 11 to 13 weeks thereafter. Injections in postpartum nonbreastfeeding women should begin within 5 days following delivery. For breastfeeding women, injections should start in the sixth week postpartum.
- Advise clients to keep follow-up appointments.
- Maintain an adequate intake of calcium and vitamin D.

ADVANTAGES
- Very effective and requires only four injections per year
- Does not impair lactation
- Possible absence of periods and decrease in bleeding
- Decreased risk of uterine cancer if used long-term

DISADVANTAGES
- Adverse effects include decrease in bone mineral density, weight gain, increase in depression, and irregular vaginal spotting or bleeding.
- Does not protect against STIs.
- Return to fertility can be delayed as long as up to 18 months after discontinuation.
- Should only be used as a long-term method of birth control (more than 2 years) if other birth control methods are inadequate.

RISKS/POSSIBLE COMPLICATIONS/CONTRAINDICATIONS
- Avoid massaging injection site following administration to avoid accelerating medication absorption, which will shorten the duration of its effectiveness.
- Contraindications include breast cancer, evidence of current cardiovascular disease, abnormal liver function, liver tumors, and unexplained vaginal bleeding.

Contraceptive vaginal ring

Contains etonogestrel and ethinyl estradiol that is delivered at continuous levels vaginally

CLIENT EDUCATION
- A client inserts the ring vaginally.
- Requires ring replacement after 3 weeks, and placement of new vaginal ring within 7 days. Insertion should occur on the same day of the week monthly.

ADVANTAGES
- Does not have to be fitted.
- Decreases the risk of forgetting to take the pill.
- Vaginal route of delivery increases bioavailability of hormones enabling lower dose and reducing adverse effects

DISADVANTAGES
- Does not protect against STIs.
- Same adverse effects as oral contraceptives.
- Some clients report discomfort during intercourse. The ring can be removed for up to 3 hr without compromising its effectiveness.

RISKS/POSSIBLE COMPLICATIONS/CONTRAINDICATIONS
- Blood clots, hypertension, stroke, heart attack
- Vaginal irritation, increased vaginal secretions, headache, weight gain, and nausea

Implantable progestin

Requires a minor surgical procedure to subdermally implant and remove a single rod containing etonogestrel on the inner side of the upper aspect of the arm

CLIENT EDUCATION: Avoid trauma to the area of implantation.

ADVANTAGES
- Effective continuous contraception for 3 years.
- Can be inserted immediately after abortion, miscarriage, childbirth, and while breastfeeding.
- Reversible.
- Can be used by mothers who are breastfeeding after 4 weeks postpartum.

DISADVANTAGES
- Etonogestrel can cause irregular menstrual bleeding.
- Does not protect against STIs.
- Adverse effects include irregular and unpredictable menstruation (most common), mood changes, headache, acne, depression, decreased bone density, and weight gain.

RISKS/POSSIBLE COMPLICATIONS/ CONTRAINDICATIONS
- Increased risk of ectopic pregnancy if pregnancy occurs.
- Contraindications include unexplained vaginal bleeding, lupus, severe cirrhosis, liver tumors, and breast cancer.

Intrauterine device (IUD)

A chemically active T-shaped device that is inserted through the cervix and placed in the uterus by the provider. Releases a chemical substance that damages sperm in transit to the uterine tubes and prevents fertilization. The most effective contraceptive methods at preventing pregnancy are the long acting reversible contraceptive (LARC) methods: implant and IUDs. IUDs can be used by nulliparous and multiparous women.

CLIENT EDUCATION: The device must be monitored monthly by clients after menstruation to ensure the presence of the small string that hangs from the device into the upper part of the vagina to rule out migration or expulsion of the device.

ADVANTAGES
- An IUD can maintain effectiveness for 1 to 10 years (hormonal IUD 3 to 5 years; copper IUD 10 years).
- Can be inserted immediately after abortion, miscarriage, childbirth, and while breastfeeding
- Contraception can be reversed with immediate return to fertility.
- Does not interfere with spontaneity.
- Safe for mothers who are breastfeeding.
- It is 99% effective in preventing pregnancy.
- Hormonal IUDs: decreased menstrual pain and heavy bleeding
- Copper IUD: no hormones so it's safe for women cautioned against hormonal birth control methods

DISADVANTAGES
- Can increase the risk of pelvic inflammatory disease, uterine perforation, or ectopic pregnancy and can be expelled.
- A client should report to the provider late or abnormal spotting or bleeding, abdominal pain or pain with intercourse, abnormal or foul-smelling vaginal discharge, fever, chills, a change in string length, or if IUD cannot be located.
- Does not protect from STIs.
- Hormonal IUD: spotting, irregular bleeding, headache, nausea, depression, breast tenderness
- Copper IUD: increase in menstrual pain and bleeding

RISKS/CONTRAINDICATIONS
- Best used by women in a monogamous relationship due to the risks of STIs
- Can cause irregular menstrual bleeding
- Risk of bacterial vaginosis, uterine perforation, or uterine expulsion
- Must be removed in the event of pregnancy

CONTRAINDICATIONS: Active pelvic infection, abnormal uterine bleeding, severe uterine distortion; for copper IUD also Wilson's diseases and copper allergy

TRANSCERVICAL STERILIZATION

- Insertion of small flexible agents through the vagina and cervix into the fallopian tubes. This results in the development of scar tissue in the tubes preventing conception.
- Examination must be done after 3 months to ensure fallopian tubes are blocked.

CLIENT EDUCATION: Normal activities can be resumed by most clients within 1 day of the procedure.

ADVANTAGES
- Quick procedure that requires no general anesthesia.
- Nonhormonal means of birth control.
- 99.8% effective in preventing pregnancy.
- Rapid return to normal activities of daily living.

DISADVANTAGES
- Not reversible.
- Not intended for use in the client who is postpartum.
- Delay in effectiveness for 3 months. An alternative means of birth control should be used until confirmation of blocked fallopian tubes occurs.
- Changes in menstrual patterns.
- Does not protect against STIs

RISKS/POSSIBLE COMPLICATIONS/CONTRAINDICATIONS
- Perforation can occur.
- Unwanted pregnancy can occur if a client has unprotected sexual intercourse during the first 3 months following the procedure.
- Increased risk of ectopic pregnancy if pregnancy occurs.

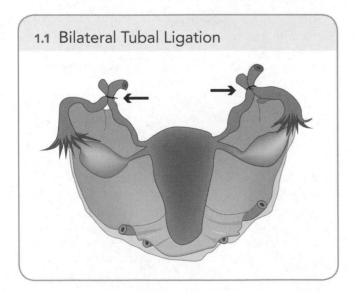

1.1 Bilateral Tubal Ligation

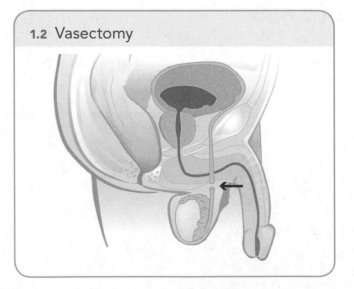

1.2 Vasectomy

SURGICAL METHODS

Female sterilization (bilateral tubal ligation)

A surgical procedure consisting of severance and/or burning or blocking the fallopian tubes to prevent fertilization

PROCEDURE: The cutting, burning, or blocking of the fallopian tubes to prevent the ovum from being fertilized by the sperm.

ADVANTAGES
- Permanent contraception.
- Can be done immediately after childbirth within 24 to 48 hr.
- Sexual function is unaffected.

DISADVANTAGES
- A surgical procedure carrying risks related to anesthesia, complications, infection, hemorrhage, or trauma
- Considered irreversible in the event that a client desires conception
- Does not protect against STIs

RISKS: Risk of ectopic pregnancy if pregnancy occurs

Male sterilization (vasectomy)

A surgical procedure consisting of ligation and severance of the vas deferens.

PROCEDURE: The cutting of the vas deferens in the male as a form of permanent sterilization. Reinforce the need for alternate forms of birth control for approximately 20 ejaculations or 1 week to several months to allow all of the sperm to clear the vas deferens. This will ensure complete male infertility.

CLIENT EDUCATION
- Following the procedure, scrotal support and moderate activity for a couple of days is recommended to reduce discomfort.
- Sterility is delayed until the proximal portion of the vas deferens is cleared of all remaining sperm (approximately 20 ejaculations).
- Alternate forms of birth control must be used until the vas deferens is cleared of sperm.
- Follow-up is important for sperm count.

ADVANTAGES
- Permanent contraceptive method.
- Procedure is short, safe, and simple.
- Sexual function is not impaired.

DISADVANTAGES
- Requires surgery.
- Reversal is possible but not always successful.
- Does not protect against STIs.

COMPLICATIONS: Rare, but can include bleeding, infection, and anesthesia reaction

Application Exercises

1. A nurse in a health clinic is reviewing contraceptive use with a group of adolescent clients. Which of the following statements by an adolescent reflects an understanding of the teaching?

   A. "A water-soluble lubricant should be used with condoms."

   B. "A diaphragm should be removed 2 hours after intercourse."

   C. "Oral contraceptives can worsen a case of acne."

   D. "A contraceptive patch is replaced once a month."

2. A nurse is instructing a client who is taking an oral contraceptive about danger signs to report to her provider. The nurse determines the client understands the teaching when the client states the need to report which of the following?

   A. Reduced menstrual flow

   B. Breast tenderness

   C. Shortness of breath

   D. Headaches

3. A nurse in an obstetrical clinic is teaching a client about using an IUD for contraception. Which of the following statements by the client indicates an understanding of the teaching?

   A. "An IUD should be replaced annually during a pelvic exam."

   B. "I cannot get an IUD until after I've had a child."

   C. "I should expect intermittent abdominal pain while the IUD is in place."

   D. "A change in the string length of my IUD is expected."

4. A nurse is teaching a client about potential adverse effects of implantable progestins. Which of the following adverse effects should the nurse include? (Select all that apply.)

   A. Tinnitus

   B. Irregular vaginal bleeding

   C. Weight gain

   D. Breast changes

   E. Gingival hyperplasia

5. A nurse in a clinic is teaching a client about her new prescription for medroxyprogesterone . Which of the following information should the nurse include in the teaching? (Select all that apply.)

   A. "Weight loss can occur."

   B. "You are protected against STIs."

   C. "You should increase your intake of calcium."

   D. "You should avoid taking antibiotics."

   E. "Irregular vaginal spotting can occur."

Application Exercises Key

1. A. **CORRECT:** Condoms are used with water-soluble lubricants.

   B. A diaphragm should be removed no sooner than 6 hr and no later than 24 hr after intercourse.

   C. Acne is reduced when taking oral contraceptives.

   D. Contraceptive patches are replaced once a week.

   Ⓝ NCLEX® Connection: Health Promotion and Maintenance, Lifestyle Choices

2. A. Reduced menstrual flow is a common adverse effect of oral contraceptives and usually subsides after a few months of use.

   B. Breast tenderness is a common adverse effect of oral contraceptives and usually subsides after a few months of use.

   C. **CORRECT:** Shortness of breath can indicate a pulmonary embolus or myocardial infarction and should be reported to the provider immediately.

   D. Headaches are a common adverse effect of oral contraceptives and usually subside after a few months of use.

   Ⓝ NCLEX® Connection: Pharmacological and Parenteral Therapies, Adverse Effects/Contraindications/Side Effects/Interactions

3. A. An IUD will be replaced every 3 to 5 years, dependent upon the type of IUD used.

   B. Clients do not have to have given birth prior to the insertion of an IUD.

   C. Abdominal pain with an IUD can indicate a potential complication and should be reported to the provider.

   D. **CORRECT:** A change in the length of the string of an IUD can indicate expulsion and should be reported to the provider.

   Ⓝ NCLEX® Connection: Pharmacological and Parenteral Therapies, Medication Administration

4. A. Tinnitus is not an adverse effect of implantable progestins.

   B. **CORRECT:** Irregular vaginal bleeding is a potential adverse effect of implantable progestins.

   C. **CORRECT:** Weight gain is a potential adverse effect of implantable progestins.

   D. **CORRECT:** Breast changes are a potential adverse effect of implantable progestins.

   E. Gingival hyperplasia is not a potential adverse effect of implantable progestins.

   Ⓝ NCLEX® Connection: Pharmacological and Parenteral Therapies, Adverse Effects/Contraindications/Side Effects/Interactions

5. A. Weight gain can occur when taking medroxyprogesterone.

   B. Medroxyprogesterone does not provide protection against STIs.

   C. **CORRECT:** Clients should take calcium and vitamin D to prevent loss of bone density, which can occur when taking medroxyprogesterone.

   D. Antibiotics are not contraindicated when taking medroxyprogesterone.

   E. **CORRECT:** Medroxyprogesterone can cause irregular vaginal bleeding.

   Ⓝ NCLEX® Connection: Pharmacological and Parenteral Therapies, Medication Administration

UNIT 1   ANTEPARTUM NURSING CARE

SECTION: HUMAN REPRODUCTION

CHAPTER 2 *Infertility*

Infertility is defined as an inability to conceive despite engaging in unprotected sexual intercourse for a prolonged period of time or at least 12 months. Common factors associated with infertility can include decreased sperm production, endometriosis, ovulation disorders, and tubal occlusions.

Partners who experience infertility can experience stress related to physical inability to conceive, expense, the effect on the couple's relationship, and lack of family support. Infertility assessments, diagnostic procedures, assisted reproductive technologies, and genetic counseling may be undertaken.

ASSESSMENT

Female

AGE: Age greater than 35 years can affect fertility.

DURATION OF INFERTILITY: More than 1 year of coitus without contraceptives. For women over the age 35 or who have a known risk factor, the recommendation is for 6 months.

MEDICAL HISTORY: Atypical secondary sexual characteristic, such as abnormal body fat distribution or hair growth, is indicative of an endocrine disorder. Assessment should include hormonal and adrenal gland disorders, as these can contribute to infertility.

SURGICAL HISTORY: Particularly pelvic and abdominal procedures.

OBSTETRIC HISTORY: Past episodes of spontaneous abortions. Other obstetric assessments should include an evaluation of hormone levels throughout the client's cycle. This can provide information about anovulation, amenorrhea, and premature ovarian failure.

GYNECOLOGIC HISTORY: Abnormal uterine contours or any history of disorders that can contribute to the formation of scar tissue that can cause blockage of ovum or sperm.

SEXUAL HISTORY: Intercourse frequency, number of partners across the lifespan, and any history of STIs.

OCCUPATIONAL/ENVIRONMENTAL EXPOSURE RISK ASSESSMENT: Exposure to hazardous teratogenic materials in the home or at a place of employment.

WEIGHT: Overweight or underweight. Nutritional deficiencies, such as anorexia, can contribute to infertility.

SUBSTANCE USE :Alcohol, tobacco, heroin, methadone.

Male

MEDICAL HISTORY: Mumps, especially after adolescence; endocrine disorders; genetic disorders; and anomalies in the reproductive system.

SEXUAL HISTORY: Intercourse frequency, and history of sexually transmitted infections.

SUBSTANCE USE: Alcohol, tobacco, heroin, methadone.

OCCUPATIONAL/ENVIRONMENTAL EXPOSURE RISK ASSESSMENT: Exposure to hazardous teratogenic materials in home or work environment, exposure of scrotum to high temperatures.

DIAGNOSTIC PROCEDURES

Female

PELVIC EXAMINATION: Assesses for uterine or vaginal anomalies.

HORMONE ANALYSIS: Evaluates hypothalamic–pituitary–ovarian axis to include serum prolactin, FSH, LH, estradiol, progesterone, and thyroid hormones.

POSTCOITAL TEST: Evaluates coital technique and mucus secretions.

ULTRASONOGRAPHY: A transvaginal or abdominal ultrasound procedure performed to visualize female reproductive organs.

HYSTEROSALPINGOGRAPHY: Outpatient radiological procedure in which dye is used to assess the patency of the fallopian tubes. Assess for history of allergies to iodine and seafood prior to beginning the procedure.

HYSTEROSCOPY: A radiographic procedure in which the uterus is examined for signs of defect, distortion, or scar tissue that can impair successful impregnation.

LAPAROSCOPY: A procedure in which gas insufflation under general anesthesia is used to observe internal organs.

Male

SEMEN ANALYSIS: In 40% of couples who are infertile, inability to conceive is due to male infertility. This test is the first in an infertility workup because it is less expensive and less invasive compared with female infertility testing. It can need to be repeated.

ULTRASONOGRAPHY: An ultrasound procedure is performed to visualize testes and abnormalities in the scrotum. A transrectal ultrasound procedure is performed to assess the ejaculatory ducts, seminal vesicles, and vas deferens.

PATIENT-CENTERED CARE

THERAPEUTIC PROCEDURES

NONMEDICAL THERAPY AND ALTERNATIVE MEASURES
- Nutritional and dietary changes
- Exercise, yoga, and stress management
- Herbal medications, only if prescribed
- Acupuncture

MEDICAL THERAPY
- Ovarian stimulation-medications are prescribed to stimulate the ovary to produce follicles.
  - Clomiphene citrate
  - Letrozole
- Other medications used to support ovulation: metformin

ASSISTED REPRODUCTIVE TECHNOLOGIES
- **Intrauterine insemination:** Procedure used to place prepared sperm in the uterus at the time of ovulation.
- **In vitro fertilization-embryo transfer (IVF-ET):** Procedure of collecting the woman's eggs from her ovaries, fertilizing the eggs in the laboratory with sperm, and transferring the embryo to her uterus.
- **Gamete intrafallopian transfer:** Oocytes are retrieved and immediately placed with prepared motile sperm. Both are placed together into a thin flexible tube (catheter). The gametes are then injected into the fallopian tubes using a surgical procedure called laparoscopy.
- **Donor oocyte:** Donated eggs are collected from a donor by an IVF procedure. The eggs are inseminated. The embryos are placed in a recipient's uterus. Prior to implantation the recipient undergoes hormonal therapy to prepare the uterus.
- **Donor embryo (embryo adoption):** Donated embryo is placed in the recipient's uterus, which is hormonally prepared.
- **Gestational carrier (embryo host):** A couple completes the process of IVF with the embryo placed in another woman, who will carry the pregnancy. This is a contract agreement with the carrier having no genetic investment with the embryo.
- **Surrogate mother:** A woman is inseminated with semen and carries the fetus until birth.
- **Therapeutic donor insemination:** Donor sperm is used to inseminate a woman.

NURSING INTERVENTIONS
- Encourage couples to express and discuss their feelings and recognize infertility as a major life stressor. Assist the couple to consider options, and provide education to assist in decision-making. Qᴘᴄᴄ
- Explain role of genetic counselor, reproductive specialist, geneticist, and pharmacist in providing psychosocial and medical care.
- Monitor for adverse effects associated with medications to treat infertility.

- Advise that the use of medications to treat female infertility can increase the risk of multiple births by more than 25%.
- Provide information regarding assisted reproductive therapies (in vitro fertilization, embryo transfer, intrafallopian gamete transfer, surrogate parenting, and reproductive alternatives such as adoption).
- Make referrals to grief and infertility support groups.

GENETIC COUNSELING

- Genetic counseling may be recommended by the provider if there is a family history of birth defects.
- Identify clients who are in need of genetic counseling, such as a client who has a sickle cell trait or sickle cell anemia, or a client older than 35. Make referrals to genetic specialists as necessary.
- Prenatal assessment of genetic disorders (amniocentesis) can pose potential risks to the fetus.
- Provide and clarify information pertaining to the risk of or the occurrence of genetic disorders within a family preceding, during, and following a genetic counseling session.

NURSING INTERVENTIONS
- Assist in the construction of family medical histories of several generations.
- Provide emotional support. Client responses vary and include denial, anger, grief, guilt, and self-blame.
- Make referrals to support groups and provide follow-up.

COMPLICATIONS

Ectopic pregnancy

- Ovum implants in the fallopian tubes or abdominal cavity due to the presence of endometrial tissue.
- As ovum increases in size, fallopian tube can rupture, and extensive bleeding occurs, resulting in surgical removal of the damaged tube.
- If ectopic pregnancy is identified prior to rupture of the tube, surgical removal of the products of conception may be performed, or methotrexate is prescribed to dissolve the pregnancy.
- Client faces increased risk of recurrence of an ectopic pregnancy and infertility.

Multiple gestation

Assisted reproductive technology is associated with an increase incidence of multiple gestations. This poses a risk for the mother and babies.

1. A nurse in a clinic is caring for a group of female clients who are being evaluated for infertility. Which of the following clients should the nurse anticipate the provider will refer to a genetic counselor?

    A. A client whose sister has alopecia

    B. A client whose partner has von Willebrand disease

    C. A client who has an allergy to sulfa

    D. A client who had rubella 3 months ago

2. A nurse is caring for a couple who is being evaluated for infertility. Which of the following statements by the nurse indicates understanding of the infertility assessment process?

    A. "You will need to see a genetic counselor as part of the assessment."

    B. "It is usually the woman who is having trouble, so the man doesn't have to be involved."

    C. "The man is the easiest to assess, and the provider will usually begin there."

    D. "Think about adopting first because there are many babies that need good homes."

3. A nurse in an infertility clinic is providing care to a couple who has been unable to conceive for 18 months. Which of the following data should be included in the assessment? (Select all that apply.)

    A. Occupation

    B. Menstrual history

    C. Childhood infectious diseases

    D. History of falls

    E. Recent blood transfusions

4. A nurse in a clinic is caring for a client who is to be seen by the provider for a postoperative appointment following a salpingectomy due to an ectopic pregnancy. Which of the following statements by the client requires clarification?

    A. "It is good to know that I won't have a tubal pregnancy in the future."

    B. "The doctor said that this surgery can affect my ability to get pregnant again."

    C. "I understand that one of my fallopian tubes had to be removed."

    D. "Ovulation can still occur because my ovaries were not affected."

5. A nurse is reviewing the health record of a client who is to undergo hysterosalpingography. Which of the following data alert the nurse that the client is at risk for a complication related to this procedure?

    VITAL SIGNS

    Temperature 37.2° C (98.9° F)
    BMI 40.3

    HISTORY AND PHYSICAL

    Employed as a radiology technician
    Allergy to shrimp
    Tonsillectomy at age 18

    LABORATORY FINDINGS

    Glucose 103 mg/dL
    Hgb 13.1 g/dL
    Total cholesterol 265 mg/dL

    MEDICATIONS

    Rosuvastatin
    Magnesium oxide
    Mafenide acetate

    A. Vital signs

    B. History and physical

    C. Laboratory findings

    D. Medications

PRACTICE Active Learning Scenario

A nurse in an infertility clinic is caring for a client and her partner. The client asks about the assessments and diagnostic procedures that are done to determine whether infertility can be identified. What is an appropriate response by the nurse? Use the ATI Active Learning Template: System Disorder to complete this item.

ALTERATION IN HEALTH (DIAGNOSIS): Define infertility.

EXPECTED FINDINGS: Describe at least three assessments.

DIAGNOSTIC PROCEDURES: Describe at least three.

Application Exercises Key

1. A. Alopecia is a nonhereditary disorder and does not warrant referral to a genetic counselor.

   B. **CORRECT:** Von Willebrand disease is a genetic bleeding disorder and warrants a client being referred to a genetic counselor.

   C. Allergy to sulfa is a nonhereditary condition and does not warrant referral to a genetic counselor.

   D. A recent episode of rubella in a nonpregnant female does not warrant a referral to a genetic counselor.

   Ⓝ NCLEX® Connection: Health Promotion and Maintenance, Health Promotion/Disease Prevention

2. A. A referral to a genetic counselor occurs if there is a reason to suspect birth defects or other physiological concerns. It is not included in all infertility assessment processes.

   B. The cause of infertility is almost evenly divided between men and women.

   C. **CORRECT:** A sperm analysis is one of the first steps in the infertility assessment process and can identify a cause of infertility in a less invasive and costly manner.

   D. Adoption is an option for the infertile couple after identifying a possible cause for the infertility.

   Ⓝ NCLEX® Connection: Health Promotion and Maintenance, Lifestyle Choices

3. A. **CORRECT:** Occupational hazards include exposure to teratogenic substances in the workplace, such as radiation, chemicals, herbicides, and pesticides.

   B. **CORRECT:** Menstrual history can identify hormone-related patterns, such as anovulation, pituitary disorders, and endometriosis.

   C. **CORRECT:** Childhood infectious diseases can identify the male partner having had the mumps.

   D. A history of falls is not a consideration in the assessment.

   E. A recent blood transfusion is not a consideration in the assessment.

   Ⓝ NCLEX® Connection: Health Promotion and Maintenance, Health Screening

4. A. **CORRECT.** The risk of recurrence of an ectopic pregnancy is increased following an ectopic pregnancy.

   B. Infertility can occur as a result of an ectopic pregnancy.

   C. A salpingectomy involves the removal of a fallopian tube.

   D. A salpingectomy does not involve the removal of the ovaries.

   Ⓝ NCLEX® Connection: Reduction of Risk Potential, Lifestyle Choices

5. A. The client is obese, but this does not place the client at risk for a complication related to the procedure.

   B. **CORRECT:** An allergy to seafood is a contraindication to the dye used in hysterosalpingography.

   C. The client's total cholesterol is elevated, but this does not place the client at risk for a complication related to the procedure.

   D. There are no contraindications related to the medications the client is taking.

   Ⓝ NCLEX® Connection: Reduction of Risk Potential, Diagnostic Tests

---

PRACTICE Answer

Using the ATI Active Learning: System Disorder

DESCRIPTION OF DISORDER/DISEASE PROCESS: Inability to conceive despite engaging in unprotected sexual intercourse for a prolonged period of time or at least 12 months. For women over the age 35 or with a known risk factor, the recommendation is for 6 months.

EXPECTED FINDINGS
- Age
- Weight
- Duration of infertility
- Medical history
- Surgical history
- Obstetric history
- Gynecologic history
- Occupational/environmental exposure risk

DIAGNOSTIC PROCEDURES
- Semen analysis
- Pelvic examination
- Hormone analysis
- Postcoital test
- Ultrasonography
- Hysterosalpingography
- Hysteroscopy
- Laparoscopy

Ⓝ NCLEX® Connection: Reduction of Risk Potential, Therapeutic Procedures

CHAPTER 3   *Expected Physiological Changes During Pregnancy*

Recognizing changes during pregnancy is helpful for both clients and nurses. The nurse and provider assess findings during the client's initial prenatal visit.

Signs of pregnancy are classified into three groups: presumptive, probable, and positive.

Calculating delivery date, number of pregnancies, and evaluating the physiological status of a client who is pregnant are performed.

SIGNS OF PREGNANCY

PRESUMPTIVE SIGNS

Presumptive signs are changes that the woman experiences that make her think that she might be pregnant. These changes might be subjective symptoms or objective signs. Signs also might be a result of physiological factors other than pregnancy (peristalsis, infections, stress).
- **Amenorrhea**
- **Fatigue**
- **Nausea and vomiting**
- **Urinary frequency**
- **Breast changes:** darkened areolae, enlarged Montgomery's glands
- **Quickening:** slight fluttering movements of the fetus felt by a woman, usually between 16 to 20 weeks of gestation
- **Uterine enlargement**

PROBABLE SIGNS

Probable signs are changes that make the examiner suspect a woman is pregnant (primarily related to physical changes of the uterus). Signs can be caused by physiological factors other than pregnancy (pelvic congestion, tumors).
- **Abdominal enlargement** related to changes in uterine size, shape, and position
- **Hegar's sign:** softening and compressibility of lower uterus
- **Chadwick's sign:** deepened violet-bluish color of cervix and vaginal mucosa
- **Goodell's sign:** softening of cervical tip
- **Ballottement:** rebound of unengaged fetus
- **Braxton Hicks contractions:** false contractions that are painless, irregular, and usually relieved by walking
- **Positive pregnancy test**

- **Fetal outline** felt by examiner

POSITIVE SIGNS

Positive signs are those that can be explained only by pregnancy.
- **Fetal heart sounds**
- **Visualization of fetus by ultrasound**
- **Fetal movement** palpated by an experienced examiner

VERIFYING PREGNANCY

Serum and urine tests provide an accurate assessment for the presence of human chorionic gonadotropin (hCG). hCG production can start as early as the day of implantation and can be detected as early as 7 to 8 days after conception.
- Production of hCG begins with implantation, peaks at about 60 to 70 days of gestation, declines until around 100 to 130 days of pregnancy, and then gradually increases until term.
- Higher levels of hCG can indicate multifetal pregnancy, ectopic pregnancy, hydatidiform mole (gestational trophoblastic disease), or a genetic abnormality such as Down syndrome.
- Lower blood levels of hCG might suggest a miscarriage or ectopic pregnancy.
- Some medications (anticonvulsants, diuretics, tranquilizers) can cause false-positive or false-negative pregnancy results.
- Home pregnancy test: Urine samples should be first-voided morning specimens and follow the directions for accuracy.

CALCULATING DELIVERY DATE AND DETERMINING NUMBER OF PREGNANCIES FOR PREGNANT CLIENT

Nägele's rule: Take the first day of the woman's last menstrual cycle, subtract 3 months, and then add 7 days and 1 year, adjusting for the year as necessary.

Measurement of fundal height in centimeters from the symphysis pubis to the top of the uterine fundus (between 18 and 32 weeks of gestation). Approximates the gestational age

Gravidity: number of pregnancies.
- Nulligravida: a woman who has never been pregnant
- Primigravida: a woman in her first pregnancy
- Multigravida: a woman who has had two or more pregnancies

Parity: number of pregnancies in which the fetus or fetuses reach 20 weeks of pregnancy, not the number of fetuses. Parity is not effected whether the fetus is born still born or alive.
- Nullipara: no pregnancy beyond the stage of viability
- Primipara: has completed one pregnancy to stage of viability
- Multipara: has completed two or more pregnancies to stage of viability

Viability: the point in time when an infant has the capacity to survive outside the uterus. There is not a specific weeks of gestation; however, infants born between 22 to 25 weeks are considered on the threshold of viability.

GTPAL acronym
- Gravidity
- Term births (38 weeks or more)
- Preterm births (from viability up to 37 weeks)
- Abortions/miscarriages (prior to viability)
- Living children

PHYSIOLOGICAL STATUS OF PREGNANT CLIENT

BODY SYSTEMS

Reproductive

Uterus increases in size and changes shape and position. Ovulation and menses cease during pregnancy.

Cardiovascular

Cardiac output increases (30% to 50%) and blood volume increases (30% to 45% at term) to meet the greater metabolic needs. Heart rate increases during pregnancy beginning around week 5 and reaches a peak (10 to 15/min above pre-pregnancy rate) around 32 weeks of pregnancy.

Respiratory

Maternal oxygen needs increase. During the last trimester, the size of the chest might enlarge, allowing for lung expansion, as the uterus pushes upward. Respiratory rate increases and total lung capacity decreases.

Musculoskeletal

Body alterations and weight increase necessitate an adjustment in posture. Pelvic joints relax.

Gastrointestinal

Nausea and vomiting might occur due to hormonal changes and/or an increase of pressure within the abdominal cavity as the pregnant client's stomach and intestines are displaced within the abdomen. Constipation might occur due to increased transit time of food through the gastrointestinal tract and, thus, increased water absorption.

Renal

Filtration rate increases secondary to the influence of pregnancy hormones and an increase in blood volume and metabolic demands. The amount of urine produced remains the same. Urinary frequency is common during pregnancy.

Endocrine

The placenta becomes an endocrine organ that produces large amounts of hCG, progesterone, estrogen, human placental lactogen, and prostaglandins. Hormones are very active during pregnancy and function to maintain pregnancy and prepare the body for delivery.

BODY IMAGE CHANGES

- Due to physical and psychological changes that occur, the pregnant woman requires support from her provider and family members.
- In the first trimester of pregnancy, physiological changes are not obvious. Many women look forward to the changes so that the pregnancy will be more noticeable.
- During the second trimester, there are rapid physical changes due to the enlargement of the abdomen and breasts. Skin changes also occur, such as stretch marks and hyperpigmentation. These changes can affect a woman's mobility. She might find herself losing her balance and feeling back or leg discomfort and fatigue. These factors might lead to a negative body image. The client might make statements of resentment toward the pregnancy and express anxiousness for the pregnancy to be over soon.

EXPECTED VITAL SIGNS Q_EBP

Blood pressure

- Blood pressure measurements are within the pre-pregnancy range during the first trimester.
- **Systolic:** slight or no increase from pre-pregnancy levels
- **Diastolic:** slight decreases around 24 to 32 weeks; will gradually return to pre-pregnancy level by the end of the pregnancy.
- The position of the pregnant woman also might affect blood pressure. In the supine position, blood pressure might appear to be lower due to the weight and pressure of the gravid uterus on the vena cava, which decreases venous blood flow to the heart. Maternal hypotension and fetal hypoxia might occur, which is referred to as supine hypotensive syndrome or supine vena cava syndrome. Signs and symptoms include dizziness, lightheadedness, and pale, clammy skin. Encourage the client to engage in maternal positioning on the left-lateral side, semi-Fowler's position, or, if supine, with a wedge placed under one hip to alleviate pressure to the vena cava.

Pulse

Pulse increases 10 to 15/min around 32 weeks of gestation and remains elevated throughout the remainder of the pregnancy.

Respirations

Respirations are unchanged or slightly increased. Respiratory changes in pregnancy are attributed to the elevation of the diaphragm by as much as 4 cm, as well as changes to the chest wall to facilitate increased maternal oxygen demands. Some shortness of breath might be noted.

EXPECTED FINDINGS Q_{EBP}

- Fetal heart tones are heard at a normal baseline rate of 110 to 160/min with reassuring FHR accelerations noted, which indicates an intact fetal CNS.
- The client's heart changes in size and shape with resulting cardiac hypertrophy to accommodate increased blood volume and increased cardiac output. Heart sounds also change to accommodate the increase in blood volume with a more distinguishable splitting of S_1 and S_2, with S_3 more easily heard following 20 weeks of gestation. Murmurs also might be auscultated. Heart size and shape should return to normal shortly after delivery.
- Uterine size changes from a uterine weight of 50 to 1,000 g (0.1 to 2.2 lb). By 36 weeks of gestation, the top of the uterus and the fundus will reach the xiphoid process. This might cause the pregnant woman to experience shortness of breath as the uterus pushes against the diaphragm.
- Cervical changes are obvious as a purplish-blue color extends into the vagina and labia, and the cervix becomes markedly soft.
- Breast changes occur due to hormones of pregnancy, with the breasts increasing in size and the areolas darkening.

SKIN CHANGES

- Chloasma: an increase of pigmentation on the face
- Linea nigra: dark line of pigmentation from the umbilicus extending to the pubic area
- Striae gravidarum: stretch marks most notably found on the abdomen and thighs

NURSING INTERVENTIONS

- Acknowledge the client's concerns about pregnancy and encourage sharing of these feelings while providing an atmosphere free of judgment.
- Discuss with the client the expected physiological changes and a possible timeline for a return to the pre-pregnant state.
- Assist the client in setting goals for the postpartum period in regard to self-care and newborn care.
- Refer the client to counseling if body image concerns appear to have a negative impact on the pregnancy.
- Provide education about the expected physiological and psychosocial changes. Common discomforts of pregnancy and ways to resolve those discomforts are reviewed during prenatal visits.
- The client is encouraged to keep all follow-up appointments and to contact the provider immediately if there is any bleeding, leakage of fluid, or contractions at any time during the pregnancy. Q_S

Application Exercises

1. A nurse is caring for a client who is pregnant and states that her last menstrual period was April 1st. Which of the following is the client's estimated date of delivery?

    A. January 8
    B. January 15
    C. February 8
    D. February 15

2. A nurse in a prenatal clinic is caring for a client who is in the first trimester of pregnancy. The client's health record includes this data: G3 T1 P0 A1 L1. How should the nurse interpret this information? (Select all that apply.)

    A. Client has delivered one newborn at term.
    B. Client has experienced no preterm labor.
    C. Client has been through active labor.
    D. Client has had two prior pregnancies.
    E. Client has one living child.

3. A nurse is reviewing the health record of a client who is pregnant. The provider indicated the client exhibits probable signs of pregnancy. Which of the following findings should the nurse expect? (Select all that apply.)

    A. Montgomery's glands
    B. Goodell's sign
    C. Ballottement
    D. Chadwick's sign
    E. Quickening

4. A nurse in a prenatal clinic is caring for a client who is pregnant and experiencing episodes of maternal hypotension. The client asks the nurse what causes these episodes. Which of the following responses should the nurse make?

    A. "This is due to an increase in blood volume."
    B. "This is due to pressure from the uterus on the diaphragm."
    C. "This is due to the weight of the uterus on the vena cava."
    D. "This is due to increased cardiac output."

5. A nurse in a clinic receives a phone call from a client who believes she is pregnant and would like to be tested in the clinic to confirm her pregnancy. Which of the following information should the nurse provide to the client?

    A. "You should wait until 4 weeks after conception to be tested."
    B. "You should be off any medications for 24 hours prior to the test."
    C. "You should be NPO for at least 8 hours prior to the test."
    D. "You should collect urine from the first morning void."

Application Exercises Key

1. A. **CORRECT:** April 1st minus 3 months plus 7 days and 1 year equals an estimated date of delivery of January. 8.

    B. This is incorrect using Nägele's rule.

    C. This is incorrect using Nägele's rule.

    D. This is incorrect using Nägele's rule.

    (N) *NCLEX® Connection: Health Promotion and Maintenance, Ante/Intra/Postpartum and Newborn Care*

2. A. **CORRECT:** T1 indicates the client has delivered one newborn at term.

    B. P0 indicates the client has had no preterm deliveries.

    C. A1 indicates the client has had one miscarriage.

    D. **CORRECT:** G3 indicates the client has had two prior pregnancies and the client is currently pregnant.

    E. **CORRECT:** L1 indicates the client has one living child.

    (N) *NCLEX® Connection: Health Promotion and Maintenance, Ante/Intra/Postpartum and Newborn Care*

3. A. Montgomery's glands are a presumptive sign of pregnancy.

    B. **CORRECT:** Goodell's sign is a probable sign of pregnancy.

    C. **CORRECT:** Ballottement is a probable sign of pregnancy.

    D. **CORRECT:** Chadwick's sign is a probable sign of pregnancy.

    E. Quickening is a presumptive sign of pregnancy.

    (N) *NCLEX® Connection: Health Promotion and Maintenance, Ante/Intra/Postpartum and Newborn Care*

4. A. An increase in blood volume during pregnancy results in cardiac hypertrophy.

    B. Pressure from the gravid uterus on the diaphragm might cause the client to experience shortness of breath.

    C. **CORRECT:** Maternal hypotension occurs when the client is lying in the supine position and the weight of the gravid uterus places pressure on the vena cava, decreasing venous blood flow to the heart.

    D. An increase in cardiac output during pregnancy results in cardiac hypertrophy.

    (N) *NCLEX® Connection: Physiological Adaptation, Alterations in Body Systems*

5. A. The production of hCG can be detected as early as 7 to 8 days after conception.

    B. The nurse should not advise the client to stop taking medications in preparation for pregnancy tests. The nurse should review the client's medications to determine whether they can affect the results.

    C. The nurse should not advise the client to remain NPO prior to pregnancy testing. Serum or blood tests are not affected by food or fluid intake.

    D. **CORRECT:** Urine pregnancy tests should be done on a first-voided morning specimen to provide the most accurate results.

    (N) *NCLEX® Connection: Reduction of Risk Potential, Laboratory Values*

A nurse is caring for a client who is in the fourth week of gestation. The client asks about skin and breast changes that can occur during pregnancy. What information should the nurse include in the teaching? Use the ATI Active Learning Template: Basic Concept to complete this item.

RELATED CONTENT: Describe at least three changes that occur to skin and breasts during pregnancy.

UNDERLYING PRINCIPLES: Describe the basis for these changes.

PRACTICE Answer

Using the ATI Active Learning Template: Basic Concept

RELATED CONTENT

- Skin changes: hyperpigmentation; linea nigra; chloasma (mask of pregnancy) on the face; striae gravidarum (stretch marks), most pronounced on abdomen and thighs
- Breast changes: darkening of the areola, enlarged Montgomery's glands, increase in size and heaviness, increased sensitivity

UNDERLYING PRINCIPLES: Increase in estrogen and progesterone occurring during pregnancy

(N) *NCLEX® Connection: Health Promotion and Maintenance, Ante/Intra/Postpartum and Newborn Care*

UNIT 1   ANTEPARTUM NURSING CARE
SECTION: CHANGES DURING PREGNANCY

CHAPTER 4 *Prenatal Care*

Prenatal care involves nursing assessments and client education for expectant mothers. When providing prenatal care, nurses must take into account cultural considerations.

Prenatal education encompasses information provided to a client who is pregnant. Major areas of focus include assisting the client in self-care of the discomforts of pregnancy, promoting a safe outcome to pregnancy, and fostering positive feelings by the pregnant woman and her family regarding the childbearing experience.

Prenatal care dramatically reduces infant and maternal morbidity and mortality rates by early detection and treatment of potential problems. A majority of birth defects occur between 2 and 8 weeks of gestation. Q̇EBP

NURSING ASSESSMENTS

Nurses play an integral role in assessing a client's current knowledge, previous pregnancies, and birthing experiences.

CLIENT HISTORY

Nursing assessment in prenatal care includes obtaining information regarding:
- **Reproductive and obstetrical history** (contraception use, gynecological diagnoses, obstetrical difficulties).
- **Medical history**, including physical preexisting conditions, surgical procedures, any handicapping conditions, and the woman's immune status (rubella and hepatitis B).
- **Nutritional history**, a complete dietary assessment can alert the practitioner to deficient practices and food allergies. Good nutrition is important and has a direct effect on the growth and development of the fetus.
- **Family history**, such as genetic disorders or conditions that could affect the mother or fetus.
- Any recent or current illnesses or infections.
- **Current medications**, including substance use and alcohol consumption. The nurse should display a nonjudgmental, matter-of-fact demeanor when interviewing a client regarding substance use and observe for clinical findings such as lack of grooming.

- **Psychosocial history** (a client's emotional response to pregnancy, adolescent pregnancy, spouse, support system, history of depression, domestic violence issues).
- Any hazardous environmental exposures; current work conditions. Q̇s
- Current exercise and lifestyle.
- **Abuse history or risk**; assess all women for all forms, including physical, sexual, or psychological abuse, because the risk increases during pregnancy.

BIRTH PLAN

A nurse ascertains what a client's goals are for the birthing process. The nurse should discuss birthing methods, such as Lamaze, and pain control options (epidural, natural childbirth). Q̇PCC

PRENATAL ASSESSMENTS

Prenatal care begins with an initial assessment (within the first 12 weeks) and continues throughout pregnancy. In an uneventful pregnancy, prenatal visits are scheduled monthly for weeks 16 through 28, every 2 weeks from 29 through 36 weeks, and every week from 36 weeks until birth.

Initial prenatal visit

- Determine the estimated date of birth based on the last menstrual period.
- Obtain medical and nursing history to include social supports and review of systems (to determine risk factors).
- Perform a physical assessment to include a client's baseline weight, vital signs, and pelvic examination.
- Obtain initial laboratory tests, including hemoglobin, hematocrit, WCB, blood type and Rh, rubella titer, urinalysis, renal function test, Pap test, cervical cultures, HIV antibody, hepatitis B surface antigen, toxoplasmosis, and RPR or VDRL.

Ongoing prenatal visits

- Monitor weight, blood pressure, and urine for glucose, protein, and leukocytes.
- Monitor for the presence of edema.
- Monitor fetal development.
  - FHR can be detected at early appointments by ultrasound. The heartbeat can be heard by Doppler late in the first trimester. Listen at the midline, right above the symphysis pubis, by holding the Doppler firmly on the abdomen.
  - Measure fundal height starting in the second trimester. From weeks 18 to 30, the fundal height in centimeters is approximately the same as the number of weeks gestation.
  - Fetal health assessment: Begin assessing for fetal movement between 16 and 20 weeks of gestation.
- Provide education for self-care to include management of common discomforts and concerns of pregnancy (nausea and vomiting, fatigue, backache, varicosities, heartburn, activity, sexuality).

Nursing care

- Perform or assist with Leopold maneuvers to palpate presentation and position of the fetus.
- Assist the provider with the gynecological examination. This examination is performed to determine the status of a client's reproductive organs and birth canal. Pelvic measurements determine whether the pelvis will allow for the passage of the fetus at delivery. Qᴛᴄ
  - The nurse has the client empty her bladder and take deep breaths during the examination to decrease discomfort.
- Administer RhO(D) immune globulin IM around 28 weeks of gestation for clients who are Rh-negative.

Routine laboratory tests

Blood type, Rh factor, and presence of irregular antibodies: Determines the risk for maternal-fetal blood incompatibility (erythroblastosis fetalis) or neonatal hyperbilirubinemia. Indirect Coombs' test identifies clients sensitized to Rh-positive blood. For clients who are Rh-negative and not sensitized, the indirect Coombs' test is repeated between 24 and 28 weeks of gestation.

CBC with differential, Hgb, and Hct: Detects infection and anemia.

Hgb electrophoresis: Identifies hemoglobinopathies (sickle cell anemia and thalassemia).

Rubella titer: Determines immunity to rubella.

Hepatitis B screen: Identifies carriers of hepatitis B.

Group B Streptococcus (GBS): Obtain a vaginal/anal culture at 35 to 37 weeks of gestation to assess for GBS infection.

Urinalysis with microscopic examination of pH, specific gravity, color, sediment, protein, glucose, albumin, RBCs, WBCs, casts, acetone, and human chorionic gonadotropin: Identifies pregnancy, diabetes mellitus, gestational hypertension, renal disease, and infection.

One-hour glucose tolerance (oral ingestion or IV administration of concentrated glucose with venous sample taken 1 hr later [fasting not necessary]): Identifies hyperglycemia; done at initial visit for at-risk clients and at 24 to 28 weeks of gestation for all pregnant women (greater than 140 mg/dL requires follow up).

Three-hour glucose tolerance (fasting overnight prior to oral ingestion or IV administration of concentrated glucose with a venous sample taken 1, 2, and 3 hr later): Used in clients who have elevated 1-hr glucose test as a screening tool for diabetes mellitus. A diagnosis of gestational diabetes requires two elevated blood-glucose readings.

Papanicolaou (Pap) test: Used as a screening tool for cervical cancer, herpes simplex type 2, and/or human papillomavirus.

Vaginal/cervical culture: Detects streptococcus β-hemolytic, bacterial vaginosis, or sexually transmitted infections (gonorrhea and chlamydia).

PPD (tuberculosis screening), chest x-ray after 20 weeks of gestation with PPD test: Identifies exposure to tuberculosis.

Venereal disease research laboratory (VDRL): Syphilis screening mandated by law.

HIV: Detects HIV infection (the Centers for Disease Control and Prevention and the American Congress of Obstetricians and Gynecologists recommend testing all clients who are pregnant unless the client refuses testing).

Toxoplasmosis, other infections, rubella, cytomegalovirus, and herpes virus (TORCH) screening when indicated: Screening for a group of infections capable of crossing the placenta and adversely affecting fetal development.

Maternal serum alpha-fetoprotein (MSAFP): Screening occurs between 15 to 22 weeks of gestation. Used to rule out Down syndrome (low level) and neural tube defects (high level). The provider might decide to use a more reliable indicator and opt for the Quad screen instead of the MSAFP at 16 to 18 weeks of gestation. This includes AFP, inhibin-A, a combination analysis of human chorionic gonadotropin, and estriol.

CLIENT EDUCATION

Prenatal education includes health promotion, preparation for pregnancy and birth, common discomforts of pregnancy, and warning/danger signs to report.

HEALTH PROMOTION

Preconception and prenatal education emphasizes healthy behaviors that promote the health of the pregnant woman and her fetus. Qᴘᴄᴄ

- A client is instructed to avoid all over-the-counter medications, supplements, and prescription medications unless the provider who is supervising her care has knowledge of this practice.
- Alcohol (birth defects) and tobacco (low birth weight) are contraindicated during pregnancy.
- Substance use of any kind is to be avoided during pregnancy and lactation. Strategies to reduce or eliminate substance use are reviewed.
- Exercise during pregnancy yields positive benefits and should consist of 30 min of moderate exercise (walking or swimming) daily if not medically or obstetrically contraindicated.
- Avoid the use of hot tubs or saunas.
- Consume at least 8 to 10 glasses (2.3 L) of water each day.

The nurse educates a client about the following:
- Need for flu immunization
- Smoking cessation
- Treatment of current infections
- Genetic testing and counseling
- Exposure to hazardous materials

PREPARATION FOR PREGNANCY AND BIRTH

- Nurses provide anticipatory teaching to the pregnant client and her family about the following:
  - Physical and emotional changes during pregnancy and interventions that can be implemented to provide relief.
  - Indications of complications to report to the provider.
  - Birthing options available to enhance the birthing process.
- Maternal adaptation to pregnancy and the attainment of the maternal role—whereby the idea of pregnancy is accepted and assimilated into the client's way of life—includes hormonal and psychological aspects.
  - Emotional lability is experienced by many women with unpredictable mood changes and increased irritability, tearfulness, and anger alternating with feelings of joy and cheerfulness. This might result from hormonal changes.
  - A feeling of ambivalence about the pregnancy, which is a normal response, might occur early in the pregnancy and resolve before the third trimester. It consists of conflicting feelings (joy, pleasure, sorrow, hostility) about the pregnancy. These feelings can occur simultaneously, whether the pregnancy was planned or not.
- The nurse anticipates reviewing prenatal education topics with a client based on her current knowledge and previous pregnancy and birth experiences. The client's readiness to learn is enhanced when the nurse provides teaching during the appropriate trimester based on learning needs. Using a variety of educational methods, such as pamphlets and videos, and having the client verbalize and demonstrate learned topics will ensure that learning has taken place. Qpcc

FIRST TRIMESTER

- Physical and psychosocial changes
- Common discomforts of pregnancy and measures to provide relief
- Lifestyle: exercise, stress, nutrition, sexual health, dental care, over-the-counter and prescription medications, tobacco, alcohol, substance use, and STIs (encourage safe sexual practices)
- Possible complications and indications to report (preterm labor)
- Fetal growth and development
- Prenatal exercise
- Expected laboratory testing

SECOND TRIMESTER

- Benefits of breastfeeding
- Common discomforts and relief measures
- Lifestyle: sex and pregnancy, rest and relaxation, posture, body mechanics, clothing, seat belt safety and travel Qs
- Fetal movement
- Complications (preterm labor, gestational hypertension, gestational diabetes mellitus, premature rupture of membranes)
- Preparation for childbirth and childbirth education classes
- Review of birthing methods
- Development of a birth plan (verbal or written agreement about what client wishes during labor and delivery)

THIRD TRIMESTER

- Childbirth preparation Qebp
  - Childbirth classes or birth plan
  - Coping methods
  - Breathing and relaxation techniques
  - Use of effleurage and counter pressure
  - Application of heat/cold, touch and massage, and water therapy
  - Use of transcutaneous electrical nerve stimulation (TENS)
  - Acupressure and acupuncture
  - Music and aromatherapy
  - Discussion regarding pain management during labor and birth (natural childbirth, epidural)
  - Use of doula during labor
  - Indications of preterm labor and labor
  - Labor process
  - Infant care
  - Postpartum care
- Fetal movement/kick counts to ascertain fetal well-being: A client should be instructed to count and record fetal movements or kicks daily. There are several different method to complete kick counts.
  - One method: Mothers should count fetal activity two or three times a day for 2 hr after meals or bedtime. Fetal movements of less than 3 per hr or movements that cease entirely for 12 hr indicate a need for further evaluation.
- Diagnostic testing for fetal well-being (nonstress test, biophysical profile, ultrasound, and contraction stress test)

COMMON DISCOMFORTS OF PREGNANCY

Nausea and vomiting might occur during the first trimester. The client should eat crackers or dry toast 30 min to 1 hr before rising in the morning to relieve discomfort. Instruct the client to avoid having an empty stomach and ingesting spicy, greasy, or gas-forming foods. Encourage the client to drink fluids between meals.

Breast tenderness might occur during the first trimester. The client should wear a bra that provides adequate support.

Urinary frequency might occur during the first and third trimesters. The client should empty her bladder frequently, decrease fluid intake before bedtime, and use perineal pads. The client is taught how to perform Kegel exercises (alternate tightening and relaxation of pubococcygeal muscles) to reduce stress incontinence (leakage of urine with coughing and sneezing).

Urinary tract infections (UTIs) are common during pregnancy because of renal changes and the vaginal flora becoming more alkaline.

- UTI risks can be decreased by encouraging the client to wipe the perineal area from front to back after voiding, avoiding bubble baths, wearing cotton underpants, avoiding tight-fitting pants, and consuming plenty of water (8 glasses per day). Qebp
- The client should urinate before and after intercourse to flush bacteria from the urethra that are present or introduced during intercourse.

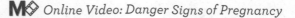

- Advise the client to urinate as soon as the urge occurs because retaining urine provides an environment for bacterial growth.
- Advise the client to notify her provider if her urine is foul-smelling, contains blood, or appears cloudy.

Fatigue might occur during the first and third trimesters. The client is encouraged to engage in frequent rest periods.

Heartburn might occur during the second and third trimesters due to the stomach being displaced by the enlarging uterus and a slowing of gastrointestinal tract motility and digestion brought about by increased progesterone levels. The client should eat small, frequent meals, not allow the stomach to get too empty or too full, sit up for 30 min after meals, and check with her provider prior to using any over-the-counter antacids.

Constipation might occur during the second and third trimesters. The client is encouraged to drink plenty of fluids, eat a diet high in fiber, and exercise regularly.

Hemorrhoids might occur during the second and third trimesters. A warm sitz bath, witch hazel pads, and application of topical ointments will help relieve discomfort.

Backaches are common during the second and third trimesters. The client is encouraged to exercise regularly, perform pelvic tilt exercises (alternately arching and straightening the back), use proper body mechanics by using the legs to lift rather than the back, and use the side-lying position.

Shortness of breath and dyspnea might occur because of the enlarged uterus, which limits inspiration. The client should maintain good posture, sleep with extra pillows, and contact her provider if symptoms worsen.

Leg cramps during the third trimester might occur due to the compression of lower-extremity nerves and blood vessels by the enlarging uterus. This can result in poor peripheral circulation, as well as an imbalance in the calcium/phosphorus ratio. The client should extend the affected leg, keeping the knee straight, and dorsiflex the foot (toes toward head). Application of heat over the affected muscle or a foot massage while the leg is extended can help relieve cramping. The client should notify her provider if frequent cramping occurs.

Varicose veins and lower-extremity edema can occur during the second and third trimesters. The client should rest with her legs elevated, avoid constricting clothing, wear support hose, avoid sitting or standing in one position for extended periods of time, and not sit with her legs crossed at the knees. She should sleep in the left-lateral position and exercise moderately with frequent walking to stimulate venous return.

Gingivitis, nasal stuffiness, and epistaxis (nosebleed) can occur as a result of elevated estrogen levels causing increased vascularity and proliferation of connective tissue. The client should gently brush her teeth, observe good dental hygiene, use a humidifier, and use normal saline nose drops or spray.

Braxton Hicks contractions, which occur from the first trimester onward, might increase in intensity and frequency during the third trimester. Inform the client that a change of position and walking should cause contractions to subside. If contractions increase in intensity and frequency (true contractions) with regularity, the client should notify her provider.

Supine hypotension occurs when a woman lies on her back and the weight of the gravid uterus compresses her vena cava. This reduces blood supply to the fetus. The client might experience feelings of lightheadedness and faintness. Teach the client to lie in a side-lying or semi-sitting position with her knees slightly flexed.

DANGER SIGNS DURING PREGNANCY

The following indicate potential dangerous situations that should be reported to the provider immediately.

FIRST TRIMESTER
- Burning on urination (infection)
- Severe vomiting (hyperemesis gravidarum)
- Diarrhea (infection)
- Fever or chills (infection)
- Abdominal cramping and/or vaginal bleeding (miscarriage, ectopic pregnancy)

SECOND AND THIRD TRIMESTER
- Gush of fluid from the vagina (rupture of amniotic fluid) prior to 37 weeks of gestation
- Vaginal bleeding (placental problems such as abruption or previa)
- Abdominal pain (premature labor, abruptio placentae, or ectopic pregnancy)
- Changes in fetal activity (decreased fetal movement might indicate fetal distress)
- Persistent vomiting (hyperemesis gravidarum)
- Severe headaches (gestational hypertension)
- Elevated temperature (infection)
- Dysuria (urinary tract infection)
- Blurred vision (gestational hypertension)
- Edema of face and hands (gestational hypertension)
- Epigastric pain (gestational hypertension)
- Concurrent occurrence of flushed dry skin, fruity breath, rapid breathing, increased thirst and urination, and headache (hyperglycemia)
- Concurrent occurrence of clammy pale skin, weakness, tremors, irritability, and lightheadedness (hypoglycemia)

Application Exercises

1. A nurse is teaching a group of women who are pregnant about measures to relieve backache during pregnancy. Which of the following measures should the nurse include in the teaching? (Select all that apply.)

    A. Avoid any lifting.

    B. Perform Kegel exercises twice a day.

    C. Perform the pelvic rock exercise every day.

    D. Use proper body mechanics.

    E. Avoid constrictive clothing.

2. A nurse is caring for a client who is pregnant and reviewing signs of complications the client should promptly report to the provider. Which of the following complications should the nurse include in the teaching?

    A. Vaginal bleeding

    B. Swelling of the ankles

    C. Heartburn after eating

    D. Lightheadedness when lying on back

3. A client who is at 7 weeks of gestation is experiencing nausea and vomiting in the morning. Which of the following information should the nurse include in the teaching?

    A. Eat crackers or plain toast before getting out of bed.

    B. Awaken during the night to eat a snack.

    C. Skip breakfast and eat lunch after nausea has subsided.

    D. Eat a large evening meal.

4. A nurse is teaching a client who is at 6 weeks of gestation about common discomforts of pregnancy. Which of the following findings should the nurse include in the teaching? (Select all that apply.)

    A. Breast tenderness

    B. Urinary frequency

    C. Epistaxis

    D. Dysuria

    E. Epigastric pain

5. A client who is at 8 weeks of gestation tells the nurse that she isn't sure she is happy about being pregnant. Which of the following responses should the nurse make?

    A. "I will inform the provider that you are having these feelings."

    B. "It is normal to have these feelings during the first few months of pregnancy."

    C. "You should be happy that you are going to bring new life into the world."

    D. "I am going to make an appointment with the counselor for you to discuss these thoughts."

PRACTICE Active Learning Scenario

A nurse is caring for a client at 14 weeks of gestation and is reviewing self-care concepts regarding the prevention of urinary tract infections (UTIs). What should the nurse include in the teaching? Use the ATI Active Learning Template: Basic Concept to complete this item.

UNDERLYING PRINCIPLES: Describe two.

NURSING INTERVENTIONS: Describe two actions that decrease the risk of UTIs as they relate to each of the following types of interventions: When? Why? and How?

1. A. Lifting may be done by using the legs rather than the back.

    B. Kegel exercises are done to strengthen the perineal muscles and do not relieve backache.

    C. **CORRECT:** The pelvic rock or tilt exercise stretches the muscles of the lower back and helps relieve lower-back pain.

    D. **CORRECT:** The use of proper body mechanics prevents back injury due to the incorrect use of muscles when lifting.

    E. Avoiding constrictive clothing helps prevent urinary tract infections, vaginal infections, varicosities, and edema of the lower extremities.

    Ⓝ *NCLEX® Connection: Basic Care and Comfort, Non–Pharmacological Comfort Interventions*

2. A. **CORRECT.** Vaginal bleeding indicates a potential complication of the placenta such as placenta previa. The nurse should instruct the client to notify the provider immediately.

    B. Swelling of the ankles is a common occurrence during pregnancy and can be relieved by sitting with the legs elevated.

    C. Heartburn occurs during pregnancy due to pressure on the stomach by the enlarging uterus. It can be relieved by eating small meals.

    D. Supine hypotension can be experienced by the client who feels lightheaded or faint when lying on her back. The nurse should instruct the client about the side-lying position to remove pressure of the uterus on the vena cava.

    Ⓝ *NCLEX® Connection: Health Promotion and Maintenance, Ante/Intra/Postpartum and Newborn Care*

3. A. **CORRECT:** Nausea and vomiting during the first trimester might be relieved by eating crackers or plain toast 30 to 60 min prior to rising in the morning.

    B. Eating during the night can cause heartburn and does not relieve nausea and vomiting during the first trimester.

    C. Instruct the client to avoid an empty stomach for prolonged periods to reduce nausea and vomiting.

    D. Eating a large meal in the evening can cause heartburn and does not relieve morning nausea and vomiting.

    Ⓝ *NCLEX® Connection: Physiological Adaptation, Alterations in Body Systems*

4. A. **CORRECT:** Breast tenderness is a common discomfort occurring during the first trimester of pregnancy.

    B. **CORRECT:** Urinary frequency is a common discomfort occurring during the first trimester of pregnancy.

    C. **CORRECT:** Epistaxis is a common discomfort occurring during the first trimester of pregnancy.

    D. Dysuria is a complication that might occur during pregnancy. The nurse should instruct the client to report this finding to the provider.

    E. Epigastric pain is a clinical finding of pregnancy-induced hypertension. The nurse should instruct the client to report this finding to the provider

    Ⓝ *NCLEX® Connection: Health Promotion and Maintenance, Ante/Intra/Postpartum and Newborn Care*

5. A. This is a nontherapeutic response by the nurse and does not acknowledge the client's concerns.

    B. **CORRECT:** Feelings of ambivalence about pregnancy are normal during the first trimester.

    C. This is a nontherapeutic response by the nurse and indicates disapproval.

    D. This is a nontherapeutic response by the nurse and does not acknowledge the client's feelings.

    Ⓝ *NCLEX® Connection: Health Promotion and Maintenance, Developmental Stages and Transitions*

PRACTICE Answer

Using ATI Active Learning Template: Basic Concept

UNDERLYING PRINCIPLES: UTIs are common because of renal changes during pregnancy and the vaginal flora becoming more alkaline.

NURSING INTERVENTIONS
Decrease risk of UTIs by:

- How, When: Encouraging client to wipe the perineal area from front to back after voiding.
- How: Avoiding bubble baths.
- How: Wearing cotton underpants, avoiding tight-fitting pants.

- How: Consuming at least 8 glasses of water per day.
- How, Why: Instructing client to urinate before and after intercourse to flush bacteria from the urethra that are present or introduced during intercourse.

- How, Why: Advising client to urinate as soon as the urge occurs because retaining urine provides an environment for bacterial growth.
- When, Why: Advising client to notify her provider if her urine is foul-smelling, contains blood, or is cloudy so evaluation and early treatment can be initiated.

Ⓝ *NCLEX® Connection: Physiological Adaptation, Illness Management*

CHAPTER 5 ## Nutrition During Pregnancy

Adequate nutritional intake during pregnancy is essential to promoting fetal and maternal health.

Recommended weight gain during pregnancy, based on a single pregnancy, is usually 11.3 to 15.9 kg (25 to 35 lb). The general rule is that clients should gain 1 to 2 kg (2.2 to 4.4 lb) during the first trimester and after that approximately 0.4 kg (1 lb) per week for the last two trimesters. Underweight women are advised to gain 28 to 40 lb; overweight women, 15 to 25 lb.

It is important for the nurse to evaluate the pregnant client's nutritional choices, possible risk factors, and diet history. The nurse also should review specific nutritional guidelines for at-risk clients. Assistance is given to clients to develop a postpartum nutritional plan.

NURSING ASSESSMENT AND INTERVENTIONS

ASSESSMENT

Obtain subjective and objective dietary information.
- Journal of the client's food habits, eating pattern, and cravings
- Nutrition-related questionnaires
- The client's weight on first prenatal visit and follow-up visits
- Laboratory findings, such as Hgb and iron levels

Determine the client's caloric intake. Qᴘᴄᴄ
Have the client record everything eaten during a 24-hr period. The nurse, dietitian, or client can identify the caloric value of each item. This record can provide better objective data about the client's nutrition status. **(5.1)**

CLIENT EDUCATION

Instruct the client to adhere to and maintain the following during pregnancy.
- **Increase calories:** An increase of 340 calories/day is recommended during the second trimester. An increase of 462 calories/day is recommended during the third trimester. If the client is breastfeeding during the postpartum period, additional caloric intake is advised. The American Academy of Pediatrics (AAP) recommends that breastfeeding women who are well nourished should add 450 to 500 calories/day to a balanced diet.
- **Increasing protein intake** is essential to basic growth. Also, the intake of foods high in folic acid is crucial for neurological development and the prevention of fetal neural tube defects. Foods high in folic acid include leafy vegetables, dried peas and beans, seeds, and orange juice. Breads, cereals, and other grains are fortified with folic acid. The March of Dimes recommends that clients who wish to become pregnant and clients of childbearing age take 400 mcg of folic acid .and clients who become pregnant take 600 mcg of folic acid. Qᴇʙᴘ
- **Iron supplements** are often added to the prenatal plan to facilitate an increase of the maternal RBC mass. Iron is best absorbed between meals and when given with a source of vitamin C. Milk and caffeine interfere with the absorption of iron supplements. Food sources of iron include beef liver, red meats, fish, poultry, dried peas and beans, and fortified cereals and breads. A stool softener might need to be added to decrease constipation experienced with iron supplements.
- **Calcium**, which is important to a developing fetus, is involved in bone and teeth formation. Sources of calcium include milk, calcium-fortified soy milk, fortified orange juice, nuts, legumes, and dark green leafy vegetables. Daily recommendation is 1,000 mg/day for pregnant and nonpregnant women 19 to 50 years of age, and 1,300 mg/day for those under 19 years of age.
- **Fluid:** 8 to 10 glasses (2.3 L) of fluid are recommended daily. Preferred fluids are water, fruit juice, and milk.
- **Limit caffeine:** The American Congress of Obstetricians and Gynecologists (ACOG) and March of Dimes recommend a daily intake of no more than 200 mg of caffeine. The equivalent of 500 to 750 mL/day of coffee could increase the risk of a spontaneous abortion or fetal intrauterine growth restriction. Qᴇʙᴘ
- It is recommended that women abstain from alcohol consumption during pregnancy.

5.1 Plan of care for a pregnant client

Expected outcomes
The client will consume the recommended dietary allowances/nutrients during her pregnancy.

Evaluation of the plan
Is there adequate weight gain?
Is the client compliant with the nursing plan of care?

Interventions
The nurse assesses the client's dietary journal on the next prenatal visit.

The nurse provides educational materials regarding nutritional benefits to the mother and her newborn.

The nurse provides encouragement and answers questions that the client has regarding her dietary plans.

The nurse weighs the client and monitors for signs of inadequate weight gain.

The nurse makes a referral if needed.

RISK FACTORS

Age, culture, education, and socioeconomic issues could affect adequate nutrition during pregnancy. Also, certain conditions specific to each client might inhibit adequate caloric intake.

- Adolescents might have poor nutritional habits (a diet low in vitamins and protein, not taking prescribed iron supplements).
- Vegetarians might have low protein, calcium, iron, zinc, and vitamin B_{12}.
- Nausea and vomiting during pregnancy
- Anemia
- Eating disorders such as anorexia nervosa or bulimia nervosa
- Pregnant clients diagnosed with the appetite disorder pica (craving to eat nonfood substances such as dirt or red clay); this disorder might diminish the amount of nutritional foods ingested.
- Excessive weight gain can lead to macrosomia and labor complications.
- Inability to gain weight could result in low birth weight of the newborn.
- Financially unable to purchase/access food; therefore, the nurse should advise the client about the Women, Infants and Children (WIC) programs, which are federally funded state programs for pregnant women and their children (up to 5 years old). Qᴛᴄ

DIETARY COMPLICATIONS DURING PREGNANCY

Nausea and constipation

Nausea and constipation are common during pregnancy.

- For nausea, tell the client to eat small amounts frequently (every 2 to 3 hr) to avoid large meals that distend the stomach and avoid alcohol, caffeine, and fried, fatty, and spicy foods. Also avoid consuming excessive amounts of fluid, and DO NOT take a medication to control nausea without first checking with her provider. Ginger (ginger ale soda, ginger tea, ginger candies) might also be helpful.
- For constipation, increase fluid consumption and include extra fiber in the diet. Fruits, vegetables, and whole grains all contain fiber.

Maternal phenylketonuria

Maternal phenylketonuria (PKU) is a maternal genetic disease in which high levels of phenylalanine pose a danger to the fetus.

- It is important for the client to resume the PKU diet for at least 3 months prior to pregnancy and continue the diet throughout pregnancy.
- The diet includes foods that are low in phenylalanine. Foods high in protein, such as fish, poultry, meat, eggs, nuts, and dairy products, must be avoided due to high phenylalanine levels. Aspartame, which contains phenylalanine, should be avoided by pregnant women who have PKU.
- The client's blood phenylalanine levels are monitored during pregnancy.
- These interventions can prevent fetal complications such as mental retardation and behavioral problems.

Diabetes mellitus

Both preexisting diabetes mellitus and gestational diabetes mellitus are complications that require nutritional interventions.

- Monitor the amount of carbohydrates in the diet and keep glucose levels within target
- Limit the amount of sweets and desserts, which typically have large amounts of carbohydrates.
- Meet with a registered dietitian.

CREATING A POSTPARTUM NUTRITIONAL PLAN

A lactating woman's nutritional plan includes the following instructions:

- Increase protein and calorie intake while adhering to a recommended, well-balanced diet.
- Increase oral fluids, but avoid alcohol and caffeine.
- Avoid food substances that do not agree with the newborn (foods that can cause altered bowel function).
- The client should take calcium supplements if she consumes an inadequate amount of dietary calcium.

A nutritional plan for a woman who is not breastfeeding should include resumption of a previously recommended well-balanced diet.

Application Exercises

1. A nurse in a prenatal clinic is providing education to a client who is in the 8th week of gestation. The client states that she does not like milk. Which of the following foods should the nurse recommend as a good source of calcium?

   A. Dark green leafy vegetables

   B. Deep red or orange vegetables

   C. White breads and rice

   D. Meat, poultry, and fish

2. A nurse in a prenatal clinic is caring for four clients. Which of the following clients' weight gain should the nurse report to the provider?

   A. 1.8 kg (4 lb) weight gain and is in her first trimester

   B. 3.6 kg (8 lb) weight gain and is in her first trimester

   C. 6.8 kg (15 lb) weight gain and is in her second trimester

   D. 11.3 kg (25 lb) weight gain and is in her third trimester

3. A nurse in a clinic is teaching a client of childbearing age about recommended folic acid supplements. Which of the following defects can occur in the fetus or neonate as a result of folic acid deficiency?

   A. Iron deficiency anemia

   B. Poor bone formation

   C. Macrosomic fetus

   D. Neural tube defects

4. A nurse is reviewing a new prescription for iron supplements with a client who is in the 8th week of gestation and has iron deficiency anemia. Which of the following beverages should the nurse instruct the client to take the iron supplements with?

   A. Ice water

   B. Low-fat or whole milk

   C. Tea or coffee

   D. Orange juice

5. A nurse is reviewing postpartum nutrition needs with a group of new mothers who are breastfeeding their newborns. Which of the following statements by a member of the group indicates an understanding of the teaching?

   A. "I am glad I can have my morning coffee."

   B. "I should take folic acid to increase my milk supply."

   C. "I will continue adding 330 calories per day to my diet."

   D. "I will continue my calcium supplements because I don't like milk."

PRACTICE Active Learning Scenario

A nurse manager in a prenatal clinic is preparing an in-service education program for a group of newly licensed nurses about risk factors preventing adequate nutrition during pregnancy. What information should the nurse include in this presentation? Use the ATI Active Learning Template: Basic Concept to answer this item.

UNDERLYING PRINCIPLES
- Identify one that is age-related.
- Identify two that are related to culture/lifestyle.
- Identify one that is related to a socioeconomic factor.
- Identify two that are related to dietary complications during pregnancy.

NURSING INTERVENTIONS: Describe a federal program that is available to woman and children to provide nutrition support.

Application Exercises Key

1. A. **CORRECT:** Good sources of calcium for bone and teeth formation include low-oxalate, dark green leafy vegetables, such as kale, artichokes, and turnip greens.

   B. Deep red or orange vegetables are good sources of vitamins C and A.

   C. White breads and rice do not contain high levels of calcium.

   D. Meat, poultry, and fish are sources of protein but do not contain high levels of calcium.

   Ⓝ *NCLEX® Connection: Basic Care and Comfort, Nutrition and Oral Hydration*

2. A. This client has gained the appropriate weight of 3 to 4 lb for a client in the first trimester.

   B. **CORRECT:** The nurse should be concerned about this client because she has exceeded the expected 3- to 4-lb weight gain of a client in the first trimester.

   C. This client has gained the appropriate weight of 3 to 4 lb. in the first trimester and approximately 1 lb per week in the second trimester.

   D. This client is within the recommended weight gain of 25 to 35 lb during the third trimester.

   Ⓝ *NCLEX® Connection: Health Promotion and Maintenance, Health Promotion/Disease Prevention*

3. A. Iron deficiency anemia is the result of a lack of iron-rich dietary sources, such as meat, chicken, and fish.

   B. Calcium deficiency can result in poor bone and teeth formation.

   C. Maternal obesity can lead to a macrosomic fetus.

   D. **CORRECT:** Neural tube defects are caused by folic acid deficiency. Food sources of folic acid include fresh green leafy vegetables, liver, peanuts, cereals, and whole-grain breads.

   Ⓝ *NCLEX® Connection: Health Promotion and Maintenance, Health Promotion/Disease Prevention*

4. A. Water does not promote absorption of iron, but drinking plenty of water can prevent constipation, which is an adverse effect of iron supplements.

   B. Milk interferes with iron absorption.

   C. Caffeine, found in tea and coffee, can interfere with iron absorption. The client should consume no more than 200 mg/day because it increases the risk of spontaneous abortion or fetal intrauterine growth restriction.

   D. **CORRECT:** Orange juice contains vitamin C, which aids in the absorption of iron.

   Ⓝ *NCLEX® Connection: Pharmacological and Parenteral Therapies, Medication Administration*

5. A. Women who are breastfeeding should avoid caffeine intake because it affects iron absorption and infant weight gain.

   B. Folic acid does not increase milk production.

   C. Women who are breastfeeding require an additional 450 to 500 calories per day to support adequate nutrition.

   D. **CORRECT:** Postpartum women who are at risk for inadequate dietary calcium should continue taking calcium supplements during lactation.

   Ⓝ *NCLEX® Connection: Health Promotion and Maintenance, Ante/Intra/Postpartum and Newborn Care*

PRACTICE Answer

Using the ATI Active Learning Template: Basic Concept

UNDERLYING PRINCIPLES
- Age-related: Adolescents may have poor nutritional habits during pregnancy.
- Culture/lifestyle: Vegetarians may have diets low in protein, calcium, zinc, and vitamin B12. Excessive weight gain can lead to macrosomia and labor complications.
- Socioeconomic factor: Inability to purchase or access foods can limit nutrition during pregnancy.
- Dietary complications: Nausea and vomiting during pregnancy, anemia, eating disorders (anorexia nervosa or bulimia nervosa), inability to gain weight, presence of the appetite disorder pica.

NURSING INTERVENTIONS: Women, Infants and Children (WIC) is a federally funded state program that provides nutritional support to pregnant women and their children (up to 5 years old).

Ⓝ *NCLEX® Connection: Health Promotion and Maintenance, Ante/Intra/Postpartum and Newborn Care*

CHAPTER 6 # Assessment of Fetal Well-Being

This chapter includes the assessments that determine the well-being of a fetus during pregnancy. Diagnostic procedures include ultrasound (abdominal, transvaginal, Doppler), biophysical profile, nonstress test, contraction stress test (nipple, oxytocin), and amniocentesis. Additional diagnostic procedures for high-risk pregnancy include percutaneous umbilical cord blood sampling, chorionic villus sampling, quad marker screening, and maternal serum alpha-fetoprotein.

Ultrasound (abdominal, transvaginal, and Doppler)

Ultrasound is a procedure lasting approximately 20 min that consists of high-frequency sound waves used to visualize internal organs and tissues by producing a real-time, three-dimensional image of the developing fetus and maternal structures (fetal heart rate [FHR], pelvic anatomy). An ultrasound allows for early diagnosis of complications, permits earlier interventions, and thereby decreases neonatal and maternal morbidity and mortality. There are three types of ultrasound: external abdominal, transvaginal, and Doppler.

External abdominal ultrasound

A safe, noninvasive, painless procedure whereby an ultrasound transducer is moved over the client's abdomen to obtain an image. An abdominal ultrasound is more useful after the first trimester when the gravid uterus is larger. The client should have a full bladder for the procedure. Q EBP

Transvaginal ultrasound

An invasive procedure in which a probe is inserted vaginally to allow for a more accurate evaluation. An advantage of this procedure is that it does not require a full bladder.
- It is especially useful in clients who are obese and those in the first trimester to detect an ectopic pregnancy, identify abnormalities, and to establish gestational age.
- A transvaginal ultrasound also can be used in the third trimester in conjunction with abdominal scanning to evaluate for preterm labor.

Doppler ultrasound blood flow analysis

A noninvasive external ultrasound method to study the maternal-fetal blood flow by measuring the velocity at which RBCs travel in the uterine and fetal vessels using a handheld ultrasound device that reflects sound waves from a moving target. It is especially useful in fetal intrauterine growth restriction (IUGR) and poor placental perfusion, and as an adjunct in pregnancies at risk because of hypertension, diabetes mellitus, multiple fetuses, or preterm labor.

Two-dimensional (2D): standard medical scan; black, white, or shades of gray

Three-dimensional (3D): multiple pictures at once; almost as clear as a photograph; images look more lifelike than standard ultrasound images

Four-dimensional (4D): like 3D but also shows fetal movements in a video

INDICATIONS

POTENTIAL DIAGNOSES

- Confirming pregnancy
- Confirming gestational age by biparietal diameter (side-to-side) measurement
- Identifying multifetal pregnancy
- Determining site of fetal implantation (uterine, ectopic)
- Assessing fetal growth and development
- Assessing maternal structures
- Confirming fetal viability or death
- Ruling out or verifying fetal abnormalities
- Locating the site of placental attachment
- Determining amniotic fluid volume
- Observing fetal movement (fetal heartbeat, breathing, and activity)
- Assessing fetal position
- Placental grading (evaluating placental maturation)
- Adjunct for other procedures (e.g., amniocentesis, biophysical profile)

CLIENT PRESENTATION

- Vaginal bleeding evaluation
- Questionable fundal height measurement in relationship to gestational weeks
- Reports of decreased fetal movements
- Preterm labor
- Questionable rupture of membranes

CONSIDERATIONS

NURSING ACTIONS

CLIENT PREPARATION

- Explain the procedure to the client and that it presents no known risk to her or her fetus.
- Advise the client to drink 1 quart of water prior to the ultrasound to fill the bladder, lift and stabilize the uterus, displace the bowel, and act as an echolucent to better reflect sound waves to obtain a better image of the fetus.
- Assist the client into a supine position with a wedge placed under her right hip to displace the uterus (prevents supine hypotension). Qs

ONGOING CARE

- Apply an ultrasonic/transducer gel to the client's abdomen before the transducer is moved over the skin to obtain a better fetal image, ensuring that the gel is at room temperature or warmer.
- Allow the client to empty her bladder at the termination of the procedure.
- Provide the client with a washcloth or tissues to wipe away gel after completion of ultrasound

Transvaginal ultrasound

CLIENT PREPARATION: Assist the client into a lithotomy position. The vaginal probe is covered with a protective device such as a condom, lubricated with a water-soluble gel, and inserted by the client or examiner.

ONGOING CARE

- During the procedure, the position of the probe or tilt of the table can be changed to facilitate the complete view of the pelvis.
- Inform the client that she might feel pressure as the probe is moved.

CLIENT EDUCATION

Fetal and maternal structures can be pointed out to the client as the ultrasound procedure is performed.

Biophysical profile

Biophysical profile (BPP) uses a real-time ultrasound to visualize physical and physiological characteristics of the fetus and observe for fetal biophysical responses to stimuli. It combines FHR monitoring (nonstress test) and fetal ultrasound.

INDICATIONS

POTENTIAL DIAGNOSES

- Nonreactive stress test
- Suspected oligohydramnios or polyhydramnios
- Suspected fetal hypoxemia or hypoxia

CLIENT PRESENTATION

- Premature rupture of membranes
- Maternal infection
- Decreased fetal movement
- Intrauterine growth restriction

CONSIDERATIONS

NURSING ACTIONS: Prepare the client following the same nursing management principles as those used for an ultrasound

INTERPRETATION OF FINDINGS

BPP assesses fetal well-being by measuring five variables with a score of 2 for each normal finding, and 0 for each abnormal finding for each variable.

VARIABLES

FHR
- Reactive (nonstress test) = 2
- Nonreactive = 0

Fetal breathing movements
- At least 1 episode of greater than 30 seconds duration in 30 min = 2
- Absent or less than 30 seconds duration = 0

Gross body movements
- At least 3 body or limb extensions with return to flexion in 30 min = 2
- Less than 3 episodes = 0

Fetal tone
- At least 1 episode of extension with return to flexion = 2
- Low extension and flexion, lack of flexion, or absent movement = 0

Qualitative amniotic fluid volume
- At least 1 pocket of fluid that measures at least 2 cm in 2 perpendicular planes = 2
- Pockets absent or less than 2 cm = 0

TOTAL SCORE FINDINGS

8 TO 10: **normal**, low risk of chronic fetal asphyxia

4 TO 6: **abnormal**, suspect chronic fetal asphyxia

LESS THAN 4: **abnormal**, strongly suspect chronic fetal asphyxia

6.1 Reactive nonstress test

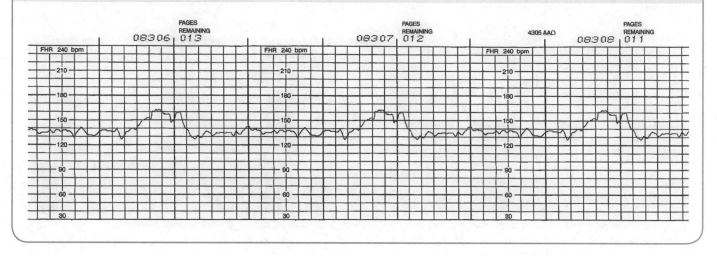

Nonstress test

Nonstress test (NST) is the most widely used technique for antepartum evaluation of fetal well-being performed during the third trimester. It is a noninvasive procedure that monitors response of the FHR to fetal movement. A Doppler transducer (used to monitor FHR) and a tocotransducer (used to monitor uterine contractions) are attached externally to a client's abdomen to obtain tracing strips. The client pushes a button attached to the monitor whenever she feels a fetal movement, which is then noted on the tracing. This allows a nurse to assess the FHR in relationship to the fetal movement.

> Disadvantages of a NST include a high rate of false nonreactive results with the fetal movement response blunted by sleep cycles of the fetus, fetal immaturity, maternal medications, and nicotine use disorder.

INDICATIONS

POTENTIAL DIAGNOSES

- Assessing for an intact fetal CNS during the third trimester.
- Ruling out the risk for fetal death in clients who have diabetes mellitus. Used twice a week starting at 28 to 32 weeks of gestation.

CLIENT PRESENTATION

- Decreased fetal movement
- Intrauterine growth restriction
- Postmaturity
- Gestational diabetes mellitus
- Gestational hypertension
- Maternal chronic hypertension
- History of previous fetal demise
- Advanced maternal age
- Sickle cell disease
- Isoimmunization

CONSIDERATIONS

NURSING ACTIONS

CLIENT PREPARATION

- Seat the client in a reclining chair, or place in a semi-Fowler's or left-lateral position.
- Apply conduction gel to the client's abdomen.
- Apply two belts to the client's abdomen, and attach the FHR and uterine contraction monitors.

ONGOING CARE

- Instruct the client to press the button on the handheld event marker each time she feels the fetus move.
- If there are no fetal movements (fetus sleeping), vibroacoustic stimulation (sound source, usually laryngeal stimulator) can be activated for 3 seconds on the maternal abdomen over the fetal head to awaken the sleeping fetus.

INTERPRETATION OF FINDINGS

- The NST is interpreted as reactive if the FHR is a normal baseline rate with moderate variability, accelerates at least 15/min (10/min prior to 32 weeks) for at least 15 seconds (10 seconds prior to 32 weeks) and occurs two or more times during a 20-min period. **(6.1)**
- Nonreactive NST is a test that does not demonstrate at least two qualifying accelerations in a 20-min window. If this is so, a further assessment, such as a contraction stress test (CST) or BPP, is indicated.

Contraction stress test

Nipple-stimulated contraction test

Consists of a woman lightly brushing her palm across her nipple for 2 min, which causes the pituitary gland to release endogenous oxytocin, and then stopping the nipple stimulation when a contraction begins. The same process is repeated after a 5-min rest period.

- Analysis of the FHR response to contractions (which decrease placental blood flow) determines how the fetus will tolerate the stress of labor. A pattern of at least three contractions within a 10-min time period with duration of 40 to 60 seconds each must be obtained to use for assessment data.
- Hyperstimulation of the uterus (uterine contraction longer than 90 seconds or five or more contractions in 10 min) should be avoided by stimulating the nipple intermittently with rest periods in between and avoiding bimanual stimulation of both nipples unless stimulation of one nipple is unsuccessful.

Oxytocin-stimulated contraction test

Also known as an oxytocin challenge test (OCT), it is used if nipple stimulation fails and consists of the IV administration of oxytocin to induce uterine contractions.

- Contractions started with oxytocin can be difficult to stop and can lead to preterm labor.
- Contraindications include placenta previa, vasa previa, preterm labor, multiple gestations, previous classic incision from a cesarean birth, and reduced cervical competence.

INDICATIONS

POTENTIAL DIAGNOSES

- High-risk pregnancies (gestational diabetes mellitus, postterm pregnancy)
- Nonreactive stress test

CLIENT PRESENTATION

- Decreased fetal movement
- Intrauterine growth restriction
- Postmaturity
- Gestational diabetes mellitus
- Gestational hypertension
- Maternal chronic hypertension
- History of previous fetal demise
- Advanced maternal age
- Sickle-cell disease

CONSIDERATIONS

NURSING ACTIONS

CLIENT PREPARATION
- Obtain and document a baseline of the FHR, fetal movement, and contractions for 10 to 20 min.
- Explain the procedure to the client, and obtain informed consent. Qpcc
- Complete an assessment without artificial stimulation if contractions are occurring spontaneously.

ONGOING CARE
- Initiate nipple stimulation if there are no contractions. Instruct the client to roll a nipple between her thumb and fingers or brush her palm across her nipple. The client should stop when a uterine contraction begins.
- Monitor and provide adequate rest periods for the client to avoid hyperstimulation of the uterus.

INTERVENTIONS
Initiate IV oxytocin administration if nipple stimulation fails to elicit a sufficient uterine contraction pattern. If hyperstimulation of the uterus or preterm labor occurs, do the following. Qebp
- Monitor for contractions lasting longer than 90 seconds or occurring more frequently than every 2 min.
- Administer tocolytics as prescribed.
- Maintain bed rest during the procedure.
- Observe the client for 30 min afterward to see that contractions have ceased and preterm labor does not begin.

INTERPRETATION OF FINDINGS

NEGATIVE CST (NORMAL FINDING): Indicated if within a 10-min period, with three uterine contractions, there are no late decelerations of the FHR.

POSITIVE CST (ABNORMAL FINDING): Indicated with persistent and consistent late decelerations with 50% or more of the contractions. This is suggestive of uteroplacental insufficiency. Variable deceleration can indicate cord compression, and early decelerations can indicate fetal head compression. Based on these findings, the provider may determine to induce labor or perform a cesarean birth. (6.2)

COMPLICATIONS

Potential for preterm labor

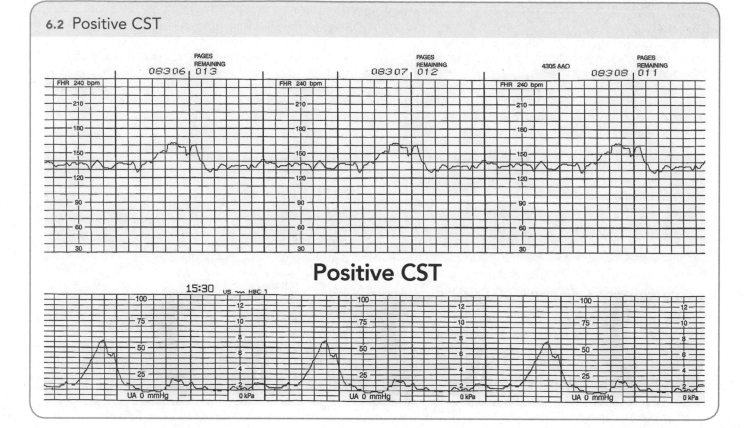

Positive CST

Amniocentesis

The aspiration of amniotic fluid for analysis by insertion of a needle transabdominally into a client's uterus and amniotic sac under direct ultrasound guidance locating the placenta and determining the position of the fetus. It may be performed after 14 weeks of gestation.

INDICATIONS

POTENTIAL DIAGNOSES

- Previous birth with a chromosomal anomaly
- A parent who is a carrier of a chromosomal anomaly
- A family history of neural tube defects
- Prenatal diagnosis of a genetic disorder or congenital anomaly of the fetus
- Alpha-fetoprotein (AFP) level for fetal abnormalities
- Lung maturity assessment
- Fetal hemolytic disease
- Meconium in the amniotic fluid

CONSIDERATIONS

PREPROCEDURE

NURSING ACTIONS: Explain the procedure to the client, and obtain informed consent.

CLIENT EDUCATION: Instruct the client to empty her bladder prior to the procedure to reduce its size and reduce the risk of inadvertent puncture. Qs

INTRAPROCEDURE

NURSING ACTIONS
- Obtain and document baseline vital signs and FHR prior to the procedure.
- Assist client into a supine position, and place a wedge under her right hip to displace the uterus off the vena cava, and place a drape over the client exposing only her abdomen.
- Prepare client for an ultrasound to locate the placenta.
- Cleanse client's abdomen with an antiseptic solution prior to the administration of a local anesthetic by the provider.

CLIENT EDUCATION: Tell the client that she will feel slight pressure as the needle is inserted. She should continue breathing because holding her breath will lower the diaphragm against the uterus and shift the intrauterine contents.

POSTPROCEDURE

NURSING ACTIONS

- Monitor vital signs, FHR, and uterine contractions throughout and 30 min following the procedure.
- Have the client rest for 30 min.
- Administer Rho(D) immune globulin to the client if she is Rh-negative (standard practice after an amniocentesis for all women who are Rh-negative to protect against Rh isoimmunization). Q_{EBP}

CLIENT EDUCATION

- Advise the client to report to her provider if she experiences fever, chills, leakage of fluid, or bleeding from the insertion site, decreased fetal movement, vaginal bleeding, or uterine contractions after the procedure.
- Encourage the client to drink plenty of liquids and rest for the 24 hr post procedure.

INTERPRETATION OF FINDINGS

AFP can be measured from the amniotic fluid between 15 and 20 weeks (16 to 18 weeks of gestation is ideal) and can be used to assess for neural tube defects in the fetus or chromosomal disorders. Can be evaluated to follow up a high level of AFP in maternal serum.

HIGH LEVELS: Associated with neural tube defects, such as anencephaly (incomplete development of fetal skull and brain), spina bifida (open spine), or omphalocele (abdominal wall defect). High AFP levels also can be present with normal multifetal pregnancies.

LOW LEVELS: Associated with chromosomal disorders (Down syndrome) or gestational trophoblastic disease (hydatidiform mole).

Fetal lung tests

Tests for fetal lung maturity can be performed if gestation is less than 37 weeks, in the event of a rupture of membranes, for preterm labor, or for a complication indicating a cesarean birth. Amniotic fluid is tested to determine whether the fetal lungs are mature enough to adapt to extrauterine life, or if the fetus will likely have respiratory distress. Determination is made whether the fetus should be removed immediately or if the fetus requires more time in utero with the administration of glucocorticoids to promote fetal lung maturity.

LECITHIN/SPHINGOMYELIN (L/S) RATIO: A 2:1 ratio indicates fetal lung maturity (2.5:1 or 3:1 for a client who has diabetes mellitus).

PRESENCE OF PHOSPHATIDYLGLYCEROL (PG): Absence of PG is associated with respiratory distress.

COMPLICATIONS

- Amniotic fluid emboli
- Maternal or fetal hemorrhage
- Fetomaternal hemorrhage with Rh isoimmunization
- Maternal or fetal infection
- Inadvertent fetal damage or anomalies involving limbs
- Fetal death
- Inadvertent maternal intestinal or bladder damage
- Miscarriage or preterm labor
- Premature rupture of membranes
- Leakage of amniotic fluid

NURSING ACTIONS

- Monitor vital signs, temperature, respiratory status, FHR, uterine contractions, and vaginal discharge for amniotic fluid or bleeding.
- Administer medication as prescribed.
- Offer support and reassurance.

High-risk pregnancy: Percutaneous umbilical blood sampling

Percutaneous umbilical blood sampling, commonly called cordocentesis, is the most common method used for fetal blood sampling and transfusion. This procedure obtains fetal blood from the umbilical cord by passing a fine-gauge, fiber-optic scope (fetoscope) into the amniotic sac using the amniocentesis technique. The needle is advanced into the umbilical cord under ultrasound guidance, and blood is aspirated from the umbilical vein. Blood studies from the cordocentesis can consist of:
- Kleihauer-Betke test that ensures that fetal blood was obtained
- CBC count with differential
- Indirect Coombs' test for Rh antibodies
- Karyotyping (visualization of chromosomes)
- Blood gases

INDICATIONS

POTENTIAL DIAGNOSES
- Fetal blood type, RBC, and chromosomal disorders
- Karyotyping of malformed fetuses
- Fetal infection
- Altered acid-base balance of fetuses with IUGR

CONSIDERATIONS

NURSING ACTIONS
- Administer medication as prescribed.
- Offer support.

INTERPRETATION OF FINDINGS

Evaluates for isoimmune fetal hemolytic anemia and assesses the need for a fetal blood transfusion.

COMPLICATIONS

- Cord laceration
- Preterm labor
- Amnionitis
- Hematoma
- Fetomaternal hemorrhage

High-risk pregnancy: Chorionic villus sampling

- Chorionic villus sampling (CVS) is assessment of a portion of the developing placenta (chorionic villi), which is aspirated through a thin sterile catheter or syringe inserted through the abdominal wall or intravaginally through the cervix under ultrasound guidance.
- CVS is a first-trimester alternative to amniocentesis with one of its advantages being an earlier diagnosis of any abnormalities. CVS is ideally performed at 10 to 13 weeks of gestation.

> The advantage of an earlier diagnosis should be weighed against the increased risk of fetal anomalies and death.

INDICATIONS

POTENTIAL DIAGNOSES: Risk for giving birth to a neonate who has a genetic chromosomal abnormality (cannot determine spina bifida or anencephaly)

CONSIDERATIONS

CLIENT EDUCATION
- Instruct the client to drink plenty of fluid to fill the bladder prior to the procedure to assist in positioning the uterus for catheter insertion.
- Provide ongoing education and support.

COMPLICATIONS

- Spontaneous abortion (higher risk with CVS than with amniocentesis)
- Risk for fetal limb loss (greatest risk prior to 9 weeks of gestation)
- Miscarriage
- Chorioamnionitis and rupture of membranes

High-risk pregnancy: Quad marker screening

A blood test that ascertains information about the likelihood of fetal birth defects. It does not diagnose the actual defect. It can be performed instead of the maternal serum AFP yielding more reliable findings. Includes testing for:
- **Human chorionic gonadotropin (hCG):** a hormone produced by the placenta
- **Alpha–fetoprotein (AFP):** a protein produced by the fetus
- **Estriol:** a protein produced by the fetus and placenta
- **Inhibin A:** a protein produced by the ovaries and placenta

INDICATIONS

CLIENT PRESENTATION
- Preferred at 16 to 18 weeks gestation
- Risk for giving birth to a neonate who has a genetic chromosomal abnormality

INTERPRETATION OF FINDINGS

- Low levels of AFP can indicate a risk for Down syndrome.
- High levels of AFP can indicate a risk for neural tube defects.
- Levels higher than the expected reference range of hCG and inhibin A indicates a risk for Down syndrome.
- Lower levels than the expected reference range of estriol can indicate a risk for Down syndrome.

High-risk pregnancy: Maternal serum alpha-fetoprotein (MSAFP)

A screening tool used to detect neural tube defects. Clients who have abnormal findings should be referred for a quad marker screening, genetic counseling, ultrasound, and an amniocentesis.

INDICATIONS

POTENTIAL DIAGNOSES: All pregnant clients, preferably between 16 and 18 weeks of gestation

CONSIDERATIONS

PREPROCEDURE NURSING ACTIONS
- Discuss testing with the client.
- Draw blood sample.
- Offer support and education as needed.

INTERPRETATION OF FINDINGS

- High levels can indicate a neural tube defect or open abdominal defect.
- Low levels can indicate Down syndrome.

Application Exercises

1. A nurse is reviewing findings of a client's biophysical profile (BPP). The nurse should expect which of the following variables to be included in this test? (Select all that apply.)

    A. Fetal weight

    B. Fetal breathing movement

    C. Fetal tone

    D. Fetal Position

    E. Amniotic fluid volume

2. A nurse is caring for a client who is in preterm labor and is scheduled to undergo an amniocentesis. The nurse should evaluate which of the following tests to assess fetal lung maturity?

    A. Alpha-fetoprotein (AFP)

    B. Lecithin/sphingomyelin (L/S) ratio

    C. Kleihauer-Betke test

    D. Indirect Coombs' test

3. A nurse is caring for a client who is pregnant and undergoing a nonstress test. The client asks why the nurse is using an acoustic vibration device. Which of the following responses should the nurse make?

    A. "It is used to stimulate uterine contractions."

    B. "It will decrease the incidence of uterine contractions."

    C. "It lulls the fetus to sleep."

    D. "It awakens a sleeping fetus."

4. A nurse is teaching a client who is pregnant about the amniocentesis procedure. Which of the following statements should the nurse include in the teaching?

    A. "You will lay on your right side during the procedure."

    B. "You should not eat anything for 24 hours prior to the procedure."

    C. "You should empty your bladder prior to the procedure."

    D. "The test is done to determine gestational age."

5. A nurse is caring for a client who is pregnant and is to undergo a contraction stress test (CST). Which of the following findings are indications for this procedure? (Select all that apply.)

    A. Decreased fetal movement

    B. Intrauterine growth restriction (IUGR)

    C. Postmaturity

    D. Placenta previa

    E. Amniotic fluid emboli

PRACTICE Active Learning Scenario

A nurse in a prenatal clinic is orienting a newly licensed nurse about how to perform a nonstress test (NST). What should the nurse include in the teaching about the procedure? Use the ATI Active Learning Template: Diagnostic Procedure to complete this item.

INDICATIONS: Identify three that relate to the status of the fetus.

INTERPRETATION OF FINDINGS: Describe a nonreactive NST.

NURSING INTERVENTIONS: Two preprocedure, one intraprocedure.

Application Exercises Key

1. A. Fetal weight is not one of the variables included in the BPP.

    B. **CORRECT:** Fetal breathing movements are included in the BPP.

    C. **CORRECT:** Fetal tone is included in the BPP.

    D. Fetal position is not included in the BPP.

    E. **CORRECT:** Amniotic fluid volume is included in the BPP.

    Ⓝ *NCLEX® Connection: Reduction of Risk Potential, Diagnostic Tests*

2. A. AFP is a test to assess for fetal neural tube defects or chromosome disorders.

    B. **CORRECT:** A test of the L/S ratio is done as a part of an amniocentesis to determine fetal lung maturity.

    C. A Kleihauer-Betke test is used to verify that fetal blood is present during a percutaneous umbilical blood sampling procedure.

    D. An indirect Coombs' test detects Rh antibodies in the mother's blood.

    Ⓝ *NCLEX® Connection: Reduction of Risk Potential, Diagnostic Tests*

3. A. The acoustic vibration device does not stimulate the uterus.

    B. The acoustic vibration device has no effect on the uterine muscles.

    C. The acoustic vibration device stimulates a sleeping fetus.

    D. **CORRECT:** The acoustic vibration device is activated for 3 seconds on the maternal abdomen over the fetal head to awaken a sleeping fetus.

    Ⓝ *NCLEX® Connection: Reduction of Risk Potential, Diagnostic Tests*

4. A. Assist the client into a supine position, place a wedge under her right hip to displace the uterus off the vena cava, and place a drape over the client, exposing only her abdomen.

    B. The client does not need to be NPO for 24 hr prior to the procedure.

    C. **CORRECT:** The client's bladder should be empty to avoid an inadvertent puncture during the procedure.

    D. Amniotic fluid is tested to identify fetal genetic defects. An amniocentesis does not determine gestational age.

    Ⓝ *NCLEX® Connection: Health Promotion and Maintenance, Ante/Intra/Postpartum and Newborn Care*

5. A. **CORRECT:** Decreased fetal movement is an indication for a CST.

    B. **CORRECT:** IUGR is an indication for a CST.

    C. **CORRECT:** Postmaturity is an indication for a CST.

    D. Placenta previa is a contraindication of a CST.

    E. Amniotic fluid emboli are a complication of an amniocentesis.

    Ⓝ *NCLEX® Connection: Reduction of Risk Potential, Diagnostic Tests*

PRACTICE Answer

Using the ATI Active Learning Template: Diagnostic Procedure

INDICATIONS

- Assessment for intact fetal CNS during the third trimester
- Rule out fetal death in a client who has diabetes mellitus
- Decreased fetal movement
- Intrauterine growth restriction
- Postmaturity

INTERPRETATION OF FINDINGS:

Nonreactive NST is a test that does not demonstrate at least two qualifying accelerations in a 20 minute window. If this is so, a further assessment, such as a contraction stress test or biophysical profile, is indicated.

NURSING INTERVENTIONS

Preprocedure

- Seat the client in a reclining chair in a semi-Fowler's or left-lateral position.
- Apply conduction gel to the client's abdomen.
- Apply the Doppler transducer and the tocotransducer.

Intraprocedure: Instruct the client to depress the event marker button each time she feels fetal movement.

Ⓝ *NCLEX® Connection: Reduction of Risk Potential, Diagnostic Tests*

UNIT 1 ANTEPARTUM NURSING CARE
SECTION: COMPLICATIONS OF PREGNANCY

CHAPTER 7 *Bleeding During Pregnancy*

Vaginal bleeding during pregnancy is always abnormal and must be investigated to determine the cause. It can impair both the outcome of the pregnancy and the mother's life. (7.1)

Spontaneous abortion

Spontaneous abortion is when a pregnancy is terminated before 20 weeks of gestation (the point of fetal viability) or a fetal weight less than 500 g.

Types of abortion are clinically classified according to manifestations and whether the products of conception are partially or completely retained or expulsed. Types of abortions include **threatened**, **inevitable**, **incomplete**, **complete**, and **missed**.

ASSESSMENT

RISK FACTORS

- Chromosomal abnormalities (account for 50%)
- Maternal illness, such as type 1 diabetes mellitus
- Advanced maternal age
- Premature cervical dilation
- Chronic maternal infections
- Maternal malnutrition
- Trauma or injury
- Anomalies in the fetus or placenta
- Substance use
- Antiphospholipid syndrome

EXPECTED FINDINGS (7.2)

- Backache and abdominal tenderness
- Rupture of membranes
- Dilation of the cervix
- Fever
- Signs and symptoms of hemorrhage, such as hypotension and tachycardia

LABORATORY TESTS

Hgb and Hct, if considerable blood loss

Clotting factors monitored for disseminated intravascular coagulopathy (DIC): a complication with retained products of conception

WBC for suspected infection

Serum human chorionic gonadotropin (hCG) levels to confirm pregnancy

DIAGNOSTIC AND THERAPEUTIC PROCEDURES

Ultrasound to determine the presence of a viable or dead fetus, or partial or complete products of conception within the uterine cavity.

Examination of the cervix to observe whether it is opened or closed.

Dilation and curettage (D&C) to dilate and scrape the uterine walls to remove uterine contents for inevitable and incomplete abortions.

Dilation and evacuation (D&E) to dilate and evacuate uterine contents after 16 weeks of gestation.

Prostaglandins and oxytocin to augment or induce uterine contractions and expulse the products of conception.

7.1 Causes of bleeding during pregnancy

First trimester
SPONTANEOUS ABORTION: Vaginal bleeding, uterine cramping, and partial or complete expulsion of products of conception

ECTOPIC PREGNANCY: Abrupt unilateral lower-quadrant abdominal pain with or without vaginal bleeding

Second trimester
GESTATIONAL TROPHOBLASTIC DISEASE: Uterine size increasing abnormally fast, abnormally high levels of hCG, nausea and increased emesis, no fetus present on ultrasound, and scant or profuse dark brown or red vaginal bleeding

Third trimester
PLACENTA PREVIA: Painless vaginal bleeding

ABRUPTIO PLACENTAE: Vaginal bleeding, sharp abdominal pain, and tender rigid uterus

VASA PREVIA: Fetal vessels are implanted into the membranes rather than the placenta.

Other causes of bleeding
RECURRENT PREMATURE DILATION OF THE CERVIX: Painless bleeding with cervical dilation leading to fetal expulsion

PRETERM LABOR: Pink-stained vaginal discharge, uterine contractions becoming regular, cervical dilation and effacement

HYDATIDIFORM MOLE: Benign proliferative growth of the placental trophoblast

PATIENT-CENTERED CARE

NURSING CARE

- Perform a pregnancy test.
- Observe color and amount of bleeding (count pads).
- Maintain client on bed rest. Inform client of risk for falls due to sedative medications if prescribed. Qs
- Avoid vaginal exams.
- Assist with an ultrasound.
- Administer medications and blood products as prescribed.
- Determine how much tissue has passed and save passed tissue for examination.
- Assist with termination of pregnancy (D&C, D&E, prostaglandin administration) as indicated.
- Use the lay term "miscarriage" with clients because the medical term "abortion" can be misunderstood.
- Provide client education and emotional support.
- Provide referral for client and partner to pregnancy loss support groups.

MEDICATIONS

- Analgesics and sedatives
- Prostaglandin, as a vaginal suppository
- Oxytocin
- Broad-spectrum antibiotics, in septic abortion
- Rho(D) immune globulin, suppresses immune response of clients who are Rh-negative

CLIENT EDUCATION

- Notify the provider of heavy, bright red vaginal bleeding; elevated temperature; or foul-smelling vaginal discharge.
- A small amount of discharge is normal for 1 to 2 weeks.
- Take prescribed antibiotics.
- Refrain from tub baths, sexual intercourse, or placing anything into the vagina for 2 weeks.
- Avoid becoming pregnant for 2 months.

Ectopic pregnancy

Ectopic pregnancy is the abnormal implantation of a fertilized ovum outside of the uterine cavity usually in the fallopian tube, which can result in a tubal rupture causing a fatal hemorrhage.

Ectopic pregnancy is the second most frequent cause of bleeding in early pregnancy and a leading cause of infertility.

ASSESSMENT

RISK FACTORS

Any factor that compromises tubal patency (STIs, assisted reproductive technologies, tubal surgery, and contraceptive intrauterine device [IUD])

EXPECTED FINDINGS

- Unilateral stabbing pain and tenderness in the lower-abdominal quadrant.
- Delayed (1 to 2 weeks), lighter than usual, or irregular menses.
- Scant, dark red, or brown vaginal spotting occurs 6 to 8 weeks after last normal menses; red, vaginal bleeding if rupture has occurred.
- Referred shoulder pain due to blood in the peritoneal cavity irritating the diaphragm or phrenic nerve after tubal rupture.
- Report of indications of shock such as faintness and dizziness related to amount of bleeding in abdominal cavity.
- Clinical findings of hemorrhage and shock (hypotension, tachycardia, pallor)

LABORATORY TESTS

Serum levels of progesterone and hCG elevated rules out ectopic pregnancy.

7.2 Spontaneous abortion assessment

	CRAMPS	BLEEDING	TISSUE PASSED	CERVICAL OPENING
THREATENED	Possible mild cramps	Spotting to moderate	None	Closed
INEVITABLE	Moderate	Mild to severe	None	Dilated with membranes or tissue bulging at cervix
INCOMPLETE	Severe	Heavy, profuse	Partial fetal tissue or placenta	Dilated with tissue in cervical canal or passage of tissue
COMPLETE	Mild	Minimal	Complete expulsion of uterine contents	Closed with no tissue in cervical canal
MISSED	None	None; brownish discharge	None, prolonged retention of tissue	Closed
SEPTIC	Varies	Varies; malodorous discharge	Varies	Usually dilated
RECURRENT	Varies	Varies	Yes	Usually dilated

DIAGNOSTIC AND THERAPEUTIC PROCEDURES

- Transvaginal ultrasound shows an empty uterus.
- Use caution if vaginal and bimanual examination are used.

RAPID TREATMENT
- **Medical management** if rupture has not occurred and tube preservation desired.
- **Methotrexate** inhibits cell division and embryo enlargement, dissolving the pregnancy
- **Salpingostomy** is done to salvage the fallopian tube if not ruptured.
- **Laparoscopic salpingectomy** (removal of the tube) is performed when the tube has ruptured.

PATIENT-CENTERED CARE

NURSING CARE

- Replace fluids, and maintain electrolyte balance.
- Provide client education and psychological support.
- Administer medications as prescribed.
- Prepare the client for surgery and postoperative nursing care.
- Provide referral for client and partner to pregnancy loss support group.
- Obtain serum hCG and progesterone levels, liver and renal function studies, CBC, and type and Rh.

CLIENT EDUCATION

- Instruct the client who is taking methotrexate to avoid alcohol consumption and vitamins containing folic acid to prevent a toxic response to the medication. Qs
- Advise the client to protect herself from sun exposure (photosensitivity).

Gestational trophoblastic disease

Gestational trophoblastic disease (GTD) is the proliferation and degeneration of trophoblastic villi in the placenta that becomes swollen, fluid-filled, and takes on the appearance of grape-like clusters. The embryo fails to develop beyond a primitive state and these structures are associated with choriocarcinoma, which is a rapidly metastasizing malignancy. Two types of molar growths are identified by chromosomal analysis.

Complete mole

- All genetic material is paternally derived.
- The ovum has no genetic material, or the material is inactive.
- The complete mole contains no fetus, placenta, amniotic membranes, or fluid.
- There is no placenta to receive maternal blood. Hemorrhage into the uterine cavity occurs, and vaginal bleeding results.
- Approximately 20% of complete moles progress toward a choriocarcinoma.

Partial mole

- Genetic material is derived both maternally and paternally.
- A normal ovum is fertilized by two sperm or one sperm in which meiosis or chromosome reduction and division did not occur.
- A partial mole often contains abnormal embryonic or fetal parts, an amniotic sac, and fetal blood, but congenital anomalies are present.
- Approximately 6% of partial moles progress toward a choriocarcinoma.

ASSESSMENT

RISK FACTORS

- Prior molar pregnancy
- Clients in early teens or older than age 40

EXPECTED FINDINGS

Excessive vomiting (hyperemesis gravidarum) due to elevated hCG levels

PHYSICAL ASSESSMENT FINDINGS
- Rapid uterine growth more than expected for the duration of the pregnancy due to the overproliferation of trophoblastic cells
- Bleeding is often dark brown resembling prune juice, or bright red that is either scant or profuse and continues for a few days or intermittently for a few weeks and can be accompanied by passage of vesicles.
- Anemia from blood loss
- Clinical findings of preeclampsia that occur prior to 24 weeks of gestation

LABORATORY TESTS

Serum level of hCG persistently high compared with expected decline after weeks 10 to 12 of pregnancy.

DIAGNOSTIC AND THERAPEUTIC PROCEDURES

- An ultrasound reveals a dense growth with characteristic vesicles, but no fetus in utero.
- Suction curettage is done to aspirate and evacuate the mole.
- Post-surgery, Rh-negative women are given Rho(D) immune globulin.
- Following mole evacuation, the client should undergo a baseline pelvic exam and ultrasound scan of the abdomen.
- Serum hCG analysis following molar pregnancy to be done weekly for 3 weeks, then monthly for 6 months up to 1 year to detect GTD.

PATIENT-CENTERED CARE

NURSING CARE

- Measure fundal height.
- Assess vaginal bleeding and discharge.
- Assess gastrointestinal status and appetite.
- Monitor for manifestations of preeclampsia.
- Administer medications as prescribed.
  - Rho(D) immune globulin to the client who is Rh-negative
  - Chemotherapeutic medications for findings of malignant cells indicating choriocarcinoma
- Advise client to save clots or tissue for evaluation.

CLIENT EDUCATION

- Provide client education and emotional support.
- Offer referral for clients and partners to pregnancy loss support groups.
- Instruct the client to use reliable contraception as a component of follow-up care.
- Reinforce the importance of follow-up due to the increased risk of choriocarcinoma.

Placenta previa

Placenta previa occurs when the placenta abnormally implants in the lower segment of the uterus near or over the cervical os instead of attaching to the fundus. The abnormal implantation results in bleeding during the third trimester of pregnancy as the cervix begins to dilate and efface. **(7.3)**

Classified into three types dependent on the degree to which the cervical os is covered by the placenta.
- **Complete or total:** The cervical os is completely covered by the placental attachment.
- **Incomplete or partial:** The cervical os is only partially covered by the placental attachment.
- **Marginal or low-lying:** The placenta is attached in the lower uterine segment but does not reach the cervical os.

ASSESSMENT

RISK FACTORS

- Previous placenta previa
- Uterine scarring (previous cesarean birth, curettage, endometritis)
- Maternal age greater than 35 years
- Multifetal gestation
- Multiple gestations or closely spaced pregnancies
- Smoking

EXPECTED FINDINGS

- Painless, bright red vaginal bleeding during the second or third trimester
- Uterus soft, relaxed, and nontender with normal tone
- Fundal height greater than usually expected for gestational age
- Fetus in a breech, oblique, or transverse position
- Reassuring FHR
- Vital signs within normal limits
- Decreasing urinary output can be a better indicator of blood loss

LABORATORY TESTS

- Hgb and Hct for blood loss assessment
- CBC
- Blood type and Rh
- Coagulation profile
- Kleihauer-Betke test (used to detect fetal blood in maternal circulation)

DIAGNOSTIC PROCEDURES

- Transabdominal or transvaginal ultrasound for placement of the placenta
- Fetal monitoring for fetal well-being assessment

PATIENT-CENTERED CARE

NURSING CARE

- Assess for bleeding, leakage, or contractions.
- Assess fundal height.
- Perform Leopold maneuvers (fetal position and presentation).
- Refrain from performing vaginal exams (can exacerbate bleeding). **Qs**
- Administer IV fluids, blood products, and medications as prescribed. Corticosteroids, such as betamethasone, promote fetal lung maturation if early delivery is anticipated (cesarean birth).
- Have oxygen equipment available in case of fetal distress.

CLIENT EDUCATION

- Bed rest
- Nothing inserted vaginally

Abruptio placentae

Abruptio placentae is the premature separation of the placenta from the uterus, which can be a partial or complete detachment. This separation occurs after 20 weeks of gestation, which is usually in the third trimester. It has significant maternal and fetal morbidity and mortality and is a leading cause of maternal death. **(7.4)**

Coagulation defect, such as disseminated intravascular coagulopathy (DIC), is often associated with moderate to severe abruption.

ASSESSMENT

RISK FACTORS

- Maternal hypertension (chronic or gestational)
- Blunt external abdominal trauma (motor-vehicle crash, maternal battering)
- Cocaine use resulting in vasoconstriction
- Previous incidents of abruptio placentae
- Cigarette smoking
- Premature rupture of membranes
- Multifetal pregnancy

EXPECTED FINDINGS

- Sudden onset of intense localized uterine pain with dark red vaginal bleeding
- Area of uterine tenderness can be localized or diffuse over uterus and boardlike
- Contractions with hypertonicity
- Fetal distress
- Clinical findings of hypovolemic shock

LABORATORY TESTS

- Hgb and Hct decreased
- Coagulation factors decreased
- Clotting defects (disseminated intravascular coagulation)
- Cross and type match for possible blood transfusions
- Kleihauer–Betke test (used to detect fetal blood in maternal circulation)

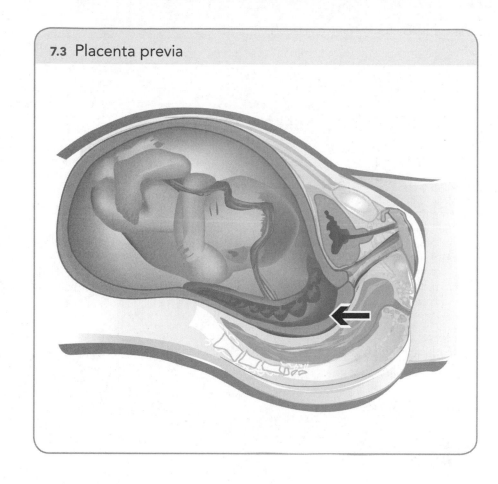

7.3 Placenta previa

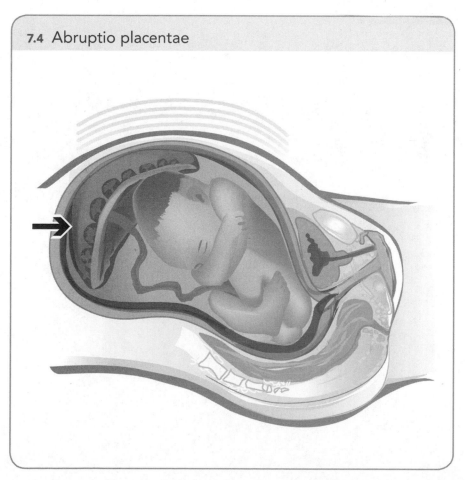

7.4 Abruptio placentae

DIAGNOSTIC PROCEDURES

- Ultrasound for fetal well-being and placental assessment
- Biophysical profile to ascertain fetal well-being

PATIENT-CENTERED CARE

NURSING CARE

- Palpate the uterus for tenderness and tone.
- Assess FHR pattern.
- Immediate birth is the management
  - Administer IV fluids, blood products, and medications as prescribed.
  - Administer oxygen 8 to 10 L/min via face mask.
  - Monitor maternal vital signs, observing for declining hemodynamic status.
  - Continuous fetal monitoring
  - Assess urinary output and monitor fluid balance.

CLIENT EDUCATION

Provide emotional support for the client and family.

Vasa previa

Vasa previa is a condition when the fetal umbilical vessels implant into the fetal membranes rather than the placenta.

There are variations of vasa previa.
- **Velamentous insertion of the cord:** Cord vessels begin in the branch at the membranes and then course to the placenta
- **Succenturiate insertion of the cord:** Placenta has divided into two or more lobes and not one mass.
- **Battledore insertion of the cord**
  - A marginal insertion
  - Increased risk of fetal hemorrhage

ASSESSMENT

DIAGNOSTIC PROCEDURES: Ultrasound for fetal well-being and vessel assessment

PATIENT-CENTERED CARE

NURSING ACTIONS: Closely monitor the patient during labor and delivery for excessive bleeding.

Application Exercises

1. A nurse in the emergency department is caring for a client who reports abrupt, sharp, right-sided lower quadrant abdominal pain and bright red vaginal bleeding. The client states she missed one menstrual cycle and cannot be pregnant because she has an intrauterine device. The nurse should suspect which of the following?

   A. Missed abortion

   B. Ectopic pregnancy

   C. Severe preeclampsia

   D. Hydatidiform mole

2. A nurse is providing care for a client who is diagnosed with a marginal abruptio placentae. The nurse is aware that which of the following findings are risk factors for developing the condition? (Select all that apply.)

   A. Fetal position

   B. Blunt abdominal trauma

   C. Cocaine use

   D. Maternal age

   E. Cigarette smoking

3. A nurse is providing care for a client who is at 32 weeks of gestation and who has a placenta previa. The nurse notes that the client is actively bleeding. Which of the following types of medications should the nurse anticipate the provider will prescribe?

   A. Betamethasone

   B. Indomethacin

   C. Nifedipine

   D. Methylergonovine

4. A nurse at an antepartum clinic is caring for a client who is at 4 months of gestation. The client reports continued nausea and vomiting and scant, prune-colored discharge. She has experienced no weight loss and has a fundal height larger than expected. Which of the following complications should the nurse suspect?

   A. Hyperemesis gravidarum

   B. Threatened abortion

   C. Hydatidiform mole

   D. Preterm labor

5. A nurse is caring for a client who has a diagnosis of ruptured ectopic pregnancy. Which of the following findings is seen with this condition?

   A. No alteration in menses

   B. Transvaginal ultrasound indicating a fetus in the uterus

   C. Serum progesterone greater than the expected reference range

   D. Report of severe shoulder pain

PRACTICE Active Learning Scenario

A nurse manager is presenting an educational program on placenta previa for a group of nurses. What should the nurse manager include in this presentation? Use the ATI Active Learning Template: System Disorder to complete this item.

ALTERATION IN HEALTH (DIAGNOSIS): Describe the three types.

RISK FACTORS: Identify three.

DIAGNOSTIC PROCEDURES: Describe two.

NURSING CARE: Describe nursing action that is contraindicated.

Application Exercises Key

1. A. A client who experienced a missed abortion would report brownish discharge and no pain.

   B. **CORRECT:** Manifestations of an ectopic pregnancy include unilateral lower quadrant pain with or without bleeding. Use of an IUD is a risk factor associated with this condition.

   C. A client who has severe preeclampsia does not have vaginal bleeding and presents with right upper quadrant epigastric pain.

   D. A client who has a hydatidiform mole usually has dark brown vaginal bleeding in the second trimester that is not accompanied by abdominal pain.

   Ⓝ NCLEX® Connection: Physiological Adaptation, Alterations in Body Systems

2. A. Fetal position is not a risk factor associated with abruptio placentae.

   B. **CORRECT:** Blunt abdominal trauma is a risk factor associated with abruptio placentae.

   C. **CORRECT:** Cocaine use is a risk factor associated with abruptio placentae.

   D. Maternal age is not a risk factor associated with abruptio placentae.

   E. **CORRECT:** Cigarette smoking is a risk factor associated with abruptio placentae.

   Ⓝ NCLEX® Connection: Health Promotion and Maintenance, Health Promotion/Disease Prevention

3. A. **CORRECT:** Betamethasone is given to promote lung maturity if delivery is anticipated.

   B. Indomethacin is prescribed for the client in preterm labor.

   C. Nifedipine is prescribed for the client in preterm labor.

   D. Methylergonovine is prescribed for the client experiencing postpartum hemorrhage.

   Ⓝ NCLEX® Connection: Pharmacological and Parenteral Therapies, Expected Actions/Outcomes

4. A. A client who has hyperemesis gravidarum will have weight loss and signs of dehydration.

   B. A client who has a threatened abortion would be in the first trimester and report spotting to moderate bleeding with no enlarged uterus.

   C. **CORRECT:** A client who has a hydatidiform mole exhibits increased fundal height that is inconsistent with the week of gestation, and excessive nausea and vomiting due to elevated hCG levels. Scant, dark discharge occurs in the second trimester.

   D. Preterm labor presents prior to 37 weeks of gestation and is accompanied by pink-stained vaginal discharge and uterine contractions that become more regular.

   Ⓝ NCLEX® Connection: Physiological Adaptation, Unexpected Response to Therapies

5. A. A client experiencing a ruptured ectopic pregnancy has delayed, scant, or irregular menses.

   B. A transvaginal ultrasound would indicate an empty uterus in a client who has a ruptured ectopic pregnancy.

   C. A serum progesterone level lower than the expected reference range is an indication of ectopic pregnancy.

   D. **CORRECT:** A client's report of severe shoulder pain is a finding associated with a ruptured ectopic pregnancy due to the presence of blood in the abdominal cavity, which irritates the diaphragm and phrenic nerve.

   Ⓝ NCLEX® Connection: Physiological Adaptation, Unexpected Response to Therapies

PRACTICE Answer

Using the ATI Active Learning Template: System Disorder

ALTERATION IN HEALTH (DIAGNOSIS):
Types of placenta previa

- Complete or total: Cervical os is covered by the placenta.
- Incomplete or partial: Cervical os is only partially covered by the placenta.
- Marginal or low-lying: Placenta is attached in the lower uterine segment but does not reach the cervical os.

RISK FACTORS

- Previous placenta previa
- Uterine scarring due to previous cesarean birth, curettage, or endometritis
- Maternal age 35 to 40 years
- Multifetal gestation
- Multiple gestations or closely spaced pregnancies
- Smoking

DIAGNOSTIC PROCEDURES

- Transabdominal or transvaginal ultrasound
- Fetal monitoring

NURSING CARE: Performing a vaginal exam

Ⓝ NCLEX® Connection: Physiological Adaptation, Unexpected Response to Therapies

CHAPTER 8 *Infections*

Maternal infections during pregnancy require prompt identification and treatment by a provider. These include human immunodeficiency virus (HIV), acquired immune deficiency syndrome (AIDS), TORCH infections, group B streptococcus (GBS), chlamydia, gonorrhea, syphilis, human papilloma virus (HPV), trichomoniasis, bacterial vaginosis (BV), and candidiasis.

HIV/AIDS

HIV is a retrovirus that attacks and causes destruction of T lymphocytes. It causes immunosuppression in a client. HIV is transmitted from the mother to a neonate perinatally through the placenta and postnatally through the breast milk.

- Routine laboratory testing in the early prenatal period includes testing for HIV. Early identification and treatment significantly decreases the incidence of perinatal transmission.
- Testing is recommended in the third trimester for clients who are at an increased risk. Rapid HIV testing should be done if a client is in labor and her HIV status is unknown.
- Procedures such as amniocentesis and episiotomy should be avoided due to the risk of maternal blood exposure.
- Use of internal fetal monitors, vacuum extraction, and forceps during labor should be avoided due to the risk of fetal bleeding. Qs
- Administration of injections and blood testing should not take place until the first bath is given to the newborn.

ASSESSMENT

RISK FACTORS

- IV drug use
- Multiple sexual partners
- Maternal history of multiple STIs
- Blood transfusion (rare occurrence)
- Men who have sex with men

EXPECTED FINDINGS

Fatigue and influenza-like findings

PHYSICAL ASSESSMENT FINDINGS
- Fever
- Diarrhea and weight loss
- Lymphadenopathy and rash
- Anemia

LABORATORY TESTS

- Obtain informed maternal consent prior to testing.
- Testing begins with an antibody screening test, such as enzyme immunoassay. Confirmation of positive results is confirmed by Western blot test or immunofluorescence assay.
- Use rapid HIV antibody test (blood or urine sample) for a client in labor.
- Screen clients for STIs such as gonorrhea, chlamydia, syphilis, and hepatitis B.
- Obtain frequent viral load levels and CD4 cell counts throughout pregnancy.

PATIENT-CENTERED CARE

NURSING CARE

- Provide counseling prior to and after testing.
- Refer the client for mental health consultation, legal assistance, and financial resources.
- Use standard precautions.
- Administer antiviral prophylaxis, triple-medication antiviral, or highly active antiretroviral therapy as prescribed.
- Obtain prescribed laboratory testing.
- Encourage immunization against hepatitis B, pneumococcal infection, *Haemophilus influenzae* type B, and viral influenza.
- Encourage use of condoms to minimize exposure if partner is the source of infection.
- Review plan for scheduled cesarean birth at 38 weeks for maternal viral load of more than 1,000 copies/mL.
- Infant should be bathed after birth before remaining with the mother.

MEDICATIONS

Retrovir

- Antiretroviral agent
- Nucleoside reverse transcriptase inhibitor

NURSING CONSIDERATIONS
- Administer retrovir at 14 weeks of gestation, throughout the pregnancy, and before the onset of labor or cesarean birth.
- Administer retrovir to the infant at delivery and for 6 weeks following birth.

CLIENT EDUCATION

DISCHARGE INSTRUCTIONS Qpcc
- Instruct the client not to breastfeed.
- Discuss HIV and safe sexual relations with the client.
- Refer the client and infant to providers specializing in care of clients who have HIV.
- All states have a reportable diseases list. HIV/AIDS is a commonly reported condition. It is the responsibility of the provider to report cases of these diseases to their local health department.

TORCH infections

Toxoplasmosis, other infections (e.g., hepatitis), rubella virus, cytomegalovirus, and herpes simplex virus are known collectively as TORCH, which is a group of infections that can negatively affect a woman who is pregnant. These infections can cross the placenta and have teratogenic effects on the fetus. TORCH does not include all the major infections that present risks to the mother and fetus.

ASSESSMENT

RISK FACTORS

- Toxoplasmosis is caused by consumption of raw or undercooked meat or handling cat feces. Manifestations are similar to influenza or lymphadenopathy.
- Other infections can include hepatitis A and B, syphilis, mumps, parvovirus B19, and varicella-zoster. These are some of the most common and can be associated with congenital anomalies.
- Rubella (German measles) is contracted through children who have rashes or neonates who are born to women who had rubella during pregnancy.
- Cytomegalovirus (member of herpes virus family) is transmitted by droplet infection from person to person, a virus found in semen, cervical and vaginal secretions, breast milk, placental tissue, urine, feces, and blood. Latent virus can be reactivated and cause disease to the fetus in utero or during passage through the birth canal.
- Herpes simplex virus (HSV) is spread by direct contact with oral or genital lesions. Transmission to the fetus is greatest during vaginal birth if the woman has active lesions.

EXPECTED FINDINGS

- Toxoplasmosis findings similar to influenza or lymphadenopathy (malaise, muscle aches flu-like symptoms)
- Rubella: symptoms of joint and muscle pain
- Cytomegalovirus: asymptomatic or mononucleosis-like manifestations
- Herpes simplex infection: symptoms consisting of painful blisters and tender lymph nodes

PHYSICAL ASSESSMENT FINDINGS
- Manifestations of toxoplasmosis include fever and tender lymph nodes.
- Manifestations of rubella include rash, mild lymphedema, fever, and fetal consequences, which include miscarriage, congenital anomalies, and death.
- HSV initially presents with lesions and tender lymph nodes. Fetal consequences include miscarriage, preterm labor, and intrauterine growth restriction. A cesarean section is recommended for all women in labor who have active genital herpes lesions or early symptoms of impending outbreak, such as vulvar pain and itching.

LABORATORY TESTS

For herpes simplex, obtain cultures from women who have HSV or are at or near term.

DIAGNOSTIC PROCEDURES

- TORCH screen: immunologic survey used to identify existence of these infections in the mother (to identify fetal risks) or newborn (detection of antibodies against infections)
- Prenatal screenings

PATIENT-CENTERED CARE

NURSING CARE

- Monitor fetal well-being.
- For rubella, immunization of women who are pregnant is contraindicated because rubella infection can develop. These women should avoid crowds of young children. Women who have low titers prior to pregnancy should receive immunizations.

MEDICATIONS

- Administer antibiotics as prescribed.
- Treatment of toxoplasmosis includes sulfonamides or a combination of pyrimethamine and sulfadiazine (potentially harmful to the fetus, but parasitic treatment is essential).

CLIENT EDUCATION Qpcc

- Educate the client on prevention practices, including correct hand hygiene and cooking meat properly. Instruct clients to avoid contact with contaminated cat litter.
- Because no treatment for cytomegalovirus exists, tell the client to prevent exposure by frequent hand hygiene before eating, and after handling infant diapers and toys.
- Emphasize to the client the importance of compliance with prescribed treatment.
- Discuss safe sexual relations with client.
- Provide client with emotional support.

Group B streptococcus

GBS is a bacterial infection that can be passed to a fetus during labor and delivery.

ASSESSMENT

RISK FACTORS

History of positive culture with previous pregnancy

RISK FACTORS FOR EARLY-ONSET NEONATAL GBS
- Maternal age less than 20 years
- African American or Hispanic ethnicity
- Positive culture with pregnancy
- Prolonged rupture of membranes
- Preterm delivery
- Low birth weight
- Use of intrauterine fetal monitoring
- Intrapartum maternal fever (38° C [100.4° F] or greater)

EXPECTED FINDINGS

PHYSICAL ASSESSMENT FINDINGS: Positive GBS can have maternal and fetal effects.
- Premature rupture of membranes
- Preterm labor and delivery
- Chorioamnionitis
- Infections of the urinary tract
- Maternal sepsis

LABORATORY TESTS

Vaginal and rectal cultures are performed at 35 to 37 weeks of gestation.

PATIENT-CENTERED CARE

NURSING CARE

Administer intrapartum antibiotic prophylaxis to the following clients.
- Client who has GBS bacteriuria during current pregnancy
- Client who has a GBS–positive screening during current pregnancy
- Client who has unknown GBS status who is delivering at less than 37 weeks of gestation
- Client who has maternal fever of 38° C (100.4° F)
- Client who has rupture of membranes for 18 hr or longer

MEDICATIONS

Penicillin G or ampicillin are most commonly prescribed for GBS.
- Administer penicillin 5 million units initially IV bolus, followed by 2.5 million units intermittent IV bolus every 4 hr. The client may receive ampicillin 2 g IV initially, followed by 1 g every 4 hr.
- Bactericidal antibiotic is used to destroy the GBS.

CLIENT EDUCATION

Instruct the client to notify the labor and delivery nurse of GBS status.

Chlamydia

Chlamydia is a bacterial infection caused by *Chlamydia trachomatis* and is the most commonly reported STI in American women.
- The infection can be difficult to diagnose because it is often asymptomatic. If chlamydia is left untreated in women, it can lead to pelvic inflammatory disease (PID), which can cause infertility.
- The Centers for Disease Control and Prevention (CDC) recommends yearly screening of all sexually active women younger than 25 years, as well as older women who have risk factors (e.g., new or multiple partners). All pregnant women should be screened at the first prenatal visit and rescreened in the third trimester if younger than 25 years and/or at high risk.

ASSESSMENT

RISK FACTORS

- Multiple sexual partners
- Unprotected sex

EXPECTED FINDINGS

Male

- Urethral discharge
- Dysuria

PHYSICAL ASSESSMENT FINDINGS: Mucoid or watery urethral discharge

Female

- Dysuria
- Urinary frequency
- Spotting or postcoital bleeding

PHYSICAL ASSESSMENT FINDINGS
- Mucopurulent endocervical discharge
- Easily induced endocervical bleeding

LABORATORY TESTS

- Urine culture preferred for male clients
- Endocervical culture preferred for female clients

PATIENT-CENTERED CARE

NURSING CARE

- Instruct the client to take the entire prescription as prescribed.
- Identify and treat all sexual partners.
- Clients who are pregnant should be retested 3 weeks after completing the prescribed regimen.

MEDICATIONS

Azithromycin or amoxicillin

- Prescribed during pregnancy
- Broad-spectrum antibiotic
- Bactericidal action

NURSING CONSIDERATIONS: Administer erythromycin to all infants following delivery. This is the medication of choice for ophthalmia neonatorum. This antibiotic is both bacteriostatic and bactericidal, and thus provides prophylaxis against *Neisseria gonorrhoeae* and *Chlamydia trachomatis.*

CLIENT EDUCATION

- Instruct the client to take all medication as prescribed.
- Educate the client about the possibility of decreasing effectiveness of oral contraceptives. Qpcc
- Educate the client regarding safe sex practices (e.g., mutual monogamy and correct, consistent condom use).
- All states have a reportable diseases list. Chlamydia is a commonly reported condition. It is the responsibility of the provider to report cases of these diseases to the local health department.

Gonorrhea

Neisseria gonorrhoeae is the causative agent of gonorrhea. Gonorrhea is a bacterial infection that is primarily spread by genital-to-genital contact. However, it also can be spread by anal-to-genital or oral-to-genital contact. It can also be transmitted to a newborn during delivery.

- Women are frequently asymptomatic. If gonorrhea is left untreated in women, it can lead to PID, which can cause infertility.
- The CDC recommends yearly screening for all sexually active women younger than 25 years as well as older women who have risk factors (e.g., new or multiple sex partners). All pregnant women at risk should be screened at the first prenatal visit and rescreened in the third trimester if at continued high risk.

ASSESSMENT

RISK FACTORS

- Multiple sexual partners
- Unprotected sexual practices

EXPECTED FINDINGS

Male

- Dysuria
- Urethral discharge

Female

- Dysuria
- Vaginal bleeding between periods and dysmenorrhea

PHYSICAL ASSESSMENT FINDINGS

- Yellowish-green vaginal discharge
- Easily induced endocervical bleeding

LABORATORY TESTS

- Urine culture preferred for male clients
- Endocervical culture preferred for female clients

PATIENT-CENTERED CARE

NURSING CARE

- Provide client education regarding disease transmission.
- Identify and treat all sexual partners.
- Administer erythromycin to all infants following delivery. This is the medication of choice for ophthalmia neonatorum. This antibiotic is both bacteriostatic and bactericidal, and thus provides prophylaxis against *Neisseria gonorrhoeae* and *Chlamydia trachomatis*.

MEDICATIONS

Ceftriaxone IM and azithromycin PO: Broad-spectrum antibiotic; bactericidal action

CLIENT EDUCATION

- Instruct the client to take all medications as prescribed.
- Instruct the client to repeat the culture to assess for medication effectiveness.
- Educate the client about the possibility of decreasing effectiveness of oral contraceptives.
- Educate the client regarding safe sex practices (e.g., mutual monogamy and correct, consistent condom use).
- All states have a reportable diseases list. Gonorrhea is a commonly reported condition. It is the responsibility of the provider to report cases of these diseases to the local health department.

Syphilis

Syphilis is an STI caused by the bacterium *Treponema pallidum*. It can have long-term complications if not adequately treated.

- Syphilis has three stages.
  - **Primary:** Characterized by presence of a chancre
  - **Secondary:** Characterized by skin rashes, such as a rash on the palms of hands and soles of feet
  - **Tertiary:** Characterized by damage to internal organs
- Black, Hispanic, and other racial/ethnic minority groups are disproportionately affected by syphilis in the U.S.
- It can be transmitted through oral, vaginal, or anal sex, as well as transmitted to an unborn child. Though the rate of congenital syphilis has recently decreased, more cases of congenital syphilis are reported in the U.S. than cases of perinatal HIV infection.
- All pregnant women should be screened at the first prenatal visit and rescreened in the third trimester if at high risk (live in areas with high numbers of syphilis cases; not previously tested; or had positive test in the first trimester).

ASSESSMENT

RISK FACTORS

- Multiple partners
- Unprotected sexual practices

EXPECTED FINDINGS

Primary stage: The client can notice a chancre or sore in the genital area.

Secondary stage: The client can notice skin rashes, such as a rash on the palmar surface of the hands and the soles of the feet.

Tertiary stage: Damage to internal organs can occur for which clients can notice the manifestations including difficulty coordinating muscle movements and blindness.

PHYSICAL ASSESSMENT FINDINGS
- **Primary stage:** Provider can observe a chancre in the genital area.
- **Secondary stage:** Provider can observe skin rashes, such as rough, red or reddish brown spots on the palms of the hands and soles of the feet.

LABORATORY TESTS

Serology tests: Nontreponemal (VDRL and rapid plasma reagin) and treponemal (enzyme immunoassay, immunoassays)
- Nontreponemal tests are often used for screening then treponemal tests to detect antibodies specific for syphilis to confirm the diagnosis.
- This sequence of nontreponemal then treponemal tests is considered the standard for testing.

PATIENT-CENTERED CARE

MEDICATIONS

Penicillin G IM in a single dose

CLIENT EDUCATION

- Instruct the client to abstain from sexual contact until sores have completely healed.
- Advise the client that partners need to be tested and treated.
- Educate the client regarding safe sex practices (e.g., mutual monogamy and correct, consistent condom use.)
- All states have a reportable diseases list. Syphilis is a commonly reported condition. It is the responsibility of the provider to report cases of these diseases to the local health department.

Human papilloma virus

HPV is the most common STI. Some types can cause genital warts (also known as *Condyloma acuminata*) and cancers.
- It is spread through oral, vaginal, and anal sex (most commonly vaginal or anal routes). When large, widespread, or occluding the birth canal, genital warts can complicate a vaginal delivery. Therefore, a cesarean section can be recommended.
- Routine screening for women 21 to 65 years old can provide early detection. Screening should occur, even during pregnancy.

ASSESSMENT

RISK FACTORS

- Multiple partners
- Unprotected sexual practices

EXPECTED FINDINGS

Client reports bumps in the genital area that might not itch or hurt.

PHYSICAL ASSESSMENT FINDINGS
- Small warts or a group of warts in the genital area that can have a cauliflower-like appearance
- Abnormal changes to the cervix that can detected by a Pap test

LABORATORY TESTS

Pap test with or without HPV co-testing per American Cancer Society and American Congress or Obstetricians and Gynecologists guidelines.
- Women 21 to 29 years old should have a Pap test every 3 years.
- Women 30 to 65 years old should have both a Pap test and an HPV test every 5 years (preferred). It is also acceptable to have a Pap test alone every 3 years.
- Women older than 65 years who have had regular screenings with normal results should not be screened for cervical cancer, unless they have cervical precancer, in which they should continue to be screened for 20 years after the precancer diagnosis.

DIAGNOSTIC PROCEDURES

- Genital warts are diagnosed by the provider based on appearance.
- Based on the Pap test result, colposcopy and biopsy can be performed to diagnose cervical precancer and cancer.

PATIENT-CENTERED CARE

MEDICATIONS

For genital warts and *Condyloma acuminata*, options include a client-applied cream, such as imiquimod, or a provider-administered therapy, such as trichloroacetic acid application.

THERAPEUTIC PROCEDURES

For precancerous changes on the cervix, the provider can perform treatments including laser therapy or cone biopsy; for a pregnant woman with an abnormal Pap that requires further follow-up, further evaluation and treatment are usually deferred until after birth.

CLIENT EDUCATION

- Vaccines are recommended to protect against low-risk types of HPV that cause genital warts and high-risk types of HPV that cause cancer. The vaccine is indicated for clients 9 to 26 years of age, though ideally given at age 11 to 12 years.
- Educate clients regarding safe sex practices (e.g., mutual monogamy and correct, consistent condom use).

Trichomoniasis

Trichomoniasis is a STI caused by the protozoan parasite *Trichomonas vaginalis*. It can be spread penis-to-vagina or vagina-to-vagina.
- If trichomoniasis is left untreated in women, it can lead to PID, which can cause infertility. All women who have clinical findings should be tested.
- Pregnant women who have trichomoniasis are more likely to have preterm delivery and babies with low birth weight (less than 5.5 lb).

ASSESSMENT

RISK FACTORS

- Multiple partners
- Unprotected sexual practices

EXPECTED FINDINGS

Male

- Penile itching or irritation
- Dysuria

PHYSICAL ASSESSMENT FINDINGS: Urethral discharge, which can be swabbed for microscopy

Female

- Yellow-green, frothy vaginal discharge with foul odor
- Dyspareunia and itching
- Dysuria

PHYSICAL ASSESSMENT FINDINGS
- Discharge in the vaginal vault, which can be sampled for microscopy
- Strawberry spots on the cervix (tiny petechiae)
- A cervix that bleeds easily

LABORATORY TESTS

A sample of the discharge is used for application to pH paper, and wet mount and whiff test performed

DIAGNOSTIC PROCEDURES

- pH greater than 4.5
- Wet mount saline prep indicates the presence of trichomonad(s).
- Whiff test can be positive or negative.

PATIENT-CENTERED CARE

MEDICATIONS

Metronidazole or tinidazole: Orally in a single dose; anti-infective

CLIENT EDUCATION

- Counsel the client to avoid alcohol while taking this medication due to the disulfiram-like reaction that occurs (severe nausea and vomiting).
- Instruct the client to take all medication as prescribed.
- Educate the client about the possibility of decreasing effectiveness of oral contraceptives.
- Identify and treat all sexual partners.
- Educate the client regarding safe sex practices (e.g., mutual monogamy and correct, consistent condom use).

Bacterial vaginosis

A bacterial infection most commonly caused by *Haemophilus vaginalis* or *Gardnerella vaginalis*. It is the most common vaginal infection in women 15 to 44 years of age. It cannot be related to sexual activity.
- If BV is left untreated, it can increase a woman's chances of developing PID, which can lead to infertility. All women who have manifestations should be tested.
- Treatment is especially important for pregnant women. BV is associated with preterm labor and babies with low birth weight (less than 5.5 lb).

ASSESSMENT

RISK FACTORS

- New or multiple sex partners
- Unprotected sexual practices
- Altered pH balance of vagina, such as caused by douching

EXPECTED FINDINGS

Thin, white or gray discharge with a fish-like odor, especially after sex

PHYSICAL ASSESSMENT FINDINGS: Discharge in the vaginal vault, which can be sampled for microscopy

LABORATORY TESTS

- Sample of the discharge used for application to pH paper
- Wet mount and whiff test performed

DIAGNOSTIC PROCEDURES

- pH greater than 4.5
- Wet mount saline prep indicates presence of clue cells
- Positive whiff test

PATIENT-CENTERED CARE

MEDICATIONS

Metronidazole: Anti-infective

CLIENT EDUCATION

- Counsel the client to avoid alcohol while taking this medication due to a disulfiram-like reaction (severe nausea and vomiting).
- Instruct the client to take all medications as prescribed.
- Educate the client about the possibility of decreasing effectiveness of oral contraceptives.
- Treatment is not usually indicated for male partners.
- Educate the client regarding safe sex practices (e.g., mutual monogamy and correct, consistent condom use).
- Instruct the client to avoid tight-fitting clothing.
- Instruct the client to wear cotton-lined underpants.
- Advise the client to avoid douching.

Candidiasis

Candidiasis, also known as vulvovaginal candidiasis or yeast infection, is a fungal infection caused by *Candida albicans*.
- It is the second most common type of vaginal infection in the U.S.
- All women who have symptoms should be tested.

ASSESSMENT

RISK FACTORS

- Pregnancy
- Diabetes mellitus
- Oral contraceptives
- Recent antibiotic treatment
- Obesity
- Diet high in refined sugars

EXPECTED FINDINGS

Vulvar and vaginal pruritus

PHYSICAL ASSESSMENT FINDINGS
- Thick, creamy, white, cottage cheese-like vaginal-discharge
- Vulvar and vaginal erythema and inflammation
- White patches on vaginal walls
- Gray-white patches on the tongue and gums (neonate)

LABORATORY TESTS

- Sample of discharge used for application to pH paper
- Wet mount and whiff test performed

DIAGNOSTIC PROCEDURES

- pH less than 4.5 (normal pH)
- Wet mount potassium hydroxide prep indicates presence of yeast buds, hyphae, and pseudohyphae.
- Negative whiff test

PATIENT-CENTERED CARE

MEDICATIONS

Fluconazole

- Can be prescribed as a single low dose
- Topical therapies recommended for use in pregnant-women
- Antifungal agent
- Fungicidal action

Over-the-counter treatments

OTC treatments, such as clotrimazole, are available to treat candidiasis. However, it is important for the provider to diagnose candidiasis initially.

CLIENT EDUCATION

- Instruct the client to avoid tight-fitting clothing.
- Instruct the client to wear cotton-lined underpants.
- Instruct the client to limit wearing damp clothing.
- Advise client to avoid douching.
- Instruct the client to increase dietary intake of yogurt with active cultures.

Application Exercises

1. A nurse is admitting a client who is in labor and has HIV. Which of the following interventions should the nurse identify as contraindicated for this client? (Select all that apply.)

   A. Episiotomy

   B. Oxytocin infusion

   C. Forceps

   D. Cesarean birth

   E. Internal fetal monitoring

2. A nurse in an antepartum clinic is assessing a client who has a TORCH infection. Which of the following findings should the nurse expect? (Select all that apply.)

   A. Joint pain

   B. Malaise

   C. Rash

   D. Urinary frequency

   E. Tender lymph nodes

3. A nurse is caring for a client who has gonorrhea. Which of the following medications should the nurse anticipate the provider will prescribe?

   A. Ceftriaxone

   B. Fluconazole

   C. Metronidazole

   D. Zidovudine

4. A nurse is caring for a client who is in labor. The nurse should identify that which of the following infections can be treated during labor or immediately following birth? (Select all that apply.)

   A. Gonorrhea

   B. Chlamydia

   C. HIV

   D. Group B streptococcus beta-hemolytic

   E. TORCH infection

5. A nurse manager is reviewing ways to prevent a TORCH infection during pregnancy with a group of newly licensed nurses. Which of the following statements by a nurse indicates understanding of the teaching?

   A. "Obtain an immunization against rubella early in pregnancy."

   B. "Seek prophylactic treatment if cytomegalovirus is detected during pregnancy."

   C. "A woman should avoid crowded places during pregnancy."

   D. "A woman should avoid consuming undercooked meat while pregnant."

PRACTICE Active Learning Scenario

A nurse is planning care for a client who is pregnant and positive for group B streptococcus beta-hemolytic. Use the ATI Active Learning Template: System Disorder to complete this item.

LABORATORY TESTS: Describe the test and when it is performed.

RISK FACTORS: Describe two maternal risk factors and three fetal risk factors.

MEDICATIONS: Describe three clients who should receive intrapartum antibiotic prophylaxis.

Application Exercises Key

1. A. **CORRECT:** An episiotomy should be avoided for a client who is HIV-positive due to the risk of maternal blood exposure.

   B. Oxytocin infusion is not contraindicated for this client.

   C. **CORRECT:** The use of forceps during delivery should be avoided due to the risk of fetal bleeding.

   D. Cesarean birth is not contraindicated for this client.

   E. **CORRECT:** Internal fetal monitoring should be avoided due to the risk of fetal bleeding.

   Ⓝ *NCLEX® Connection: Reduction of Risk Potential, Potential for Complications from Surgical Procedures and Health Alterations*

2. A. **CORRECT:** TORCH infections are flu-like in presentation, such as joint pain.

   B. **CORRECT:** TORCH infections are flu-like in presentation, such as malaise.

   C. **CORRECT:** TORCH infections can include findings such as a rash.

   D. Urinary frequency is not a clinical finding associated with a TORCH infection.

   E. **CORRECT:** TORCH infections are flu-like in presentation, such as tender lymph nodes.

   Ⓝ *NCLEX® Connection: Reduction of Risk Potential, Potential for Complications from Surgical Procedures and Health Alterations*

3. A. **CORRECT:** Ceftriaxone IM or doxycycline orally for 7 days is prescribed for the treatment of gonorrhea.

   B. Fluconazole is used to treat candidiasis.

   C. Metronidazole is used in the treatment of bacterial vaginosis and trichomoniasis.

   D. Zidovudine is used to treat HIV/AIDS.

   Ⓝ *NCLEX® Connection: Pharmacological and Parenteral Therapies, Medication Administration*

4. A. **CORRECT:** Erythromycin is administered to the infant immediately following delivery to prevent *Neisseria gonorrhoeae*.

   B. **CORRECT:** Erythromycin is administered to the infant immediately following delivery to prevent *Chlamydia trachomatis*.

   C. **CORRECT:** Retrovir is prescribed to a client in labor who is HIV-positive.

   D. **CORRECT:** Penicillin G or ampicillin may be prescribed to treat positive GBS.

   E. A TORCH infection can be treated during pregnancy depending upon the infection.

   Ⓝ *NCLEX® Connection: Health Promotion and Maintenance, Ante/Intra/Postpartum and Newborn Care*

5. A. Immunization against rubella is contraindicated during pregnancy due to the risk of fetal congenital anomalies.

   B. There is no treatment for cytomegalovirus.

   C. A TORCH infection cannot be transmitted by being in areas where large crowds are present.

   D. **CORRECT:** Toxoplasmosis, a TORCH infection, is contracted by consuming undercooked meat.

   Ⓝ *NCLEX® Connection: Reduction of Risk Potential, Potential for Complications from Surgical Procedures and Health Alterations*

PRACTICE Answer

Using the ATI Active Learning Template: System Disorder

LABORATORY TESTS: Vaginal and rectal cultures performed at 36 to 37 weeks of gestation

RISK FACTORS

Maternal
- History of positive culture with previous pregnancy
- Maternal age less than 20 years
- African American or Hispanic ethnicity

Fetal
- Positive during pregnancy
- Prolonged rupture of membranes
- Preterm delivery
- Low birth weight
- Use of intrauterine fetal monitoring
- Intrapartum maternal fever (38° C [100.4° F])

MEDICATIONS
- Client who has GBS bacteriuria during current pregnancy
- Client who has a GBS-positive screen during current pregnancy
- Client who has unknown GBS status who is delivering at less than 37 weeks of gestation
- Client who has maternal fever of 38° C (100.4° F)
- Client who has rupture of membranes for 18 hr or longer

Ⓝ *NCLEX® Connection: Reduction of Risk Potential, Potential for Complications from Surgical Procedures and Health Alterations*

CHAPTER 9 *Medical Conditions*

Unexpected medical conditions can occur during pregnancy. Awareness, early detection, and interventions are crucial components to ensure fetal well-being and maternal health.

Unexpected medical conditions include cervical insufficiency, hyperemesis gravidarum, anemia, gestational diabetes mellitus, and gestational hypertension.

Cervical insufficiency (premature cervical dilatation)

Cervical insufficiency is a variable condition whereby expulsion of the products of conception occurs. It is thought to be related to tissue changes and alterations in the length of the cervix.

ASSESSMENT

RISK FACTORS

- History of cervical trauma (cervical tears from previous deliveries, excessive dilations, curettage for biopsy, and surgical procedures involving the cervix), short labors, pregnancy loss in early gestation, or advanced cervical dilation at earlier weeks of gestation
- In utero exposure to diethylstilbestrol, ingested by the client's mother during pregnancy
- Congenital structural defects of the uterus or cervix

EXPECTED FINDINGS

Increase in pelvic pressure or urge to push

PHYSICAL ASSESSMENT FINDINGS
- Pink-stained vaginal discharge or bleeding
- Possible gush of fluid (rupture of membranes)
- Uterine contractions with the expulsion of the fetus
- Postoperative (cerclage) monitoring for uterine contractions, rupture of membranes, and signs of infection

DIAGNOSTIC AND THERAPEUTIC PROCEDURES

- An **ultrasound** showing a short cervix (less than 25 mm in length), presence of cervical funneling (beaking), or effacement of the cervical os indicates reduced cervical competence.
- **Prophylactic cervical cerclage** is the surgical reinforcement of the cervix with a heavy ligature that is placed submucosally around the cervix to strengthen it and prevent premature cervical dilation. Best results occur if this is done at 12 to 14 weeks of gestation. The cerclage is removed at 37 weeks of gestation or when spontaneous labor occurs.

PATIENT-CENTERED CARE

NURSING CARE

- Evaluate the client's support systems and availability of assistance if activity restrictions or bed rest are prescribed.
- Assess vaginal discharge.
- Monitor client reports of pressure and contractions.
- Check vital signs.

MEDICATIONS

Administer tocolytics prophylactically to inhibit uterine contractions.

CLIENT EDUCATION

DISCHARGE INSTRUCTIONS
- Place the client on activity restriction or bed rest.
- Encourage hydration to promote a relaxed uterus. (Dehydration stimulates uterine contractions.)
- Advise the client to avoid intercourse, tampons, and douching, and to monitor for cervical/uterine changes.
- The client can require cervical cerclage (indicated for women who have singleton pregnancy), often placed at 12 to 14 weeks gestation and removed at 37 weeks gestation

HEALTH PROMOTION AND DISEASE PREVENTION
- Provide education about clinical findings to report to the provider for preterm labor, rupture of membranes, infection, strong contractions less than 5 min apart, severe perineal pressure, and an urge to push.
- Instruct the client about using the home uterine activity monitor to evaluate uterine contractions.

NURSING ACTIONS
- Arrange for the client to follow up with a home health agency for close observation and supervision.
- Plan for removal of the cerclage around 37 weeks of gestation.

Hyperemesis gravidarum

- Hyperemesis gravidarum is excessive nausea and vomiting (possibly related to elevated hCG levels) that is prolonged past 12 weeks of gestation and results in a 5% weight loss from prepregnancy weight, electrolyte imbalance, acetonuria, and ketosis.
- There is a risk to the fetus for intrauterine growth restriction or preterm birth if the condition persists.

ASSESSMENT

RISK FACTORS

- Maternal age younger than 30 years
- History of migraines
- Obesity
- First pregnancy
- Multifetal gestation
- Gestational trophoblastic disease or fetus with chromosomal anomaly
- Psychosocial issues and high levels of emotional stress
- Clinical hyperthyroid disorders
- Diabetes
- Gastrointestinal disorders
- Family history of hyperemesis

EXPECTED FINDINGS

PHYSICAL ASSESSMENT FINDINGS
- Excessive vomiting for prolonged periods
- Dehydration with possible electrolyte imbalance
- Weight loss
- Increased pulse rate
- Decreased blood pressure
- Poor skin turgor and dry mucous membranes

LABORATORY TESTS

- **Urinalysis** for ketones and acetones (breakdown of protein and fat) is the most important initial laboratory test: Elevated urine specific gravity
- **Chemistry profile** revealing electrolyte imbalances
  - Sodium, potassium, and chloride reduced from low intake
  - Metabolic acidosis (secondary to starvation)
  - Metabolic alkalosis due to excessive vomiting
  - Elevated liver enzymes
  - Bilirubin level
- **Thyroid test** indicating hyperthyroidism.
- **Complete blood count** (CBC): Hct concentration is elevated because inability to retain fluid results in hemoconcentration.

PATIENT-CENTERED CARE

NURSING CARE

- Monitor I&O.
- Assess skin turgor and mucous membranes.
- Monitor vital signs.
- Monitor weight.
- Have the client remain NPO for 24 to 48 hr.

MEDICATIONS

- Give the client IV lactated Ringer's for hydration.
- Give pyridoxine (vitamin B_6) and other vitamin supplements as tolerated. American Congress of Obstetricians and Gynecologists recommend the use of pyridoxine alone or in combination with doxylamine as the initial medication management because these medications are considered both safe and effective.
- Use antiemetic medications (ondansetron, metoclopramide) cautiously for uncontrollable nausea and vomiting.
- Use corticosteroids to treat refractory hyperemesis gravidarum.

CLIENT EDUCATION

DISCHARGE INSTRUCTIONS
- Advance the client to clear liquids after 24 hr if no vomiting.
- Advance the client's diet as tolerated, with frequent small meals. Start with dry toast, crackers, or cereal; then move to a soft diet; and finally to a normal diet as tolerated. Q**EBP**
- In severe cases, or if vomiting returns, enteral nutrition per feeding tube or total parental nutrition can be considered.

Iron-deficiency anemia

Iron-deficiency anemia occurs during pregnancy due to inadequacy in maternal iron stores and consuming insufficient amounts of dietary iron.

ASSESSMENT

RISK FACTORS

- Less than 2 years between pregnancies
- Heavy menses
- Diet low in iron
- Multifetal gestation
- Vomiting frequently due to morning sickness

EXPECTED FINDINGS

- Fatigue and weakness
- Irritability
- Headache
- Feeling dizzy or lightheaded
- Shortness of breath with exertion
- Palpitations
- Craving unusual food (pica)

PHYSICAL ASSESSMENT FINDINGS
- Pallor
- Brittle nails
- Shortness of breath

LABORATORY TESTS

- **Hgb** less than 11 mg/dL in the first and third trimesters and less than 10.5 mg/dL in the second trimester
- **Hct** less than 3%

PATIENT-CENTERED CARE

NURSING CARE

- The recommended iron intake for pregnant women is 27 mg/day. Prenatal vitamins typically contain 30 mg iron. If maternal iron deficiency anemia is present, increased dosages of 60 to 120 mg/day can be required.
- Increase dietary intake of foods rich in iron (legumes, fruit, green leafy vegetables, and meat).
- Educate the client about ways to minimize gastrointestinal adverse effects.

MEDICATIONS

Ferrous sulfate iron supplements

CLIENT EDUCATION
- Instruct the client to take the supplement on an empty stomach and take with orange juice to increase absorption.
- Encourage a diet rich in vitamin C-containing foods to increase absorption.
- Suggest that the client increase roughage and fluid intake in diet to assist with discomforts of constipation.

Iron dextran

Used in the treatment of iron-deficiency anemia when oral iron supplements cannot be tolerated by the client who is pregnant.

Gestational diabetes mellitus

- Gestational diabetes mellitus (GDM) is an impaired tolerance to glucose with the first onset or recognition during pregnancy. The ideal blood glucose level during pregnancy should range between 70 and 110 mg/dL.
- Symptoms of diabetes mellitus can disappear a few weeks following delivery. However, approximately 50% of women will develop Type II diabetes mellitus within 5 years.

INCREASED RISKS TO FETUS
- **Spontaneous abortion**, related to poor glycemic control
- **Infections** (urinary and vaginal), related to increased glucose in the urine and decreased resistance because of altered carbohydrate metabolism
- **Hydramnios**, which can cause overdistention of the uterus, premature rupture of membranes, preterm labor, and hemorrhage

- **Ketoacidosis** from diabetogenic effect of pregnancy (increased insulin resistance), untreated hyperglycemia, or inappropriate insulin dosing
- **Hypoglycemia**, caused by overdosing in insulin, skipped or late meals, or increased exercise
- **Hyperglycemia**, which can cause excessive fetal growth (macrosomia)

ASSESSMENT

RISK FACTORS

- Obesity
- Hypertension
- Glycosuria
- Maternal age older than 25 years
- Family history of diabetes mellitus
- Previous delivery of an infant that was large or stillborn

EXPECTED FINDINGS

Hypoglycemia: nervousness, headache, weakness, irritability, hunger, blurred vision, tingling of mouth or extremities

Hyperglycemia: polydipsia, polyphagia, polyuria, nausea, abdominal pain, flushed dry skin, fruity breath

PHYSICAL ASSESSMENT FINDINGS
- Hypoglycemia
- Shaking
- Clammy pale skin
- Shallow respirations
- Rapid pulse
- Hyperglycemia
- Vomiting
- Excess weight gain during pregnancy

LABORATORY TESTS

- **Routine urinalysis** with glycosuria
- **Glucola screening test/1-hr glucose tolerance test:** 50 g oral glucose load, followed by plasma glucose analysis 1 hr later performed at 24 to 28 weeks of gestation; fasting not necessary; a positive blood glucose screening is 130 to 140 mg/dL or greater; additional testing with a 3-hr oral glucose tolerance test (OGTT) is indicated **Q**EBP
- **Oral glucose tolerance test** following overnight fasting, avoidance of caffeine, and abstinence from smoking for 12 hr prior to testing; a fasting glucose is obtained, a 100 g glucose load is given, and serum glucose levels are determined at 1, 2, and 3 hr following glucose ingestion
- **Presence of ketones in urine** to assess severity of ketoacidosis

DIAGNOSTIC PROCEDURES

- Biophysical profile to ascertain fetal well-being
- Amniocentesis with alpha-fetoprotein
- Nonstress test to assess fetal well-being

PATIENT-CENTERED CARE

NURSING CARE

- Monitor the client's blood glucose.
- Monitor the fetus.

MEDICATIONS

In contrast to women who have type I diabetes mellitus, women who have GDM are managed initially with diet and exercise alone. If glucose levels are persistently high, insulin is begun.

Oral hypoglycemic therapy is an alternative to insulin in women who have GDM who require medication in addition to diet for blood glucose control. Most oral hypoglycemic agents are contraindicated for gestational diabetes mellitus, but there is limited use of glyburide. The provider will need to make the determination if these medications can be used.

CLIENT EDUCATION

- Instruct the client to perform daily kick counts.
- Educate the client about diet, including standard diabetic diet and restricted carbohydrate intake. Dietary counseling by a registered dietitian should occur.
- Educate the client about exercise.
- Instruct the client about self-administration of insulin.
- Educate the client about the need for postpartum laboratory testing to include OGTT and blood glucose levels.

Gestational hypertension

- Hypertensive disease in pregnancy is divided into clinical subsets of the disease based on end-organ effects and progresses along a continuum from mild gestational hypertension; mild and severe preeclampsia; eclampsia; and hemolysis, elevated liver enzymes, and low platelets (HELLP) syndrome.
- Vasospasm contributing to poor tissue perfusion is the underlying mechanism for the manifestations of pregnancy hypertensive disorders.
- Gestational hypertensive disease and chronic hypertension can occur simultaneously.
- Gestational hypertensive diseases are associated with placental abruption, kidney failure, hepatic rupture, preterm birth, and fetal and maternal death.

Gestational hypertension (GH), which begins after the 20th week of pregnancy, describes hypertensive disorders of pregnancy whereby the woman has an elevated blood pressure at 140/90 mm Hg or greater recorded on two different occasions, at least 4 hr. apart. There is no proteinuria. The presence of edema is no longer considered in the definition of hypertensive disease of pregnancy. Blood pressure returns to baseline by 6 weeks postpartum.

Mild preeclampsia is GH with the addition of proteinuria of greater than or equal to 1+. Report of transient headaches might occur along with episodes of irritability. Edema can be present.

Severe preeclampsia consists of blood pressure that is 160/110 mm Hg or greater, proteinuria greater than 3+, oliguria, elevated serum creatinine greater than 1.1 mg/dL, cerebral or visual disturbances (headache and blurred vision), hyperreflexia with possible ankle clonus, pulmonary or cardiac involvement, extensive peripheral edema, hepatic dysfunction, epigastric and right upper-quadrant pain, and thrombocytopenia.

Eclampsia is severe preeclampsia manifestations with the onset of seizure activity or coma. Eclampsia is usually preceded by headache, severe epigastric pain, hyperreflexia, and hemoconcentrations, which are warning signs of probable convulsions.

HELLP syndrome is a variant of GH in which hematologic conditions coexist with severe preeclampsia involving hepatic dysfunction. HELLP syndrome is diagnosed by laboratory tests, not clinically.
- **H: Hemolysis** resulting in anemia and jaundice
- **EL: Elevated liver enzymes** resulting in elevated alanine aminotransferase (ALT) or aspartate transaminase (AST), epigastric pain, and nausea and vomiting
- **LP: Low platelets** (less than 100,000/mm³), resulting in thrombocytopenia, abnormal bleeding and clotting time, bleeding gums, petechiae, and possibly disseminated intravascular coagulopathy

ASSESSMENT

RISK FACTORS

No single profile identifies risks for gestational hypertensive disorders, but some high risks include the following.
- Maternal age younger than 19 or older than 40 years
- First pregnancy
- Morbid obesity
- Multifetal gestation
- Chronic renal disease
- Chronic hypertension
- Familiar history of preeclampsia
- Diabetes mellitus
- Rheumatoid arthritis
- Systemic lupus erythematosus

EXPECTED FINDINGS

- Severe continuous headache
- Nausea
- Blurring of vision
- Flashes of lights or dots before the eyes

PHYSICAL ASSESSMENT FINDINGS
- Hypertension
- Proteinuria
- Periorbital, facial, hand, and abdominal edema
- Pitting edema of lower extremities
- Vomiting
- Oliguria
- Hyperreflexia
- Scotoma
- Epigastric pain
- Right upper quadrant pain
- Dyspnea
- Diminished breath sounds
- Seizures
- Jaundice
- Signs of progression of hypertensive disease with indications of worsening liver involvement, kidney failure, worsening hypertension, cerebral involvement, and developing coagulopathies

ABNORMAL LABORATORY FINDINGS
- Elevated liver enzymes (LDH, AST)
- Increased creatinine
- Increased plasma uric acid
- Thrombocytopenia
- Decreased Hgb
- Hyperbilirubinemia

LABORATORY TESTS

- Liver enzymes
- Serum creatinine, BUN, uric acid, and magnesium increase as renal function decreases
- CBC
- Clotting studies
- Chemistry profile

DIAGNOSTIC PROCEDURES

- Dipstick testing of urine for proteinuria
- 24-hr urine collection for protein and creatinine clearance
- Nonstress test, contraction stress test, biophysical profile, and serial ultrasounds to assess fetal status
- Doppler blood flow analysis to assess fetal well-being

PATIENT-CENTERED CARE

NURSING CARE

- Assess level of consciousness.
- Obtain pulse oximetry.
- Monitor urine output, and obtain a clean-catch urine sample to assess for proteinuria.
- Obtain daily weights.
- Monitor vital signs with careful attention to blood pressure measurement (e.g., using proper size cuff and avoiding talking to client during measurement).
- Encourage lateral positioning.
- Perform NST and daily kick counts.
- Instruct the client to monitor I&O.

MEDICATIONS

It is recommended that daily low dose aspirin therapy be initiated late in the first trimester for women who have a history of early onset preeclampsia.

ANTIHYPERTENSIVE MEDICATIONS
- **Methyldopa**
- **Nifedipine**
- **Hydralazine**
- **Labetalol**
- Avoid ACE inhibitors and angiotensin II receptor blockers.

ANTICONVULSANT MEDICATIONS: **Magnesium sulfate**
- Medication of choice for prophylaxis or treatment to lower blood pressure and depress the CNS.
- Nursing Considerations
  - Use an infusion control device to maintain a regular flow rate.
  - Inform the client that she can initially feel flushed, hot, and sedated with the magnesium sulfate bolus.
  - Monitor blood pressure, pulse, respiratory rate, deep-tendon reflexes, level of consciousness, urinary output (indwelling urinary catheter for accuracy), presence of headache, visual disturbances, epigastric pain, uterine contractions, and fetal heart rate and activity.
  - Place the client on fluid restriction of 100 to 125 mL/hr, and maintain a urinary output of 30 mL/hr or greater.
  - Monitor for signs of magnesium sulfate toxicity. Qs
    - Absence of patellar deep tendon reflexes
    - Urine output less than 30 mL/hr
    - Respirations less than 12/min
    - Decreased level of consciousness
    - Cardiac dysrhythmias
  - If magnesium toxicity is suspected:
    - Immediately discontinue infusion.
    - Administer antidote calcium gluconate or calcium chloride. Qs
    - Prepare for actions to prevent respiratory or cardiac arrest.

CLIENT EDUCATION

DISCHARGE INSTRUCTIONS
- Maintain the client on bed rest and encourage side-lying position.
- Promote diversional activities (e.g., TV, visits from family or friends, gentle exercise).
- Have the client avoid foods that are high in sodium.
- Have the client avoid alcohol and tobacco and limit caffeine intake.
- Instruct the client to drink six to eight 8-ounce glasses of water a day.
- Maintain a dark quiet environment to avoid stimuli that can precipitate a seizure.
- Maintain a patent airway in the event of a seizure.
- Administer antihypertensive medications as prescribed.

Application Exercises

1. A nurse is caring for a client who is at 14 weeks of gestation and has hyperemesis gravidarum. The nurse should identify that which of the following are risk factors for the client? (Select all that apply.)

   A. Obesity

   B. Multifetal pregnancy

   C. Maternal age greater than 40

   D. Migraine headache

   E. Oligohydramnios

2. A nurse is caring for a client who has suspected hyperemesis gravidarum and is reviewing the client's laboratory reports. Which of the following findings is a manifestation of this condition?

   A. Hgb 12.2 g/dL

   B. Urine ketones present

   C. Alanine aminotransferase 20 IU/L

   D. Serum glucose 114 mg/dL

3. A nurse is administering magnesium sulfate IV to a client who has severe preeclampsia for seizure prophylaxis. Which of the following indicates magnesium sulfate toxicity? (Select all that apply.)

   A. Respirations less than 12/min

   B. Urinary output less than 30 mL/hr

   C. Hyporreflexic deep-tendon reflexes

   D. Decreased level of consciousness

   E. Flushing and sweating

4. A nursing is caring for a client who is receiving IV magnesium sulfate. Which of the following medications should the nurse anticipate administering if magnesium sulfate toxicity is suspected?

   A. Nifedipine

   B. Pyridoxine

   C. Ferrous sulfate

   D. Calcium gluconate

5. A nurse is reviewing a new prescription for ferrous sulfate with a client who is at 12 weeks of gestation. Which of the following statements by the client indicates understanding of the teaching?

   A. "I will take this pill with my breakfast."

   B. "I will take this medication with a glass of milk."

   C. "I plan to drink more orange juice while taking this pill."

   D. "I plan to add more calcium-rich foods to my diet while taking this medication."

PRACTICE Active Learning Scenario

A nurse is preparing to teach a client who is at 20 weeks of gestation and is scheduled to undergo a prophylactic cervical cerclage. What information should the nurse include in the teaching? Use the ATI Active Learning Template: Therapeutic Procedure to complete this item.

DESCRIPTION OF PROCEDURE

POTENTIAL COMPLICATIONS: Identify two.

CLIENT EDUCATION: Describe at least four instructions to give the client.

Application Exercises Key

1. A. **CORRECT:** Obesity is a risk factor for hyperemesis gravidarum.

   B. **CORRECT:** Multifetal pregnancy is a risk factor for hyperemesis gravidarum.

   C. Maternal age less than 30 is a risk factor for hyperemesis gravidarum.

   D. **CORRECT:** Migraine headache is a risk factor for hyperemesis gravidarum.

   E. Oligohydramnios is not a risk factor for hyperemesis gravidarum.

   (N) *NCLEX® Connection: Health Promotion and Maintenance, Health Promotion/Disease Prevention*

2. A. Altered hematocrit is a manifestation of hyperemesis gravidarum due to the hemoconcentration that occurs with dehydration.

   B. **CORRECT:** The presence of ketones in the urine is associated with the breakdown of proteins and fats that occurs in a client who has hyperemesis gravidarum.

   C. Liver enzymes are elevated in a client who has hyperemesis gravidarum. This finding is within the expected reference range.

   D. Decreased serum glucose is anticipated in a client who has hyperemesis gravidarum. This result is within the expected reference range.

   (N) *NCLEX® Connection: Reduction of Risk Potential, Laboratory Values*

3. A. **CORRECT:** A respiratory rate less than 12/min is a sign of magnesium sulfate toxicity.

   B. **CORRECT:** Urinary output less than 30 mL/hr is a sign of magnesium sulfate toxicity.

   C. The absence of patellar deep-tendon reflexes is a sign of magnesium sulfate toxicity.

   D. **CORRECT:** Decreased level of consciousness is a sign of magnesium sulfate toxicity.

   E. Flushing and sweating are adverse effects of magnesium sulfate but are not signs of toxicity.

   (N) *NCLEX® Connection: Pharmacological and Parenteral Therapies, Expected Actions/Outcomes*

4. A. Nifedipine is an antihypertensive medication that can be administered to women who have gestational hypertension.

   B. Pyridoxine (vitamin B$_6$) is a vitamin supplement prescribed for clients who have hyperemesis gravidarum.

   C. Ferrous sulfate is a medication used in the treatment of iron deficiency anemia.

   D. **CORRECT:** Calcium gluconate is the antidote for magnesium sulfate.

   (N) *NCLEX® Connection: Physiological Adaptation, Expected Actions/Outcomes*

5. A. Ferrous sulfate should be taken on an empty stomach.

   B. Milk will decrease the absorption of ferrous sulfate.

   C. **CORRECT:** A diet with increased vitamin C improves the absorption of ferrous sulfate.

   D. Although a diet of calcium-rich foods is appropriate for the client during pregnancy, it does not improve the effectiveness of ferrous sulfate.

   (N) *NCLEX® Connection: Pharmacological and Parenteral Therapies, Medication Administration*

PRACTICE Answer

Using the ATI Active Learning Template: Therapeutic Procedure

DESCRIPTION OF PROCEDURE: Surgical reinforcement of the cervix with a heavy ligature (suture) that is placed submucosally around the cervix to strength it and prevent premature cervical dilation.

POTENTIAL COMPLICATIONS
- Uterine contractions
- Rupture of membranes
- Infection

CLIENT EDUCATION
- Remain on activity restrictions/bed rest as prescribed.
- Increase hydration to promote a relaxed uterus.
- Refrain from sexual intercourse.
- Clinical findings to report to the provider: preterm labor, rupture of membranes, signs of infection, strong contractions less than 5 min apart, perineal pressure, and the urge to push.
- Use of home uterine activity monitor.
- Home health agency to follow up.
- Plan for removal of the cerclage at 37 weeks of gestation.

(N) *NCLEX® Connection: Reduction of Risk Potential, Therapeutic Procedures*

CHAPTER 10 *Early Onset of Labor*

Understanding the importance of identifying the onset of early labor in a client who is pregnant is crucial for maternal and fetal well-being. This chapter includes preterm labor, premature rupture of membranes, and preterm premature rupture of membranes.

Preterm labor

Preterm labor is uterine contractions and cervical changes that occur between 20 and 37 weeks of gestation.

ASSESSMENT

RISK FACTORS

- Infections of the urinary tract, vagina, or chorioamnionitis (infection of the amniotic sac)
- Previous preterm birth
- Multifetal pregnancy
- Hydramnios (excessive amniotic fluid)
- Age below 17 or above 35
- Low socioeconomic status
- Smoking
- Substance use
- Intimate partner violence
- History of multiple miscarriages or abortions
- Diabetes mellitus
- Chronic hypertension
- Preeclampsia
- Lack of prenatal care
- Recurrent premature dilation of the cervix
- Placenta previa or abruptio placentae
- Preterm premature rupture of membranes
- Short interval between pregnancies
- Uterine abnormalities
- Second trimester bleeding
- Low prepregnancy weight

EXPECTED FINDINGS

- Uterine contractions
- Pressure in the pelvis and menstrual-like cramping
- Persistent low backache
- Gastrointestinal cramping, sometimes with diarrhea
- Urinary frequency
- Vaginal discharge

PHYSICAL ASSESSMENT FINDINGS

- Increase, change, odor or blood in vaginal discharge
- Change in cervical dilation
- Regular uterine contractions with a frequency of every 10 min or greater, lasting 1 hr or longer
- Premature rupture of membranes

LABORATORY TESTS

- Fetal fibronectin
- Cervical cultures
- CBC
- Urinalysis

DIAGNOSTIC PROCEDURES

- Obtain swab of vaginal secretions for fetal fibronectin between 24 and 34 weeks of gestation. This protein can be found in vaginal secretions and can be related to inflammation of the placenta that can lead to preterm birth. This test is used to determine preterm labor.
- Measure endocervical length with an ultrasound to assess for a shortened cervix, which is suggested in certain studies to precede preterm labor.
- Use home uterine activity monitoring (HUAM), which is a uterine contraction monitor that can be used by the client at home. HUAM is not considered to be effective in preventing preterm labor.
- Obtain cervical cultures to detect if there is a presence of infectious organisms. Culture and sensitivity results guide prescription of an appropriate antibiotic, if indicated.
- Perform a biophysical profile and/or a nonstress test to provide information about the fetal well-being.

PATIENT-CENTERED CARE

NURSING CARE

Management of a client who is in preterm labor includes focusing on stopping uterine contractions.

Activity restriction
- Instruct the client on ways to modify her environment to allow for modified bed rest, yet have the ability to fulfill role responsibilities. Strict bed rest can have adverse effects. Q EBP
- Encourage the client to rest in the left lateral position to increase blood flow to the uterus and decrease uterine activity. Q EBP
- Tell the client to avoid sexual intercourse.

Ensuring hydration: Dehydration stimulates the pituitary gland to secrete an antidiuretic hormone and oxytocin. Preventing dehydration prevents the release of oxytocin, which stimulates uterine contractions.

Identifying and treating an infection
- Have the client report any vaginal discharge, noting amount, color, consistency, and odor.
- Monitor vital signs and temperature.

Chorioamnionitis should be suspected with the occurrence of elevated temperature and tachycardia.

Monitor FHR and contraction pattern.

Fetal tachycardia, which is a prolonged increase in the FHR greater than 160/min can indicate infection, is frequently associated with preterm labor.

MEDICATIONS

Nifedipine

CLASSIFICATION AND THERAPEUTIC INTENT: A calcium channel blocker that is used to suppress contractions by inhibiting calcium from entering smooth muscles

NURSING CONSIDERATIONS
- Monitor for headache, flushing, dizziness, and nausea. These usually are related to orthostatic hypotension that occurs with administration.
- Should not be administered concurrent with magnesium sulfate, or concurrent or immediately following a beta$_2$-adrenergic agonist. Q$_s$

CLIENT EDUCATION Q$_s$
- Instruct the client to slowly change positions from supine to upright, and to sit until dizziness disappears.
- Tell the client to maintain adequate hydration to counter hypotension.

Magnesium sulfate

CLASSIFICATION AND THERAPEUTIC INTENT: A commonly used tocolytic that relaxes the smooth muscle of the uterus and thus inhibits uterine activity by suppressing contractions.

NURSING CONSIDERATIONS
- Contraindications for tocolysis include active vaginal bleeding, dilation of the cervix greater than 6 cm, chorioamnionitis, greater than 34 weeks of gestation, and acute fetal distress.
- Monitor the client closely. Discontinue tocolytic therapy immediately if the client exhibits manifestations of pulmonary edema, which includes chest pain, shortness of breath, respiratory distress, audible wheezing and crackles, and a productive cough containing blood-tinged sputum.
- Monitor for adverse effects.
- Monitor for magnesium sulfate toxicity, and discontinue for any of the following adverse effects: loss of deep tendon reflexes, urinary output less than 30 mL/hr, respiratory depression (less than 12/min), pulmonary edema, and chest pain. Q$_s$
- Administer calcium gluconate or calcium chloride as an antidote for magnesium sulfate toxicity.

CLIENT EDUCATION: Instruct the client to notify the nurse of blurred vision, headache, nausea, vomiting, or difficulty breathing.

Indomethacin

CLASSIFICATION AND THERAPEUTIC INTENT: Indomethacin is a nonsteroidal anti-inflammatory drug (NSAID) that suppresses preterm labor by blocking the production of prostaglandins. This inhibition of prostaglandins suppresses uterine contractions.

NURSING CONSIDERATIONS
- Monitor the client closely. Discontinue tocolytic therapy immediately if the client exhibits manifestations of pulmonary edema, which include chest pain, shortness of breath, respiratory distress, audible wheezing and crackles, and a productive cough containing blood-tinged sputum.
- Indomethacin treatment should not exceed 48 hr.
- Indomethacin should only be used if gestational age is less than 32 weeks of gestation.
- Monitor for postpartum hemorrhage related to reduced platelet aggregation.
- Administer indomethacin with food or rectally to decrease gastrointestinal distress.
- Notify the provider if the client reports blurred vision, headache, nausea, vomiting, or difficulty breathing.
- Monitor the neonate at birth.

Betamethasone

CLASSIFICATION AND THERAPEUTIC INTENT: A glucocorticoid that is administered IM in two injections 24 hr apart, and requires 24 hr to be effective. The therapeutic action is to enhance fetal lung maturity and surfactant production in fetuses between 24 to 34 weeks gestation.

NURSING CONSIDERATIONS
- Administer the medication deep into the gluteal muscle 24 and 48 hr prior to birth of a preterm neonate.
- Monitor the client and neonate for pulmonary edema by assessing lung sounds.
- Monitor for maternal and neonate hyperglycemia.
- Monitor the neonate for heart rate changes.

CLIENT EDUCATION: Educate the client regarding signs of pulmonary edema (chest pain, shortness of breath, and crackles).

Premature rupture of membranes and preterm premature rupture of membranes

Premature rupture of membranes (PROM) is the spontaneous rupture of the amniotic membranes 1 hr or more prior to the onset of true labor. For most women, PROM signifies the onset of true labor if gestational duration is at term.

Preterm premature rupture of membranes (PPROM) is the premature spontaneous rupture of membranes after 20 weeks of gestation and prior to 37 weeks of gestation.

ASSESSMENT

RISK FACTORS

- Infection is a major risk of PROM and PPROM for the client and the fetus. Once the amniotic membranes have ruptured, micro-organisms can ascend from the vagina into the amniotic sac. Infection often precedes PPROM.
- Chorioamnionitis is an infection of the amniotic membranes.
  - There is an increased risk of infection if there is a lag period over the 24-hr period from when the membranes rupture to delivery.
  - History of prior preterm birth
  - Second and third trimester bleeding

EXPECTED FINDINGS

Client reports a gush or leakage of clear fluid from the vagina.

PHYSICAL ASSESSMENT FINDINGS
- Temperature elevation
- Increased maternal heart rate or FHR
- Foul-smelling fluid or vaginal discharge
- Abdominal tenderness

Assess for a prolapsed umbilical cord. Qs
- Abrupt FHR variable or prolonged deceleration
- Visible or palpable cord at the introitus

LABORATORY TESTS

A positive nitrazine paper test (blue, pH 6.5 to 7.5) or positive ferning test is conducted on amniotic fluid to verify rupture of membranes.

PATIENT-CENTERED CARE

NURSING CARE

- Prepare for birth if indicated.
- Nursing management depends on gestational duration, if there is evidence of infection, or an indication of fetal or maternal compromise.
- Obtain vaginal/rectal cultures for streptococcus β-hemolytic.
- Obtain vaginal cultures for chlamydia, and *Neisseria gonorrhoeae*.
- Avoid vaginal exams.
- Provide reassurance to reduce anxiety.
- Assess vital signs every 2 hr. Notify the provider of a temperature greater than 38° C (100° F).
- Assess FHR and uterine contractions.
- Advise the client to adhere to bed rest with bathroom privileges.
- Encourage hydration.
- Obtain a CBC.
- Instruct the client to perform daily fetal kick counts and to notify the nurse of uterine contractions.

MEDICATIONS

Ampicillin

CLASSIFICATION AND THERAPEUTIC INTENT: Ampicillin is an antibiotic used to treat infection. It is commonly used to treat chorioamnionitis.

NURSING CARE: Obtain vaginal, urine, and blood cultures prior to administration of antibiotic.

Betamethasone

CLASSIFICATION AND THERAPEUTIC INTENT
- Betamethasone is a glucocorticoid administered IM in two injections, 24 hr apart, and requires 24-hr to be effective. The therapeutic action is to enhance fetal lung maturity and surfactant production.
- A single dose is given with PROM at 24 to 31 weeks of gestation to reduce the risk of perinatal mortality, respiratory distress syndrome, and other morbidities.

NURSING CONSIDERATIONS
- Administer the medication deep into the gluteal muscle 24 and 48 hr prior to birth of a preterm neonate.
- Monitor the client and neonate for pulmonary edema by assessing lung sounds.
- Monitor for maternal and neonate hyperglycemia.
- Monitor the neonate for heart rate changes.

CLIENT EDUCATION: Educate the client regarding indications of pulmonary edema (chest pain, shortness of breath, and crackles).

CLIENT EDUCATION

- Expect that the client will be discharged home if dilation is less than 3 cm, no evidence of infection, no contractions, and no malpresentation.
- Advise the client to adhere to limited activity with bathroom privileges.
- Encourage hydration.
- Instruct the client to conduct a self-assessment for uterine contractions.
- Tell the client to record daily kick counts for fetal movement.
- Instruct the client to monitor for foul-smelling vaginal discharge.
- Remind the client to refrain from inserting anything into the vagina.
- Instruct the client to abstain from intercourse.
- Tell the client to avoid tub baths.
- Teach the client to wipe her perineal area from front to back after voiding and fecal elimination.
- Instruct the client to take her temperature every 4 hr when awake and report a temperature that is greater than 38° C (100° F).

1. A nurse is caring for a client who reports indications of preterm labor. Which of the following findings are risk factors of this condition? (Select all that apply).

    A. Urinary tract infection

    B. Multifetal pregnancy

    C. Oligohydramnios

    D. Diabetes mellitus

    E. Uterine abnormalities

2. A nurse in labor and delivery is providing care for a client who is in preterm labor at 32 weeks of gestation. Which of the following medications should the nurse anticipate the provider will prescribe to hasten fetal lung maturity?

    A. Calcium gluconate

    B. Indomethacin

    C. Nifedipine

    D. Betamethasone

3. A nurse is caring for a client who is receiving nifedipine for prevention of preterm labor. The nurse should monitor the client for which of the following manifestations?

    A. Blood-tinged sputum

    B. Dizziness

    C. Pallor

    D. Somnolence

4. A nurse is caring for a client who has a prescription for magnesium sulfate. The nurse should recognize that which of the following are contraindications for use of this medication? (Select all that apply.)

    A. Fetal distress

    B. Preterm labor

    C. Vaginal bleeding

    D. Cervical dilation greater than 6 cm

    E. Severe gestational hypertension

5. A nurse is reviewing discharge teaching with a client who has premature rupture of membranes at 26 weeks of gestation. Which of the following instructions should the nurse include in the teaching?

    A. Use a condom with sexual intercourse.

    B. Avoid bubble bath solution when taking a tub bath.

    C. Wipe from the back to front when performing perineal hygiene.

    D. Keep a daily record of fetal kick counts.

PRACTICE Active Learning Scenario

A nurse in a prenatal clinic is reviewing preterm labor with a newly hired nurse. What should the nurse include in the discussion? Use the ATI Active Learning Template: System Disorder to complete this item.

ALTERATION IN HEALTH (DIAGNOSIS)

EXPECTED FINDINGS: Describe at least six manifestations.

DIAGNOSTIC PROCEDURES: Describe at least three.

Application Exercises Key

1. A. **CORRECT:** A urinary tract infection is a risk factor of preterm labor.

    B. **CORRECT:** Multifetal pregnancy is a risk factor of preterm labor.

    C. Hydramnios (excessive amniotic fluid) is a risk factor for preterm labor.

    D. **CORRECT:** Diabetes mellitus is a risk factor of preterm labor.

    E. **CORRECT:** Uterine abnormalities are a risk factor of preterm labor.

    Ⓝ *NCLEX® Connection: Health Promotion and Maintenance, Health Promotion/Disease Prevention*

2. A. Calcium gluconate is administered as an antidote for magnesium sulfate toxicity.

    B. Indomethacin is an NSAID used to suppress preterm labor by blocking prostaglandin production.

    C. Nifedipine is a calcium channel blocker used to suppress uterine contractions.

    D. **CORRECT:** Betamethasone is a glucocorticoid given to clients in preterm labor to hasten surfactant production.

    Ⓝ *NCLEX® Connection: Pharmacological and Parenteral Therapies, Medication Administration*

3. A. Blood-tinged sputum production is an adverse effect associated with indomethacin.

    B. **CORRECT:** Dizziness and lightheadedness are associated with orthostatic hypotension, which occurs when taking nifedipine.

    C. Facial flushing and heat sensation are adverse effects associated with nifedipine.

    D. Nervousness, jitteriness, and sleep disturbances are adverse effects associated with nifedipine.

    Ⓝ *NCLEX® Connection: Pharmacological and Parenteral Therapies, Adverse Effects/Contraindications/Side Effects/Interactions*

4. A. **CORRECT:** Acute fetal distress is a complication that is a contraindication for use of magnesium sulfate therapy.

    B. Preterm labor is an indication for use of magnesium sulfate.

    C. **CORRECT:** Vaginal bleeding is a complication that is a contraindication for magnesium sulfate therapy.

    D. **CORRECT:** Cervical dilation greater than 6 cm is a complication that is a contraindication for magnesium sulfate therapy.

    E. Severe gestational hypertension is an indication for the use of magnesium sulfate.

    Ⓝ *NCLEX® Connection: Pharmacological and Parenteral Therapies, Adverse Effects/Contraindications/Side Effects/Interactions*

5. A. The client who has ruptured membranes should not insert anything into her vagina.

    B. The nurse should instruct the client to avoid tub baths and take showers.

    C. The nurse should instruct the client to wipe from front to back when performing perineal hygiene.

    D. **CORRECT:** The client should record daily fetal kick counts.

    Ⓝ *NCLEX® Connection: Physiological Adaptation, Illness Management*

PRACTICE Answer

Using the ATI Active Learning Template: System Disorder

ALTERATION IN HEALTH (DIAGNOSIS): Uterine contractions and cervical changes that occur between 20 and 37 weeks of gestation

EXPECTED FINDINGS

- Persistent low backache
- Pressure in the pelvis and cramping
- Gastrointestinal cramping, sometimes with diarrhea
- Urinary frequency
- Vaginal discharge
- Increase, change, or blood in vaginal discharge
- Change in cervical dilation
- Regular uterine contractions with a frequency of every 10 min or greater, lasting 1 hr or longer
- Premature rupture of membranes

DIAGNOSTIC PROCEDURES

- Test for fetal fibronectin
- Ultrasound to measure endocervical length
- Cervical culture to detect presence of infectious organisms
- Biophysical profile
- Nonstress test
- Home uterine activity monitoring for uterine contractions

Ⓝ *NCLEX® Connection: Physiological Adaptation, Illness Management*

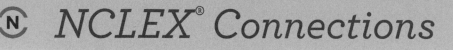
When reviewing the following chapters, keep in mind the relevant topics and tasks of the NCLEX outline, in particular:

Client Needs: Health Promotion and Maintenance

ANTE/INTRA/POSTPARTUM AND NEWBORN CARE: Provide care and education to client in labor or an antepartum client.

Client Needs: Pharmacological and Parenteral Therapies

ADVERSE EFFECTS/CONTRAINDICATIONS/SIDE EFFECTS/INTERACTIONS: Identify a contraindication to the administration of a medication to the client.

DOSAGE CALCULATION: Use clinical decision making/ critical thinking when calculating dosages.

MEDICATION ADMINISTRATION: Educate client about medications.

Client Needs: Physiological Adaptation

ALTERATIONS IN BODY SYSTEMS: Provide care for client experiencing complications of pregnancy/labor and/or delivery.

Client Needs: Basic Care and Comfort

NON-PHARMACOLOGICAL COMFORT INTERVENTIONS: Incorporate alternative/complementary therapies into client plan of care.

Client Needs: Reduction of Risk Potential

POTENTIAL FOR COMPLICATIONS OF DIAGNOSTIC TESTS/TREATMENTS/PROCEDURES: Evaluate responses to procedures and treatments.

THERAPEUTIC PROCEDURES: Assess client response to recovery from local, regional, or general anesthesia.

CHAPTER 11 # Labor and Delivery Processes

An intrapartum nurse should care for three clients during each labor and delivery: the fetus, mother, and family unit. (11.1)

ASSESSMENT

An intrapartum nurse should collect assessment data on maternal and fetal well-being during labor, the progress of labor, and psychosocial and cultural factors that affect labor. Q𝗣𝗖𝗖

PHYSIOLOGIC CHANGES PRECEDING LABOR (PREMONITORY SIGNS)

Backache: Constant low, dull backache caused by pelvic muscle relaxation

Weight loss: 0.5 to 1.5 kg (1 to 3.5 lb) weight loss

Lightening: Fetal head descends into true pelvis about 14 days before labor; feeling that the fetus has "dropped"; easier breathing, but more pressure on bladder, resulting in urinary frequency; more pronounced in clients who are primigravida

Contractions: Begin with irregular uterine contractions (Braxton Hicks) that eventually progress in strength and regularity

Increased vaginal discharge or bloody show: Expulsion of the cervical mucus plug may occur. Brownish or blood-tinged mucus plug resulting from the onset of cervical dilation and effacement.

Energy burst: Sometimes called "nesting" response

Gastrointestinal changes: Less common; include nausea, vomiting, and indigestion

---

11.1 Stages of labor

FIRST STAGE 12.5 hr duration			SECOND STAGE P: 30 min to 2 hr M: 5 to 30 min	THIRD STAGE 5 to 30 min	FOURTH STAGE 1 to 4 hr
LATENT PHASE P: 6 hr M: 4 hr	*ACTIVE PHASE* P: 3 hr M: 2 hr	*TRANSITION* 20 to 40 min			
Cervical dilation: P: 1 cm/hr M: 1.5 cm/hr					
0 cm 3 cm	4 cm 7 cm	8 cm 10 cm			
Onset of labor Contractions • Irregular, mild to moderate • Frequency: 5 to 30 min • Duration: 30 to 45 seconds	Contractions • More regular, moderate to strong • Frequency: 3 to 5 min • Duration: 40 to 70 seconds	Contractions • Strong to very strong • Frequency: 2 to 3 min • Duration: 45 to 90 seconds Complete dilation	Full dilation Progresses to intense contractions every 1 to 2 min Birth	Delivery of the neonate Delivery of placenta	Delivery of placenta Maternal stabilization of vital signs
MATERNAL CHARACTERISTICS Some dilation and effacement Talkative and eager	Rapid dilation and effacement Some fetal descent Feelings of helplessness Anxiety and restlessness increase as contractions become stronger	Tired, restless, and irritable Feeling out of control, client often states, "cannot continue" Can have nausea and vomiting Urge to push Increased rectal pressure and feelings of needing to have a bowel movement Increased bloody show Most difficult part of labor	Pushing results in birth of fetus	Placental separation and expulsion Schultz presentation: shiny fetal surface of placenta emerges first Duncan presentation: dull maternal surface of placenta emerges firs	Achievement of vital sign homeostasis Lochia scant to moderate rubra

P = primigravida   M = multigravida

Cervical ripening: Cervix becomes soft (opens) and partially effaced, and can begin to dilate

Rupture of membranes: Spontaneous rupture of membranes can initiate labor or can occur anytime during labor, most commonly during the transition phase.

- Labor usually occurs within 24 hr of the rupture of membranes.
- Prolonged rupture of membranes greater than 24 hr before delivery of fetus can lead to an infection.
- Immediately following the rupture of membranes, a nurse should assess the FHR for abrupt decelerations, which are indicative of fetal distress to rule out umbilical cord prolapse. Qs

Assessment of amniotic fluid: Completed once the membranes rupture

- Should be watery, clear, and pale- to straw-yellow in color.
- Odor should not be foul.
- Volume is between 500 and 1,200 mL.
- Use nitrazine paper to confirm that amniotic fluid is present.
  - **Amniotic fluid is alkaline:** Nitrazine paper is deep blue, indicating pH of 6.5 to 7.5.
  - **Urine is slightly acidic:** Nitrazine paper remains yellow.

FIVE P'S

There are five factors that affect and define the labor and birth process: **passenger** (fetus and placenta), **passageway** (birth canal), **powers** (contractions), **position** (of the woman), and **psychological** response.

Passenger

Consists of the fetus and the placenta. The size of the fetal head, fetal presentation, fetal lie, fetal attitude, and fetal position affect the ability of the fetus to navigate the birth canal. The placenta can be considered a passenger because it also must pass through the canal.

Presentation: The part of the fetus that is entering the pelvic inlet first and leads through the birth canal during labor. It can be the back of the head (occiput), chin (mentum), shoulder (scapula), or breech (sacrum or feet).

Lie: The relationship of the maternal longitudinal axis (spine) to the fetal longitudinal axis (spine)

- **Transverse:** Fetal long axis is horizontal, forms a right angle to maternal axis, and will not accommodate vaginal birth. The shoulder is the presenting part and can require delivery by cesarean birth if the fetus does not rotate spontaneously.
- **Parallel or longitudinal:** Fetal long axis is parallel to maternal long axis, either a cephalic or breech presentation. Breech presentation can require a cesarean birth.

Attitude: Relationship of fetal body parts to one another
- **Fetal flexion:** Chin flexed to chest, extremities flexed into torso
- **Fetal extension:** Chin extended away from chest, extremities extended

Fetopelvic or fetal position: The relationship of the presenting part of the fetus (sacrum, mentum, or occiput), preferably the occiput, in reference to its directional position as it relates to one of the four maternal pelvic quadrants. It is labeled with three letters
- **Right (R) or left (L):** The first letter references either the side of the maternal pelvis.
- **Occiput (O), sacrum (S), mentum (M), or scapula (Sc):** The second letter references the presenting part of the fetus.
- **Anterior (A), posterior (P), or transverse (T):** The third letter references the part of the maternal pelvis.

Station: Measurement of fetal descent in centimeters with station 0 being at the level of an imaginary line at the level of the ischial spines, minus stations superior to the ischial spines, and plus stations inferior to the ischial spines.

Passageway

The birth canal that is composed of the bony pelvis, cervix, pelvic floor, vagina, and introitus (vaginal opening). The size and shape of the bony pelvis must be adequate to allow the fetus to pass through it. The cervix must dilate and efface in response to contractions and fetal descent.

Powers

Uterine contractions cause effacement (shortening and thinning of the cervix) during the first stage of labor and dilation of the cervix (enlargement or widening of the cervical opening and canal) that occurs once labor has begun and the fetus is descending. Involuntary urge to push and voluntary bearing down in the second stage of labor helps in the expulsion of the fetus.

Position

The client should engage in frequent position changes during labor to increase comfort, relieve fatigue, and promote circulation. Position during the second stage is determined by maternal preference, provider preference, and the condition of the mother and the fetus.

Gravity can aid in the fetal descent in upright, sitting, kneeling, and squatting positions.

Psychological response

Maternal stress, tension, and anxiety can produce physiological changes that impair the progress of labor.

PATIENT-CENTERED CARE

PREPROCEDURE

NURSING CARE

- **Leopold maneuvers:** Abdominal palpation of the number of fetuses, the fetal presenting part, lie, attitude, descent, and the probable location where fetal heart tones can be best auscultated on the woman's abdomen
- **External electronic monitoring (tocotransducer):** Separate transducer applied to the maternal abdomen over the fundus that measures uterine activity
  - Displays uterine contraction patterns
  - Easily applied by the nurse but must be repositioned with maternal movement to ensure proper placement
- **External fetal monitoring (EFM):** Transducer applied to the abdomen of the client to assess FHR patterns during labor and birth

LABORATORY ANALYSIS

- **Group B streptococcus:** Culture is obtained if results are not available from screening at 35 to 37 weeks. If positive, intravenous prophylactic antibiotic is prescribed. (Exceptions are planned cesarean birth and membranes intact.) Qs
- **Urinalysis:** Clean-catch urine sample obtained to ascertain maternal:
  - Hydration status via specific gravity
  - Nutritional status via ketones
  - Proteinuria, which can be indicative of gestational hypertension or preeclampsia
  - Glucosuria which can be indicative of gestational diabetes
  - Urinary tract infection (UTI) via bacterial count (UTIs are common in a diabetic pregnancy)
- **Blood tests**
  - CBC level
  - ABO typing and Rh-factor if not previously done

CLIENT EDUCATION: Provide the client and her partner with ongoing education regarding the labor and delivery process and procedures.

INTRAPROCEDURE

NURSING CARE

- **Assess maternal vital signs** per agency protocol. Check maternal temperature every 1 to 2 hr if membranes are ruptured.
- **Assess FHR** to determine fetal well-being. This can be performed by use of EFM or spiral electrode that is applied to the fetal scalp. Prior to electrode placement, cervical dilation and rupture of membranes must occur.
- **Assess uterine labor contraction characteristics** by palpation (placing a hand over the fundus to assess contraction frequency, duration, and intensity) or by the use of external or internal monitoring. **(11.2)**
  - **Frequency:** Established from the beginning of one contraction to the beginning of the next
  - **Duration:** Time between the beginning of a contraction to the end of that same contraction
  - **Intensity:** Strength of the contraction at its peak, described as mild (slightly tense, like pressing finger to tip of nose), moderate (firm, like pressing finger to chin), or strong (rigid, like pressing finger to forehead)
  - **Resting tone of uterine contractions:** Tone of the uterine muscle in between contractions. A prolonged contraction duration (greater than 90 seconds) or too frequent contractions (more than five in a 10-min period) without sufficient time for uterine relaxation (less than 30 seconds) in between can reduce blood flow to the placenta. This can result in fetal hypoxia and decreased FHR. Qs
- **Intrauterine pressure catheter:** Insert a solid, sterile, water-filled intrauterine pressure catheter inside the uterus to measure intrauterine pressure.
  - Displays uterine contraction patterns on monitor
  - Requires the membranes to be ruptured and the cervix to be sufficiently dilated

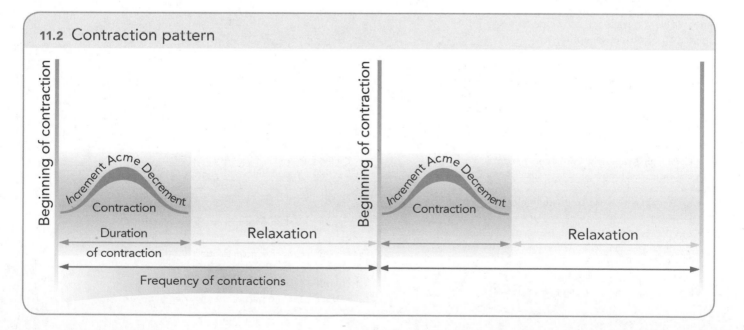

11.2 Contraction pattern

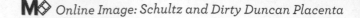

- **Vaginal examination:** Performed digitally by the provider or qualified nurse to assess for the following:
  ○ Cervical dilation (stretching of cervical os adequate to allow fetal passage) and effacement (cervical thinning and shortening) **(11.3)**
  ○ Descent of the fetus through the birth canal as measured by fetal station in centimeters
  ○ Fetal position, presenting part, and lie
  ○ Membranes that are intact or ruptured
- **Mechanism of labor in vertex presentation:** The adaptations the fetus makes as it progresses through the birth canal during the birthing process
  ○ **Engagement:** Occurs when the presenting part, usually biparietal (largest) diameter of the fetal head passes the pelvic inlet at the level of the ischial spines, referred to as station 0.
  ○ **Descent:** The progress of the presenting part (preferably the occiput) through the pelvis. Measured by station during a vaginal examination as either negative (–) station measured in centimeters if superior to station 0 and not yet engaged, or positive (+) station measured in centimeters if inferior to station 0.
  ○ **Flexion:** When the fetal head meets resistance of the cervix, pelvic wall, or pelvic floor. The head flexes, bringing the chin close to the chest, presenting a smaller diameter to pass through the pelvis.
  ○ **Internal rotation:** The fetal occiput ideally rotates to a lateral anterior position as it progresses from the ischial spines to the lower pelvis in a corkscrew motion to pass through the pelvis.
  ○ **Extension:** The fetal occiput passes under the symphysis pubis, and then the head is deflected anteriorly and is born by extension of the chin away from the fetal chest.
  ○ **External rotation (restitution):** After the head is born, it rotates to the position it occupied as it entered the pelvic inlet (restitution) in alignment with the fetal body and completes a quarter turn to face transverse as the anterior shoulder passes under the symphysis.
  ○ **Birth by expulsion:** After birth of the head and shoulders, the trunk of the neonate is born by flexing it toward the symphysis pubis.

POSTPROCEDURE

NURSING ASSESSMENTS DURING THE FOURTH STAGE
- Maternal vital signs
- Fundus
- Lochia
- Perineum
- Urinary output
- Maternal/newborn baby-friendly activities

NURSING INTERVENTIONS DURING THE FOURTH STAGE
- American Academy of Pediatrics and American Congress of Obstetricians and Gynecologists recommend that blood pressure and pulse be assessed at least every 15 min for the first 2 hr after birth, and that temperature be assessed every 4 hr for the first 8 hr after birth and then at least every 8 hr.
- Assess fundus and lochia every 15 min for the first hour and then according to facility protocol.
- Massage the uterine fundus and/or administer oxytocics as prescribed to maintain uterine tone to prevent hemorrhage. **Qs**
- Assess the client's perineum, and provide comfort measures as indicated.
- Encourage voiding to prevent bladder distention.
- Promote an opportunity for maternal/newborn bonding.

CLIENT EDUCATION: Instruct the client to notify the nurse of increased vaginal bleeding or passage of blood clots. Offer assistance with breastfeeding, and provide reassurance.

11.3 Characteristics of true vs. false labor

True labor leads to cervical dilation and effacement.

True labor

CONTRACTIONS
- Can begin irregularly, but become regular in frequency
- Stronger, last longer, and are more frequent
- Felt in lower back, radiating to abdomen
- Walking can increase contraction intensity
- Continue despite comfort measures

CERVIX (assessed by vaginal exam)
- Progressive change in dilation and effacement
- Moves to anterior position
- Bloody show

FETUS: Presenting part engages in pelvis

False labor

CONTRACTIONS
- Painless, irregular frequency, and intermittent
- Decrease in frequency, duration, and intensity with walking or position changes
- Felt in lower back or abdomen above umbilicus
- Often stop with sleep or comfort measures such as oral hydration or emptying of the bladder

CERVIX (assessed by vaginal exam)
- No significant change in dilation or effacement
- Often remains in posterior position
- No significant bloody show

FETUS: Presenting part is not engaged in pelvis

Application Exercises

1. A nurse in the labor and delivery unit receives a phone call from a client who reports that her contractions started about 2 hr ago, did not go away when she had two glasses of water and rested, and became stronger since she started walking. Her contractions occur every 10 min and last about 30 seconds. She hasn't had any fluid leak from her vagina. However, she saw some blood when she wiped after voiding. Based on this report, which of the following clinical findings should the nurse recognize that the client is experiencing?

   A. Braxton Hicks contractions

   B. Rupture of membranes

   C. Fetal descent

   D. True contractions

2. A nurse in the labor and delivery unit is caring for a client in labor and applies an external fetal monitor and tocotransducer. The FHR is around 140/min. Contractions are occurring every 8 min and 30 to 40 seconds in duration. The nurse performs a vaginal exam and finds the cervix is 2 cm dilated, 50% effaced, and the fetus is at a -2 station. Which of the following stages and phases of labor is this client experiencing?

   A. First stage, latent phase

   B. First stage, active phase

   C. First stage, transition phase

   D. Second stage of labor

3. A client experiences a large gush of fluid from her vagina while walking in the hallway of the birthing unit. Which of the following actions should the nurse take first?

   A. Check the amniotic fluid for meconium.

   B. Monitor FHR for distress.

   C. Dry the client and make her comfortable.

   D. Monitor uterine contractions.

4. A nurse in labor and delivery unit is completing an admission assessment for a client who is at 39 weeks of gestation. The client reports that she has been leaking fluid from her vagina for 2 days. Which of the following conditions is the client at risk for developing?

   A. Cord prolapse

   B. Infection

   C. Postpartum hemorrhage

   D. Hydramnios

5. A nurse is caring for a client who is in active labor and becomes nauseous and vomits. The client is very irritable and feels the urge to have a bowel movement. She states, "I've had enough. I can't do this anymore. I want to go home right now." Which of the following stages of labor is the client experiencing?

   A. Second stage

   B. Fourth stage

   C. Transition phase

   D. Latent phase

PRACTICE Active Learning Scenario

A manager of a labor and delivery unit is reviewing the procedure for vaginal examination with a group of newly hired nurses. What interventions should be included in this discussion? Use the ATI Active Learning Template: Therapeutic Procedure to complete this item.

NURSING INTERVENTIONS: Describe four actions that are preprocedure, intraprocedure, and postprocedure.

OUTCOMES/EVALUATION: Describe three assessment findings that can be determined by the procedure.

Application Exercises Key

1.   A. Braxton Hicks contractions decrease with hydration and walking.

    B. Rupture of membranes would be indicated by the presence of a gush of fluid that is unrelated to the client's activity.

    C. Fetal descent is the downward movement of the fetus in the birth canal and cannot be evaluated based on the client's report.

    D. **CORRECT:** True contractions do not go away with hydration or walking. They are regular in frequency, duration, and intensity and become stronger with walking.

    Ⓝ *NCLEX® Connection: Health Promotion and Maintenance, Ante/Intra/Postpartum and Newborn Care*

2.   A. **CORRECT:** In stage 1, latent phase, the cervix dilates from 0 to 3 cm, and contraction duration ranges from 30 to 45 seconds.

    B. In stage 1, active phase, the cervix dilates from 4 to 7 cm, and contraction duration ranges from 40 to 70 seconds.

    C. In stage 1, transition phase, the cervix dilates from 8 to 10 cm, and contraction duration ranges from 45 to 90 seconds.

    D. The second stage of labor consists of the expulsion of the fetus.

    Ⓝ *NCLEX® Connection: Health Promotion and Maintenance, Ante/Intra/Postpartum and Newborn Care*

3.   A. The nurse assesses color, clarity, odor, and amount of amniotic fluid, but this is not the first action the nurse should take.

    B. **CORRECT:** The greatest risk to the client and fetus is umbilical cord prolapse, leading to fetal distress following rupture of membranes. The first action by the nurse is to monitor the FHR for clinical findings of distress.

    C. The nurse should provide comfort by drying the client following rupture of the membranes, but this is not the first action the nurse should take.

    D. The nurse monitors the client's uterine contraction pattern after rupture of the membranes, but this is not the first action the nurse should take.

    Ⓝ *NCLEX® Connection: Health Promotion and Maintenance, Ante/Intra/Postpartum and Newborn Care*

4.   A. Although cord prolapse is a risk with rupture of membranes, it occurs when the fluid rushes out, rather than trickling or leaking out.

    B. **CORRECT:** Rupture of membranes for longer than 24 hr prior to delivery increases the risk that infectious organisms will enter the vagina and then eventually into the uterus.

    C. The risk for postpartum hemorrhage by this client is not any greater than other clients who are pregnant.

    D. This client is more likely to have oligohydramnios or insufficient amniotic fluid, rather than hydramnios, or excess amniotic fluid.

    Ⓝ *NCLEX® Connection: Physiological Adaptation, Alterations in Body Systems*

5.   A. The second stage of labor occurs with the expulsion of the fetus.

    B. The fourth stage of labor is the recovery period, following the delivery of the placenta.

    C. **CORRECT:** The transition phase of labor occurs when the client becomes irritable, feels rectal pressure similar to the need to have a bowel movement, and can become nauseous with emesis.

    D. The latent phase of labor occurs in stage one, and coincides with mild contractions. The client is more relaxed, talkative, and eager for labor to progress.

    Ⓝ *NCLEX® Connection: Health Promotion and Maintenance, Ante/Intra/Postpartum and Newborn Care*

PRACTICE Answer

Using the ATI Active Learning Template: Therapeutic Procedure

NURSING ACTIONS

- Explain procedure, and obtain client's permission for the examination.
- Don sterile glove with antiseptic solution or soluble gel for lubrication.
- Position the client to avoid supine hypotension.
- Provide for privacy.

- Cleanse the vulva or perineum if needed.
- Insert index and middle finger into the client's vagina.
- Explain findings to the client.
- Document findings, and report to the provider.

OUTCOMES/EVALUATION

- Cervical dilation, effacement, and position
- Fetal presenting part, position, and station
- Status of membranes
- Characteristics of amniotic fluid if membranes ruptured

Ⓝ *NCLEX® Connection: Health Promotion and Maintenance, Ante/Intra/Postpartum and Newborn Care*

CHAPTER 12 *Pain Management*

Pain is a subjective and individual experience, and each client's response to the pain of labor is unique. Safety for the mother and fetus must be the first consideration of the nurse when planning pain management measures. Qs

SOURCES OF PAIN DURING LABOR

First stage

Internal visceral pain that can be felt as back and leg pain.

PAIN CAUSES
- Dilation, effacement, and stretching of the cervix
- Distention of the lower segment of the uterus
- Contractions of the uterus with resultant uterine ischemia

Second stage

Pain that is somatic and occurs with fetal descent and expulsion.

PAIN CAUSES
- Pressure and distention of the vagina and the perineum, described by the client as "burning," "splitting," and "tearing"
- Pressure and pulling on the pelvic structures (ligaments, fallopian tubes, ovaries, bladder, and peritoneum)
- Lacerations of soft tissues (cervix, vagina, and perineum)

Third stage

Pain with the expulsion of the placenta is similar to the pain experienced during the first stage.

PAIN CAUSES
- Uterine contractions
- Pressure and pulling of pelvic structures

Fourth stage

Pain is caused by distention and stretching of the vagina and perineum incurred during the second stage with a splitting, burning, and tearing sensation.

PAIN ASSESSMENT

- Pain level cannot always be assessed by monitoring the outward expressions of a client. Client pain assessment can require persistent questioning and astute observation by the nurse. Cultural beliefs and behaviors of women during labor and delivery can affect the client's pain management.
- Anxiety and fear are associated with pain. As fear and anxiety increase, muscle tension increases, and thus the experience of pain increases, becoming a cycle of pain. Fear, tension, and pain slow the progression of labor.
- Assess beliefs and expectations related to discomfort, pain relief, and birth plans regarding pain relief methods for clients in labor.
- Assess level, quality, frequency, duration, intensity, and location of pain through verbal and nonverbal cues. Use an appropriate pain scale allowing the client to indicate the severity of her pain on a scale of 0 to 10, with 10 representing the most severe pain.
- INDICATIONS OF PAIN
  - Behavioral manifestations such as crying, moaning, screaming, gesturing, writhing, avoidance or withdrawal, and inability to follow instructions
  - Increasing blood pressure, tachycardia, and hyperventilation
- The nurse is responsible for helping the client maintain the proper position during administration of pharmacological interventions. The nurse is also responsible for assisting the client with positioning for comfort during labor and birth, and following pharmacological interventions.
- A nurse should provide client safety after any pharmacological intervention by putting the bed in a low position, maintaining side rails in the up position, placing the call light within the client's reach, and advising the client and her partner to call for assistance if she needs to leave the bed or ambulate. Qs
- Evaluate the client's response to pain relief methods used (verbal report that pain is relieved or being relieved, appears relaxed between contractions). (12.1)

12.1 Appropriate pain relief measures during labor

	FIRST STAGE	SECOND STAGE	VAGINAL BIRTH	CESAREAN BIRTH
Opioid agonist analgesics	✓			
Opioid agonist-antagonist analgesics	✓			
Epidural (block) analgesia	✓	✓	✓	
Epidural (block) anesthesia			✓	✓
Combined spinal-epidural (CSE) analgesia	✓		✓	
Nitrous oxide	✓	✓	✓	
Local infiltration anesthesia		✓	✓	
Nerve block analgesia and anesthesia		✓		
Pudendal block		✓	✓	
Spinal (block) anesthesia	✓	✓		✓
General anesthesia				✓

NONPHARMACOLOGICAL PAIN MANAGEMENT

Nonpharmacological pain management measures reduce anxiety, fear, and tension, which are major contributing factors to pain in labor.

GATE-CONTROL THEORY OF PAIN

- Based on the concept that the sensory nerve pathways that pain sensations use to travel to the brain will allow only a limited number of sensations to travel at any given time. By sending alternate signals through these pathways, the pain signals can be blocked from ascending the neurological pathway and inhibit the brain's perception and sensation of pain.
- Assists in the understanding of how nonpharmacological pain techniques can work to relieve pain.

INTERVENTIONS

Cognitive strategies

- Childbirth education
- Childbirth preparation methods, such as Lamaze and patterned breathing exercises, promote relaxation and pain management.
- Doulas can assist clients using methods for nonpharmacological pain management.
- Nursing implications include assessing for signs of hyperventilation (caused by low blood levels of PCO_2 from blowing off too much CO_2), such as lightheadedness and tingling of the fingers. If this occurs, have the client breathe into a paper bag or her cupped hands.
- Hypnosis
- Biofeedback

Sensory stimulation strategies

Based on the gate-control theory to promote relaxation and pain relief
- Aromatherapy
- Breathing techniques
- Imagery
- Music
- Use of focal points
- Subdued lighting

Cutaneous stimulation strategies

Based on the gate-control theory to promote relaxation and pain relief
- Therapeutic touch and massage: back rubs and massage
- Walking
- Rocking
- Effleurage: Light, gentle circular stroking of the client's abdomen with the fingertips in rhythm with breathing during contractions
- Sacral counterpressure: Consistent pressure is applied by the support person using the heel of the hand or fist against the client's sacral area to counteract pain in the lower back
- Application of heat or cold

- Transcutaneous electrical nerve stimulation (TENS) therapy
- Hydrotherapy (whirlpool or shower) increases maternal endorphin levels
- Acupressure
- Frequent maternal position changes to promote relaxation and pain relief
  - Semi-sitting
  - Squatting
  - Kneeling
  - Kneeling and rocking back and forth
  - Supine position only with the placement of a wedge under one of the client's hips to tilt the uterus and avoid supine hypotension syndrome

CLIENT EDUCATION: Teach the client who is in labor about techniques to promote pain management, such as patterned breathing and progressive relaxation exercises.

PHARMACOLOGICAL PAIN MANAGEMENT

Includes analgesia and local/regional analgesics. To avoid slowing the progress of labor, prior to administering analgesic medications, the nurse should verify that labor is well established by performing a vaginal exam and evaluating uterine contraction pattern. Q_EBP

Alleviates pain sensations or raises the threshold for pain perception

ANALGESIA

Sedatives (barbiturates)

Sedatives such as secobarbital pentobarbital and phenobarbital are not typically used during birth, but they can be used during the early or latent phase of labor to relieve anxiety and induce sleep.

ADVERSE EFFECTS
- Neonate respiratory depression secondary to the medication crossing the placenta and affecting the fetus. These medications should not be administered if birth is anticipated within 12 to 24 hr. Q_EBP
- Unsteady ambulation of the client.
- Inhibition of the mother's ability to cope with the pain of labor. Sedatives should not be given if the client is experiencing pain because apprehension can increase and cause the client to become hyperactive and disoriented.

CLIENT EDUCATION
- Explain to the client that the medication will cause drowsiness.
- Instruct the client to request assistance with ambulation.

NURSING ACTIONS
- Dim the lights, and provide a quiet atmosphere.
- Provide safety for the client by lowering the position of the bed and elevating the side rails.
- Assist the mother to cope with labor. Q_s
- Assess the neonate for respiratory depression.

Opioid analgesics

Opioid analgesics such as meperidine hydrochloride, fentanyl, butorphanol, and nalbuphine act in the CNS to decrease the perception of pain without the loss of consciousness. The client can receive opioid analgesics IM or IV, but the IV route is recommended during labor because the action is quicker. These are usually given during the early part of active labor.

Butorphanol and nalbuphine provide pain relief without causing significant respiratory depression in the mother or fetus. Both IM and IV routes are used.

ADVERSE EFFECTS
- Crosses the placental barrier. If given to the mother too close to the time of delivery, opioid analgesics can cause respiratory depression in the neonate.
- Reduces gastric emptying; increases the risk for nausea and emesis
- Increases the risk for aspiration of food or fluids in the stomach
- Bladder and bowel elimination can be inhibited
- Sedation
- Altered mental status
- Tachycardia
- Hypotension
- Decreased FHR variability
- Allergic reaction

CLIENT EDUCATION
- Explain to the client that the medication will cause drowsiness.
- Instruct the client to request assistance with ambulation.

NURSING ACTIONS
- Prior to administering analgesic medication, verify that labor is well established by performing a vaginal exam that reveals cervical dilation of at least 4 cm with a fetus that is engaged.
- Administer antiemetics as prescribed.
- Monitor maternal vital signs, uterine contraction pattern, continuous FHR monitoring. Assess maternal vital signs and fetal heart rate and pattern and documented before and after administration of opioids for pain relief.
- Assess for adverse reactions (e.g., difficulty breathing) and be prepared to administer antidotes whenever medications are administered.

> Naloxone, an opioid antagonist, should be readily available for reversal of opioid-induced respiratory depression. Qs

Ondansetron and metoclopramide

Can control nausea and anxiety. They do not relieve pain and are used as an adjunct with opioids.

ADVERSE EFFECTS: Dry mouth and sedation

NURSING ACTIONS
- Provide ice chips or mouth swabs.
- Provide safety measures for the client.

Epidural and spinal regional analgesia

Consists of using analgesics such as fentanyl and sufentanil, which are short-acting opioids that are administered as a motor block into the epidural or intrathecal space without anesthesia. These opioids produce regional analgesia, providing rapid pain relief while still allowing the client to sense contractions and maintain the ability to bear down.

ADVERSE EFFECTS
- Decreased gastric emptying resulting in nausea and vomiting
- Inhibition of bowel and bladder elimination sensations
- Bradycardia or tachycardia
- Hypotension
- Respiratory depression
- Allergic reaction and pruritus
- Elevated temperature

CLIENT EDUCATION: Provide the client with ongoing education related to expectations for procedure.

NURSING ACTIONS
- Institute safety precautions, such as putting side rails up on the client's bed. The client can experience dizziness and sedation, which increases maternal risk for injury. Qs
- Assess for nausea and emesis, and administer antiemetics as prescribed.
- Monitor maternal vital signs per facility protocol.
- Monitor for allergic reaction.
- Continue FHR pattern monitoring.

PHARMACOLOGICAL ANESTHESIA

- Pharmacological anesthesia eliminates pain perceptions by interrupting the nerve impulses to the brain.
- Anesthesia used in childbirth includes regional blocks and general anesthesia.

Regional blocks

Regional blocks are most commonly used and consist of pudendal, epidural, spinal, and paracervical nerve block.

Pudendal block
Consists of a local anesthetic, such as lidocaine or bupivacaine, administered transvaginally into the space in front of the pudendal nerve. This type of block has no maternal or fetal systemic effects, but it does provide local anesthesia to the perineum, vulva, and rectal areas during delivery, episiotomy, and episiotomy repair. It is administered during the late second stage of labor 10 to 20 min before delivery, providing analgesia prior to spontaneous expulsion of the fetus or forceps-assisted or vacuum-assisted birth. It is suitable during the second and third stages of labor and for repair of episiotomy and lacerations.
- ADVERSE EFFECTS
  - Broad ligament hematoma
  - Compromise of maternal bearing down reflex
- NURSING ACTIONS
  - Instruct the client about the method.
  - Coach the client about when to bear down.
  - Assess the perineal and vulvar area postpartum for hematoma.

Epidural block

Consists of a local anesthetic, bupivacaine, along with an analgesic, morphine or fentanyl, injected into the epidural space at the level of the fourth or fifth vertebrae. This eliminates all sensation from the level of the umbilicus to the thighs, relieving the discomfort of uterine contractions, fetal descent, and pressure and stretching of the perineum. It is administered when the client is in active labor and dilated to at least 4 cm. Continuous infusion or intermittent injections can be administered through an indwelling epidural catheter. Patient-controlled epidural analgesia is a technique for labor analgesia and is a favored method of pain management for labor and birth. It is suitable for all stages of labor and types of birth and for repair of episiotomy and lacerations.

- ADVERSE EFFECTS
  ○ Maternal hypotension
  ○ Fetal bradycardia
  ○ Inability to feel the urge to void
  ○ Loss of the bearing down reflex
- NURSING ACTIONS
  ○ Administer a bolus of IV fluids to help offset maternal hypotension as prescribed. **Q**ᴇʙᴘ
  ○ Help position and steady the client into a sitting or side-lying modified Sims' position with her back curved to widen the intervertebral space for insertion of the epidural catheter.
  ○ Encourage the client to remain in the side-lying position after insertion of the epidural catheter to avoid supine hypotension syndrome with compression of the vena cava.
  ○ Coach the client in pushing efforts, and request an evaluation of epidural pain management by anesthesia personnel if pushing efforts are ineffective.
  ○ Monitor maternal blood pressure and pulse, and observe for hypotension, respiratory depression, and decreased oxygen saturation.
  ○ Assess FHR patterns continuously.
  ○ Maintain the IV line, and have oxygen and suction available.
  ○ Assess for orthostatic hypotension. If present, be prepared to administer an IV vasopressor such as ephedrine, position the client laterally, increase rate of IV fluid administration, and initiate oxygen. **Q**ˢ
  ○ Provide for client safety, such as by raising the side rails of the bed. Do not allow the client to ambulate unassisted.
  ○ Assess the bladder for distention at frequent intervals, and catheterize if necessary to prevent discomfort and interference with uterine contractions.
  ○ Monitor for the return of sensation and motor control in the client's legs after delivery but prior to standing. Assist the client with standing and walking for the first time after a delivery that included epidural anesthesia.
- CLIENT EDUCATION
  ○ Provide ongoing instructions related to the procedure and nursing actions.
  ○ Provide client education regarding patient-controlled analgesia, if used.

Spinal anesthesia (block)

Consists of a local anesthetic that is injected into the subarachnoid space into the spinal fluid at the third, fourth, or fifth lumbar interspace. This can be done alone or in combination with an analgesic such as fentanyl. The spinal block eliminates all sensations from the level of the nipples to the feet. It is commonly used for cesarean births. A low spinal block can be used for a vaginal birth, but it is not used for labor. A spinal block is administered in the late second stage or before cesarean birth.

- ADVERSE EFFECTS
  ○ Maternal hypotension
  ○ Fetal bradycardia
  ○ Loss of the bearing down reflex in the mother with a higher incidence of operative births
  ○ Potential headache from leakage of cerebrospinal fluid at the puncture site
  ○ Higher incidence of maternal bladder and uterine atony following birth
- NURSING ACTIONS
  ○ Assess maternal vital signs every 10 min.
  ○ Manage maternal hypotension by administering an IV fluid bolus as prescribed, positioning the mother laterally, increasing the rate of IV fluid administration, and initiating oxygen. **Q**ˢ
  ○ Assess uterine contractions.
  ○ Assess level of anesthesia.
  ○ Assess FHR patterns.
  ○ Provide client safety to prevent injury by raising the side rails of the bed, and assisting the client with repositioning.
  ○ Recognize signs of impending birth, including sitting on one buttock, making grunting sounds, and bulging of the perineum.
  ○ Encourage interventions to relieve a postpartum headache resulting from a cerebrospinal fluid leak. Interventions include placing the client in a supine position, promoting bed rest in a dark room, and administering oral analgesics, caffeine, and fluids. An autologous blood patch is the most beneficial and reliable relief measure for cerebrospinal fluid leaks.
- CLIENT EDUCATION
  ○ Instruct the client about the method.
  ○ Instruct the client to bear down for expulsion of the fetus because during a vaginal birth, the mother will not feel her contractions.

General anesthesia

Rarely used for vaginal or cesarean births when there are no complications present. It is used only in the event of a delivery complication or emergency when there is a contraindication to nerve block analgesia or anesthesia. General anesthesia produces unconsciousness.

NURSING ACTIONS
- Monitor maternal vital signs.
- Monitor FHR patterns.
- Ensure that the client has had nothing by mouth.
- Ensure that the IV infusion is in place.
- Apply antiembolic stockings or sequential compression devices.

- Premedicate the client with oral antacid to neutralize acidic stomach contents.
- Administer a histamine$_2$-receptor antagonist, such as ranitidine, to decrease gastric acid production.
- Administer metoclopramide to increase gastric emptying as prescribed.
- Place a wedge under one of the client's hips to displace the uterus.
- Maintain an open airway and cardiopulmonary function.
- Assess the client postpartum for decreased uterine tone, which can lead to hemorrhage and be produced by pharmacological agents used in general anesthesia. Qs

CLIENT EDUCATION: Facilitate parent–newborn attachment as soon as possible.

PRACTICE Active Learning Scenario

A nurse in a prenatal clinic is teaching a childbirth education class on methods to promote relaxation and pain management to a group of women in the third trimester. What nonpharmacological pain management strategies should the nurse include in the discussion? Use the ATI Active Learning Template: Basic Concept to complete this item.

UNDERLYING PRINCIPLES: Describe the underlying principle for the use of sensory stimulation and cutaneous strategies.

RELATED CONTENT
- Describe three sensory stimulation strategies.
- Describe three cutaneous strategies.

Application Exercises

1. A nurse is caring for a client who is at 40 weeks of gestation and experiencing contractions every 3 to 5 min and becoming stronger. A vaginal exam reveals that the client's cervix is 3 cm dilated, 80% effaced, and -1 station. The client asks for pain medication. Which of the following actions should the nurse take? (Select all that apply.)

   A. Encourage use of patterned breathing techniques.

   B. Insert an indwelling urinary catheter.

   C. Administer opioid analgesic medication.

   D. Suggest application of cold.

   E. Provide ice chips.

2. A nurse is caring for a client who is in active labor. The client reports lower-back pain. The nurse suspects that this pain is related to a persistent occiput posterior fetal position. Which of the following nonpharmacological nursing interventions should the nurse recommend to the client?

   A. Abdominal effleurage

   B. Sacral counterpressure

   C. Showering if not contraindicated

   D. Back rub and massage

3. A nurse is caring for a client following the administration of an epidural block and is preparing to administer an IV fluid bolus. The client's partner asks about the purpose of the IV fluids. Which of the following is an appropriate response for the nurse to make?

   A. "It is needed to promote increased urine output."

   B. "It is needed to counteract respiratory depression."

   C. "It is needed to counteract hypotension."

   D. "It is needed to prevent oligohydramnios."

4. A nurse is caring for a client who is in the second stage of labor. The client's labor has been progressing, and she is expected to deliver vaginally in 20 min. The provider is preparing to administer lidocaine for pain relief and perform an episiotomy. The nurse should know that which of the following types of regional anesthetic block is to be administered?

   A. Pudendal

   B. Epidural

   C. Spinal

   D. Paracervical

5. A nurse is caring for a client who is using patterned breathing during labor. The client reports numbness and tingling of the fingers. Which of the following actions should the nurse take?

   A. Administer oxygen via nasal cannula at 2 L/min.

   B. Apply a warm blanket.

   C. Assist the client to a side-lying position.

   D. Place an oxygen mask over the client's nose and mouth.

Application Exercises Key

1. A. **CORRECT:** The use of patterned breathing techniques can assist with pain management at this time.

   B. There is no indication for the insertion of an indwelling urinary catheter at this time.

   C. **CORRECT:** An opioid analgesic can be safely administered at this time.

   D. **CORRECT:** The use of a nonpharmacological approach, such as the application of cold, is an appropriate intervention at this time.

   E. This action does not address the client's request for assistance with pain management.

   (N) *NCLEX® Connection: Health Promotion and Maintenance, Ante/Intra/Postpartum and Newborn Care*

2. A. Abdominal effleurage is an appropriate pain management technique but does not address the pressure on the pelvis due to the fetal position.

   B. **CORRECT:** Sacral counterpressure to the lower back relieves the pressure exerted on the pelvis and spinal nerves by the fetus.

   C. A shower is an appropriate pain management strategy but does not address the pressure on the pelvis due to the fetal position.

   D. A back rub with massage is an appropriate pain management strategy but does not address the pressure on the pelvis due to the fetal position.

   (N) *NCLEX® Connection: Basic Care and Comfort, Non-Pharmacological Comfort Interventions*

3. A. Urinary output is not affected by an epidural block.

   B. Oxygen is administered to counteract respiratory depression that can occur following an epidural block.

   C. **CORRECT:** Maternal hypotension can occur following an epidural block and can be offset by administering an IV fluid bolus.

   D. Oligohydramnios does not occur as a result of an epidural block.

   (N) *NCLEX® Connection: Pharmacological and Parenteral Therapies, Medication Administration*

4. A. **CORRECT:** A pudendal block is a transvaginal injection of local anesthetic that anesthetizes the perineal area for the episiotomy and repair, and the expulsion of the fetus.

   B. Epidural blocks are administered during labor and allow the client to participate in the second stage while remaining comfortable.

   C. Spinal blocks are administered in the late second stage but most commonly preceding a cesarean birth.

   D. Paracervical blocks are used early in labor to block pain of uterine contractions but are rarely used today.

   (N) *NCLEX® Connection: Reduction of Risk Potential, Therapeutic Procedures*

5. A. The client is experiencing hyperventilation caused by low levels of serum PCO_2. Supplying additional oxygen will not resolve this issue.

   B. The client is experiencing hyperventilation caused by low levels of serum PCO_2. Applying a warm blanket will not resolve this issue.

   C. The client is experiencing hyperventilation caused by low serum levels of PCO_2. Assisting the client to a side-lying position will not resolve this issue.

   D. **CORRECT:** The client is experiencing hyperventilation caused by low serum levels of PCO_2. Placing an oxygen mask over the client's nose and mouth or having the client breathe into a paper bag will reduce the intake of oxygen, allowing the PCO_2 to rise and alleviate the numbness and tingling.

   (N) *NCLEX® Connection: Reduction of Risk Potential, Potential for Complications from Surgical Procedures and Health Alterations*

PRACTICE Answer

Using the ATI Active Learning Template: Basic Concept

UNDERLYING PRINCIPLES: Gate control theory of pain is based on the concept that the sensory nerve pathways that pain sensations use to travel to the brain will allow only a limited number of sensations to travel at any given time. By sending alternate signals through these pathways, the pain signals can be blocked from ascending the neurological pathway and inhibit the brain's perception and sensation of pain.

RELATED CONTENT

Sensory stimulation strategies
- Aromatherapy
- Breathing techniques
- Imagery
- Music
- Use of focal points

Cutaneous strategies
- Back rubs and massage
- Effleurage
- Sacral counterpressure
- Heat or cold therapy
- Hydrotherapy
- Acupressure

(N) *NCLEX® Connection: Basic Care and Comfort, Non-Pharmacological Comfort Interventions*

CHAPTER 13 *Fetal Assessment During Labor*

The diagnostic procedures mentioned in this chapter include Leopold maneuvers, and fetal heart rate (FHR) pattern and uterine contraction monitoring.

Leopold maneuvers

Leopold maneuvers consist of performing external palpations of the maternal uterus through the abdominal wall to determine the following.
- Number of fetuses
- Presenting part, fetal lie, and fetal attitude
- Degree of descent of the presenting part into the pelvis
- Location of the fetus's back to assess for fetal heart tones
  - **Vertex presentation:** Fetal heart tones should be assessed below the mother's umbilicus in either the right- or left-lower quadrant of the abdomen.
  - **Breech presentation:** Fetal heart tones should be assessed above the mother's umbilicus in either the right- or left-upper quadrant of the abdomen.

CONSIDERATIONS

PREPARATION OF THE CLIENT
- Ask the client to empty her bladder before beginning the assessment.
- Place the client in the supine position with a pillow under her head, and have her knees slightly flexed.
- Place a small, rolled towel under the client's right or left hip to displace the uterus off the major blood vessels to prevent supine hypotensive syndrome.

ONGOING CARE
- Identify the fetal part occupying the fundus. The head should feel round, firm, and move freely. The breech should feel irregular and soft. This maneuver identifies the fetal lie (longitudinal or transverse) and presenting part (cephalic or breech).
- Locate and palpate the smooth contour of the fetal back using the palm of one hand and the irregular small parts of the hands, feet, and elbows using the palm of the other hand. This maneuver validates the presenting part.

- Determine the part that is presenting over the true pelvis inlet by gently grasping the lower segment of the uterus between the thumb and fingers. If the head is presenting and not engaged, determine whether the head is flexed or extended. This maneuver assists in identifying the descent of the presenting part into the pelvis.
- Face the client's feet and outline the fetal head using the palmar surface of the fingertips on both hands to palpate the cephalic prominence. If the cephalic prominence is on the same side as the small parts, the head is flexed with vertex presentation. If the cephalic prominence is on the same side as the back, the head is extended with a face presentation. This maneuver identifies the fetal attitude.

INTERVENTIONS
- Auscultate the FHR post-maneuvers to assess the fetal tolerance to the procedure.
- Document the findings from the maneuvers.

Intermittent auscultation and uterine contraction palpation

Intermittent auscultation of the FHR is a low-technology method that can be performed during labor using a hand-held Doppler ultrasound device, ultrasound stethoscope, or fetoscope to assess FHR. In conjunction, palpation of contractions at the fundus for frequency, intensity, duration, and resting tone is used to evaluate fetal well-being. During labor, uterine contractions compress the uteroplacental arteries, temporarily stopping maternal blood flow into the uterus and intervillous spaces of the placenta, decreasing fetal circulation and oxygenation. Circulation to the uterus and placenta resumes during uterine relaxation between contractions. For low-risk labor and delivery, this procedure allows the woman freedom of movement and can be done at home or a birthing center.

Guidelines for intermittent auscultation or continuous electronic fetal monitoring
- During latent phase: every 30 to 60 min
- During active phase: every 15 to 30 min
- During second stage: every 5 to 15 min

INDICATIONS

- Determine active labor
- Rupture of membranes, spontaneously or artificially
- Preceding and subsequent to ambulation
- Prior to and following administration of or a change in medication analgesia
- At peak action of anesthesia
- Following vaginal examination
- Following expulsion of an enema
- After urinary catheterization
- Abnormal or excessive uterine contractions

CONSIDERATIONS

PREPARATION OF THE CLIENT
- Based on findings obtained using Leopold maneuvers, auscultate the FHR using listening device.
- Palpate the uterine fundus to assess uterine activity.
- Count FHR for 30 to 60 seconds between contractions to determine baseline rate.
- Auscultate FHR before, during and after a contraction to determine FHR in response to the contractions.

ONGOING CARE
Identify FHR patterns and characteristics of uterine contractions.

INTERVENTIONS
- It is the responsibility of the nurse to assess FHR patterns and characteristics of uterine contractions, implement nursing interventions, and report nonreassuring patterns or abnormal uterine contractions to the provider.
- Cultural considerations, as well as the emotional, educational, and comfort needs of the mother and the family, must be incorporated into the plan of care while continuing to assess the FHR pattern's response to uterine contractions during the labor process. Qpcc

> The method and frequency of fetal surveillance during labor will vary and depend on maternal/fetal risk factors as well as the preference of the facility, provider, and client.

INTERPRETATION OF FINDINGS

- A normal, reassuring FHR is 110 to 160/min with increases and decreases from baseline.
- Tachycardia is a FHR greater than 160/min for 1 min or longer.
- Bradycardia is a FHR less than 110/min for 1 min or longer.

Continuous electronic fetal monitoring

Continuous external fetal monitoring is accomplished by securing an ultrasound transducer over the client's abdomen, which records the FHR pattern, and a tocotransducer on the fundus that records the uterine contractions.

ADVANTAGES
- Noninvasive and reduces risk for infection.
- Membranes do not have to be ruptured.
- Cervix does not have to be dilated.
- Placement of transducers can be performed by the nurse.
- Provides permanent record of FHR and uterine contraction tracing.

DISADVANTAGES
- Contraction intensity is not measurable.
- Movement of the client requires frequent repositioning of transducers
- Quality of recording is affected by client obesity and fetal position

INDICATIONS

- Multiple gestations
- Oxytocin infusion (augmentation or induction of labor)
- Placenta previa
- Fetal bradycardia
- Maternal complications (gestational diabetes mellitus, gestational hypertension, kidney disease)
- Intrauterine growth restriction
- Post–date gestation
- Active labor
- Meconium–stained amniotic fluid
- Abruptio placentae: suspected or actual
- Abnormal nonstress test or contraction stress test
- Abnormal uterine contractions
- Fetal distress

CONSIDERATIONS

PREPARATION OF THE CLIENT
- Based on findings obtained using Leopold maneuvers, auscultate FHR using listening device.
- Palpate the fundus to identify uterine activity for proper placement of the tocotransducer to monitor uterine contractions.

ONGOING CARE
- Provide education regarding the procedure to the client and the client's partner during placement and adjustments of the fetal monitor equipment. Client and family teaching is important when an electronic fetal monitor is used. Explain the purpose and reassure that use of monitoring does not necessarily imply fetal jeopardy.
- Encourage frequent maternal position changes, which can require adjustments of the transducers with position changes.
- If the client needs to void and can ambulate, and it is not contraindicated, the nurse can disconnect the external monitor for the client to use the bathroom.
- If disconnecting the FHR monitor is contraindicated or an internal FHR monitor is being used, the nurse can bring the client a bedpan.

INTERPRETATION OF FINDINGS

- A normal fetal heart rate baseline at term is 110 to 160/min excluding accelerations, decelerations, and periods of marked variability within a 10 min window. At least 2 min of baseline segments in a 10 min window should be present. A single number should be documented instead of a baseline range.
- Fetal heart rate baseline variability is described as fluctuations in the FHR baseline that are irregular in frequency and amplitude. Expected variability should be moderate variability. Classification of variability is as follows.
  - Absent or undetectable variability (considered nonreassuring)
  - Minimal variability (detectable but equal to or less than 5/min)
  - Moderate variability (6 to 25/min)
  - Marked variability (greater than 25/min)

- Changes in fetal heart rate patterns are categorized as episodic or periodic changes. Episodic changes are not associated with uterine contractions, and periodic changes occur with uterine contractions. These changes include accelerations and decelerations.

THREE-TIER SYSTEM

Current recommendations for fetal monitoring include a three-tier fetal heart rate interpretation system.

Category I

All of the following are included in the fetal heart rate tracing:
- Baseline fetal heart rate of 110 to 160/min
- Baseline fetal heart rate variability: moderate
- Accelerations: present or absent
- Early decelerations: present or absent
- Variable or late decelerations: absent

Category II

Category II tracings include all fetal heart rate tracings not categorized as Category I or Category III. Examples of Category II fetal heart rate tracings contain any of the following:

Baseline rate
- Tachycardia
- Bradycardia not accompanied by absent baseline variability

Baseline FHR variability
- Minimal baseline variability
- Absent baseline variability not accompanied by recurrent decelerations
- Marked baseline variability

Episodic or periodic decelerations
- Prolonged fetal heart rate deceleration equal or greater than 2 min but less than 10 min
- Recurrent late decelerations with moderate baseline variability
- Recurrent variable decelerations with minimal or moderate baseline variability
- Variable decelerations with additional characteristics, including "overshoots," "shoulders," or slow return to baseline fetal heart rate

Accelerations: Absence of induced accelerations after fetal stimulation

Category III

Category III fetal heart rate tracings include either:
- Sinusoidal pattern
- Absent baseline fetal heart rate variability and any of the following.
  - Recurrent variable decelerations
  - Recurrent late decelerations
  - Bradycardia

Each uterine contraction is comprised of the following.
- **Increment:** the beginning of the contraction as intensity is increasing
- **Acme:** the peak intensity of the contraction
- **Decrement:** the decline of the contraction intensity as the contraction is ending

Nonreassuring FHR patterns are associated with fetal hypoxia and include the following.
- Fetal bradycardia
- Fetal tachycardia
- Absence of FHR variability
- Late decelerations
- Variable decelerations

FHR PATTERNS

Accelerations

Variable transitory increase in the FHR above baseline

CAUSES/COMPLICATIONS
- Healthy fetal/placental exchange
- Intact fetal central nervous system (CNS) response to fetal movement
- Vaginal exam
- Uterine contractions
- Fundal pressure

NURSING INTERVENTIONS
- Reassuring.
- No interventions required.
- Indicate reactive nonstress test.

Fetal bradycardia

FHR less than 110/min for 10 min or more

CAUSES/COMPLICATIONS
- Uteroplacental insufficiency
- Umbilical cord prolapse
- Maternal hypotension
- Prolonged umbilical cord compression
- Fetal congenital heart block
- Anesthetic medications
- Viral infection
- Maternal hypoglycemia
- Fetal heart failure
- Maternal hypothermia

NURSING INTERVENTIONS
- Discontinue oxytocin if being administered.
- Assist the client to a side-lying position.
- Administer oxygen by mask at 10 L/min via nonrebreather face mask.
- Insert an IV catheter if one is not in place and administer maintenance IV fluids.
- Administer a tocolytic medication as prescribed.
- Notify the provider.

Fetal tachycardia

FHR greater than 160/min for 10 min or more

CAUSES/COMPLICATIONS
- Maternal infection, chorioamnionitis
- Fetal anemia
- Fetal cardiac dysrhythmias
- Maternal use of cocaine or methamphetamines
- Maternal dehydration
- Maternal or fetal infection
- Maternal hyperthyroidism

NURSING INTERVENTIONS
- Administer prescribed antipyretics for maternal fever, if present.
- Administer oxygen by mask at 10 L/min via nonrebreather face mask.
- Administer IV fluid bolus.

Decrease or loss of FHR variability

Decrease or loss of irregular fluctuations in the baseline of the FHR

CAUSES/COMPLICATIONS
- Medications that depress the CNS, such as narcotics, barbiturates, tranquilizers, or general anesthetics
- Fetal hypoxemia and metabolic acidemia
- Fetal sleep cycle (minimal variability sleep cycles usually do not last longer than 30 min)
- Congenital abnormalities

NURSING INTERVENTIONS
- Stimulate the fetal scalp.
- Assist provider with application of scalp electrode.
- Place client in left-lateral position.

Early deceleration of FHR

Slowing of FHR with start of contraction with return of FHR to baseline at end of contraction

CAUSES/COMPLICATIONS
- Compression of the fetal head resulting from uterine contraction
- Uterine contractions
- Vaginal exam
- Fundal pressure

NURSING INTERVENTIONS. No intervention required.

Late deceleration of FHR

Slowing of FHR after contraction has started with return of FHR to baseline well after contraction has ended

CAUSES/COMPLICATIONS
- Uteroplacental insufficiency causing inadequate fetal oxygenation
- Maternal hypotension, placenta previa, abruptio placentae, uterine hyperstimulation with oxytocin
- Preeclampsia
- Late- or post-term pregnancy
- Maternal diabetes mellitus

NURSING INTERVENTIONS
- Place client in side-lying position.
- Insert an IV catheter if not in place, and increase rate of IV fluid administration.
- Discontinue oxytocin if being infused.
- Administer oxygen by mask at 8 to 10 L/min via nonrebreather face mask.
- Elevate the clients legs
- Notify the provider.
- Prepare for an assisted vaginal birth or cesarean birth.

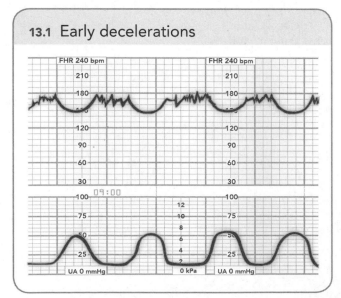

13.1 Early decelerations

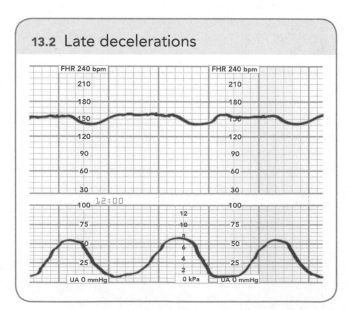

13.2 Late decelerations

Variable deceleration of FHR

Transitory, abrupt slowing of FHR less than 110/min, variable in duration, intensity, and timing in relation to uterine contraction)

CAUSES/COMPLICATIONS
- Umbilical cord compression
- Short cord
- Prolapsed cord
- Nuchal cord (around fetal neck)

NURSING INTERVENTIONS
- Reposition client from side to side or into knee-chest.
- Discontinue oxytocin if being infused.
- Administer oxygen by mask at 8 to 10 L/min via nonrebreather face mask.
- Perform or assist with a vaginal examination.
- Assist with an amnioinfusion if prescribed.

Continuous internal fetal monitoring

Continuous internal fetal monitoring with a scalp electrode is performed by attaching a small spiral electrode to the presenting part of the fetus to monitor the FHR. The electrode wires are then attached to a leg plate that is placed on the client's thigh and then attached to the fetal monitor.

INDICATIONS

Continuous internal fetal monitoring can be used in conjunction with an intrauterine pressure catheter (IUPC), which is a solid or fluid-filled transducer placed inside the client's uterine cavity to monitor the frequency, duration, and intensity of contractions. The average pressure is usually 50 to 85 mm Hg.

ADVANTAGES
- Early detection of abnormal FHR patterns suggestive of fetal distress.
- Accurate assessment of FHR variability.
- Accurate measurement of uterine contraction intensity.
- Allows greater maternal freedom of movement because tracing is not affected by fetal activity, maternal position changes, or obesity.

DISADVANTAGES
- Membranes must have ruptured to use internal monitoring.
- Cervix must be adequately dilated to a minimum of 2 to 3 cm.
- Presenting part must have descended to place electrode.
- Potential risk of injury to fetus if electrode is not properly applied.
- A provider, nurse practitioner/midwife, or specially trained registered nurse must perform this procedure.
- Potential risk of infection to the client and the fetus.

CONSIDERATIONS

PREPARATION OF THE CLIENT
- Ensure electronic fetal monitoring equipment is functioning properly.
- Use aseptic techniques when assisting with procedures.

ONGOING CARE
- Monitor maternal vital signs, and obtain maternal temperature every 1 to 2 hr.
- Encourage frequent repositioning of the client. If the client is lying supine, place a wedge under one of the client's hips to tilt her uterus.

COMPLICATIONS

- Misinterpretation of FHR patterns
- Maternal or fetal infection
- Fetal trauma if fetal monitoring electrode or IUPC are inserted into the vagina improperly
- Supine hypotension secondary to internal monitor placement

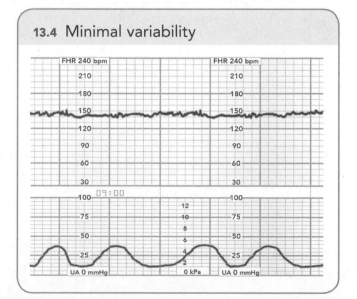

13.3 Variable decelerations

13.4 Minimal variability

Application Exercises

1. A nurse is providing care for a client who is in active labor. Her cervix is dilated to 5 cm, and her membranes are intact. Based on the use of external electronic fetal monitoring, the nurse notes a FHR of 115 to 125/min with occasional increases up to 150 to 155/min that last for 25 seconds, and have beat-to-beat variability of 20/min. There is no slowing of FHR from the baseline. The nurse should recognize that this client is exhibiting signs of which of the following? (Select all that apply.)

   A. Moderate variability
   B. FHR accelerations
   C. FHR decelerations
   D. Normal baseline FHR
   E. Fetal tachycardia

2. A nurse is teaching a client about the benefits of internal fetal heart monitoring. Which of the following should statements the nurse include in the teaching? (Select all that apply.)

   A. "It is considered a noninvasive procedure."
   B. "It can detect abnormal fetal heart tones early."
   C. "It can determine the amount of amniotic fluid you have."
   D. "It allows for accurate readings with maternal movement."
   E. "It can measure uterine contraction intensity."

3. A nurse is reviewing the electronic monitor tracing of a client who is in active labor. The nurse should know that a fetus receives more oxygen when which of the following appears on the tracing?

   A. Peak of the uterine contraction
   B. Moderate variability
   C. FHR acceleration
   D. Relaxation between uterine contractions

4. A nurse is caring for a client who is in labor and observes late decelerations on the electronic fetal monitor. Which of the following is the first action the nurse should take?

   A. Assist the client into the left-lateral position.
   B. Apply a fetal scalp electrode.
   C. Insert an IV catheter.
   D. Perform a vaginal exam.

5. A nurse is performing Leopold maneuvers on a client who is in labor. Which of the following techniques should the nurse use to identify the fetal lie?

   A. Apply palms of both hands to sides of uterus.
   B. Palpate the fundus of the uterus.
   C. Grasp lower uterine segment between thumb and fingers.
   D. Stand facing client's feet with fingertips outlining cephalic prominence.

PRACTICE Active Learning Scenario

A nurse in labor and delivery is reviewing intermittent fetal auscultation and uterine contraction palpation with a recently hired nurse. What should be included in the review? Use the ATI Active Learning Template: Therapeutic Procedure to complete this item.

INDICATIONS: Describe four situations when this procedure should be performed.

OUTCOMES/EVALUATION: Describe normal expected FHR findings.

NURSING INTERVENTIONS
• Preprocedure: Describe the three types of devices that are used to auscultate FHR.
• Intraprocedure: Identify the time frame for counting FHR to determine the baseline rate and when auscultation should take place.

Application Exercises Key

1. A. **CORRECT:** There is moderate variability of 20/min (6 to 25/min is expected reference range).

   B. **CORRECT:** FHR accelerations are present with increases up to 150 to 155/min lasting for 25 seconds.

   C. There are no FHR decelerations because the FHR does not slow down.

   D. **CORRECT:** There is a normal baseline FHR of 115 to 125/min falls within the expected reference range of 110 to 160/min.

   E. There is no evidence of fetal tachycardia because the FHR is within the expected reference range of 115 to 125/min.

   Ⓝ *NCLEX® Connection: Reduction of Risk Potential, Diagnostic Tests*

2. A. A disadvantage of internal fetal monitoring is that it is an invasive procedure.

   B. **CORRECT:** A benefit of internal fetal monitoring is that it can detect abnormal fetal heart tones early.

   C. Internal fetal monitoring cannot determine the amount of amniotic fluid.

   D. **CORRECT:** A benefit of internal fetal monitoring is that it allows for accurate readings with maternal movement which external monitoring needs adjusting when the client moves.

   E. **CORRECT:** A benefit of internal fetal monitoring is that it can measure uterine contraction intensity which external monitoring cannot.

   Ⓝ *NCLEX® Connection: Reduction of Risk Potential, Diagnostic Tests*

3. A. Compression of the arteries to the uteroplacental intervillous spaces is most acute at the peak (acme) of the uterine contraction, resulting in a decrease in fetal circulation and oxygenation.

   B. Moderate variability indicates fluctuations in the fetal heart and is not an indication the fetus is receiving more oxygen.

   C. FHR accelerations indicate an intact fetal CNS and is not an indication the fetus is receiving more oxygen.

   D. **CORRECT:** A fetus is most oxygenated during the relaxation period between contractions. During contractions, the arteries to the uteroplacental intervillous spaces are compressed, resulting in a decrease in fetal circulation and oxygenation.

   Ⓝ *NCLEX® Connection: Reduction of Risk Potential, Diagnostic Tests*

4. A. **CORRECT:** The greatest risk to the fetus during late decelerations is uteroplacental insufficiency. The initial nursing action should be to place the client into the left-lateral position to increase uteroplacental perfusion.

   B. The application of a fetal scalp electrode will assist in the assessment of fetal well-being, but this is not the first action the nurse should take.

   C. Inserting an IV catheter is an intervention for late decelerations, but this is not the first action the nurse should take.

   D. The nurse may perform a vaginal exam to assess dilation, but this is not the first action the nurse should take.

   Ⓝ *NCLEX® Connection: Health Promotion and Maintenance, Ante/Intra/Postpartum and Newborn Care*

5. A. Using the palms of the hands on the sides of the uterus to identify the fetal back and small body parts verifies the presenting part.

   B. **CORRECT:** Palpating the fundus of the uterus identifies the fetal part that is present, indicating the fetal lie (longitudinal or transverse).

   C. The descent of the presenting part into the pelvis is determined by gently grasping the lower uterine segment between the thumb and fingers.

   D. Fetal attitude is identified by facing the client's feet and outlining the cephalic prominence (fetal head) using the fingertips of both hands.

   Ⓝ *NCLEX® Connection: Health Promotion and Maintenance, Ante/Intra/Postpartum and Newborn Care*

PRACTICE Answer

Using the ATI Active Learning Template: Therapeutic Procedure

INDICATIONS

- Determine active labor
- Rupture of membranes, spontaneously or artificially
- Preceding and subsequent to ambulation
- Prior to and following administration of or a change in medication analgesia
- At the peak action of anesthesia
- Following vaginal examination
- Following expulsion of an enema
- After urinary catheterization
- Abnormal or excessive uterine contractions

OUTCOMES/EVALUATION: A normal, reassuring FHR is 110 to 160/min with increases and decreases from baseline.

NURSING INTERVENTIONS

Preprocedure
- Hand-held Doppler ultrasound
- Ultrasound stethoscope
- Fetoscope

Intraprocedure
- Count FHR for 30 to 60 seconds between contractions to determine baseline rate.
- Auscultate FHR before, during and after a contraction to determine FHR in response to the contractions.

Ⓝ *NCLEX® Connection: Reduction of Risk Potential, Diagnostic Tests*

CHAPTER 14 Nursing Care During Stages of Labor

Labor occurs in four stages. It is the responsibility of a nurse to care for, monitor, and provide interventions for the client during each stage.

NURSING RESPONSIBILITIES

ASSESSMENT

- Assess the client prior to admission to the birthing facility.
- Orient the client and her partner to the unit during admission.
  - Conduct an admission history, review of antepartum care, and review of the birth plan.
  - Obtain laboratory reports.
  - Monitor baseline fetal heart tones and uterine contraction patterns for 20 to 30 min.
  - Obtain maternal vital signs.
  - Check the status of the amniotic membranes.
- Perform maternal and fetal assessments continuously throughout the labor process and immediately after birth.
- Avoid vaginal examinations in the presence of vaginal bleeding or until placenta previa or abruptio placentae is ruled out. If necessary, vaginal examinations should be done by the provider.
- Cervical dilation is the single most important indicator of the progress of labor.
- Progress of labor is affected by size of fetal head, fetal presentation, fetal lie, fetal attitude, and fetal position.
- The frequency, duration, and strength (intensity) of the uterine contractions cause fetal descent and cervical dilation.

PATIENT-CENTERED CARE

Provide culturally competent care that respects and is compatible with the client's culture. (These are commonalities, and not meant to overgeneralize.) Qᴘᴄᴄ

Hispanic: Prefer mother to be present rather than partner

African American: Prefer female family members for support

Asian American: Might prefer mother to be present; partner not an active participant; labor in silence; cesarean birth undesirable

Native American: Prefer female nursing personnel; family involved in birth; use of herbs during labor; squatting position for birth

European American: Birth is public concern; focus on technology; partner expected to be involved; provider seen as head of health care team

FIRST STAGE

Lasts from onset of regular uterine contractions to full effacement and dilation of cervix (longer than second and third stages combined)

ASSESSMENT

- Perform Leopold maneuvers.
- Perform a vaginal examination as indicated (if no evidence of progress) to allow the examiner to assess whether client is in true labor and whether membranes have ruptured.
  - Encourage the client to take slow, deep breaths prior to the vaginal exam.
  - Monitor cervical dilation and effacement.
  - Monitor station and fetal presentation.
  - Prepare for impending delivery as the presenting part moves into positive stations and begins to push against the pelvic floor (crowning).

14.1 Stages of labor

FIRST STAGE			SECOND STAGE	THIRD STAGE	FOURTH STAGE
LATENT PHASE	*ACTIVE PHASE*	*TRANSITION*			
Onset of labor Contractions • Irregular, mild to moderate • Frequency: 5 to 30 min • Duration: 30 to 45 seconds	Contractions • More regular, moderate to strong • Frequency: 3 to 5 min • Duration: 40 to 70 seconds	Contractions • Strong to very strong • Frequency: 2 to 3 min • Duration: 45 to 90 seconds Complete dilation	Full dilation Progresses to intense contractions every 1 to 2 min Birth	Delivery of the neonate Delivery of placenta	Delivery of placenta Maternal stabilization of vital signs

- Assessments related to possible rupture of membranes
  - When there is suspected rupture of membranes, the nurse should first assess the FHR to ensure there is no fetal distress from possible umbilical cord prolapse, which can occur with the gush of amniotic fluid. Qs
  - Verify presence of alkaline amniotic fluid using nitrazine paper (turns blue, pH 6.5 to 7.5).
  - A sample of the fluid may be obtained and viewed on a slide under a microscope. Amniotic fluid will exhibit a frond-like ferning pattern. Assess the amniotic fluid for color and odor.
    - Expected findings are clear, straw color, and free of odor.
    - Abnormal findings include the presence of meconium, abnormal color (yellow or port wine), and a foul odor.
- Perform bladder palpation on a regular basis to prevent bladder distention, which can impede fetal descent through the birth canal and cause trauma to the bladder.
  - Clients might not feel the urge to void secondary to the labor process or anesthesia.
  - Encourage the client to void frequently.
- Temperature assessment every 4 hr (every 1 to 2 hr if membranes have ruptured)

NURSING ACTIONS

Teach the client and her partner about what to expect during labor and implementing relaxation measures: breathing (deep cleansing breaths help divert focus away from contractions), effleurage (gentle circular stroking of the abdomen in rhythm with breathing during contractions), diversional activities (distraction, concentration on a focal point, or imagery).

- Encourage upright positions, application of warm/cold packs, ambulation, or hydrotherapy if not contraindicated to promote comfort.
- Encourage voiding every 2 hr.

DURING THE ACTIVE PHASE
- Provide client/fetal monitoring.
- Encourage frequent position changes.
- Encourage voiding at least every 2 hr.
- Encourage deep cleansing breaths before and after modified paced breathing.
- Encourage relaxation.
- Provide nonpharmacological comfort measures.
- Provide pharmacological pain relief as prescribed.

DURING THE TRANSITION PHASE
- Continue to encourage voiding every 2 hr.
- Continue to monitor and support the client and fetus.
- Encourage a rapid pant-pant-blow breathing pattern if the client has not learned a particular breathing pattern.
- Discourage pushing efforts until the cervix is fully dilated.
- Listen for client statements expressing the need to have a bowel movement. This sensation is a finding of complete dilation and fetal descent.
- Prepare the client for the birth.
- Observe for perineal bulging or crowning (appearance of the fetal head at the perineum).
- Encourage the client to begin bearing down with contractions once the cervix is fully dilated.

SECOND STAGE

Lasts from the time the cervix is fully dilated to the birth of the fetus

ASSESSMENT

Begins with complete dilation and effacement
- Blood pressure, pulse, and respiration measurements every 5 to 30 min
- Uterine contractions
- Pushing efforts by client
- Increase in bloody show
- Shaking of extremities
- FHR every 15 min and immediately following birth

Assessment for perineal lacerations, which usually occur as the fetal head is expulsed. Perineal lacerations are defined in terms of depth.
- **First degree:** Laceration extends through the skin of the perineum and does not involve the muscles.
- **Second degree:** Laceration extends through the skin and muscles into the perineum but not the anal sphincter.
- **Third degree:** Laceration extends through the skin, muscles, perineum, and external anal sphincter muscle.
- **Fourth degree:** Laceration extends through skin, muscles, anal sphincter, and the anterior rectal wall.

14.2 Assessment in the first stage

	LATENT PHASE	ACTIVE PHASE	TRANSITIONAL PHASE
Blood pressure, pulse, and respiration measurements	every 30 to 60 min	every 30 min	every 15 to 30 min
Contraction monitoring	every 30 to 60 min	every 15 to 30 min	every 10 to 15 min
FHR monitoring (normal range 110 to 160/min)	every 30 to 60 min	every 15 to 30 min	every 15 to 30 min

NURSING ACTIONS

- Continue to monitor the client/fetus.
- Assist in positioning the client for effective pushing.
- Assist in partner involvement with pushing efforts and in encouraging bearing down efforts during contractions.
- Promote rest between contractions.
- Provide comfort measures such as cold compresses.
- Cleanse the client's perineum as needed if fecal material is expelled during pushing.
- Prepare for episiotomy, if needed.
- Provide feedback on labor progress to the client.
- Prepare for care of neonate. A nurse trained in neonatal resuscitation should be present at delivery.
  - Check oxygen flow and tank on warmer.
  - Preheat radiant warmer.
  - Lay out newborn stethoscope and bulb syringe.
  - Have resuscitation equipment in working order (resuscitation bag, laryngoscope) and emergency medications available.
  - Check suction apparatus.

THIRD STAGE

Lasts from the birth of the fetus until the placenta is delivered

ASSESSMENT

- Blood pressure, pulse, and respiration measurements every 15 min
- Clinical findings of placental separation from the uterus as indicated by
  - Fundus firmly contracting
  - Swift gush of dark blood from introitus
  - Umbilical cord appears to lengthen as placenta descends
  - Vaginal fullness on exam
- Assignment of 1 and 5 min Apgar scores to the neonate

NURSING ACTIONS

- Instruct the client to push once findings of placental separation are present. Keep mother/parents informed of progress of placental expulsion and perineal repair if appropriate.
- Administer oxytocics expulsion of the placenta to occurs to stimulate the uterus to contract and thus prevent hemorrhage.
- Administer analgesics as prescribed.
- Gently cleanse the perineal area with warm water and apply a perineal pad or ice pack to the perineum.
- Promote baby-friendly activities between the family and the newborn, which facilitates the release of endogenous maternal oxytocin. Examples of such activities include introducing the parents to the baby and facilitating the attachment process by promoting skin-to-skin contact immediately following the birth. Allow private time and encourage breastfeeding. Qᴘᴄᴄ

FOURTH STAGE

Begins with the delivery of the placenta and includes at least the first 2 hr after birth

ASSESSMENT

- Maternal vital signs
- Fundus
- Lochia
- Urinary output
- Baby-friendly activities of the family

NURSING ACTIONS

- Assess maternal blood pressure and pulse every 15 min for the first 2 hr and determine the temperature at the beginning of the recovery period, then assess every 4 hr for the first 8 hr after birth, then at least every 8 hr.
- Assess fundus and lochia every 15 min for the first hour and then according to facility protocol.
- Massage the uterine fundus and/or administer oxytocics as prescribed to maintain uterine tone and to prevent hemorrhage. Qs
- Encourage voiding to prevent bladder distention.
- Assess episiotomy or laceration repair for erythema
- Promote an opportunity for parental-newborn bonding.
- After they have had a chance to bond with their baby and eat, most new mothers are ready for a nap or at least a quiet period of rest

Application Exercises

1. A nurse is caring for a client and her partner during the second stage of labor. The client's partner asks the nurse to explain how he will know when crowning occurs. Which of the following responses should the nurse make?

   A. "The placenta will protrude from the vagina."

   B. "Your partner will report a decrease in the intensity of contractions."

   C. "The vaginal area will bulge as the baby's head appears."

   D. "Your partner will report less rectal pressure."

2. A nurse is caring for a client who is in the transition phase of labor and reports that she needs to have a bowel movement with the peak of contractions. Which of the following actions should the nurse make?

   A. Assist the client to the bathroom.

   B. Prepare for an impending delivery.

   C. Prepare to remove a fecal impaction.

   D. Encourage the client to take deep, cleansing breaths.

3. A nurse is caring for a client in the third stage of labor. Which of the following findings indicate that placental separation? (Select all that apply.)

   A. Lengthening of the umbilical cord

   B. Swift gush of clear amniotic fluid

   C. Softening of the lower uterine segment

   D. Appearance of dark blood from the vagina

   E. Fundus firm upon palpation

4. A nurse in labor and delivery is planning care for a newly admitted client who reports she is in labor and has been having vaginal bleeding for 2 weeks. Which of the following should the nurse include in the plan of care?

   A. Inspect the introitus for a prolapsed cord.

   B. Perform a test to identify the ferning pattern.

   C. Monitor station of the presenting part.

   D. Defer vaginal examinations.

5. A nurse is caring for a client who is in the first stage of labor and is encouraging the client to void every 2 hr. Which of the following statements should the nurse make?

   A. "A full bladder increases the risk for fetal trauma."

   B. "A full bladder increases the risk for bladder infections."

   C. "A distended bladder will be traumatized by frequent pelvic exams."

   D. "A distended bladder reduces pelvic space needed for birth."

PRACTICE Active Learning Scenario

A nurse is caring for a client in the fourth stage of labor. What actions should the nurse take? Use the ATI Active Learning Template: Basic Concept to complete this item.

UNDERLYING PRINCIPLES: Describe.

NURSING INTERVENTIONS: Describe four.

Application Exercises Key

1. A. The appearance of the placenta occurs after crowning and the birth of the neonate.

    B. Crowning occurs with an increase in the intensity of contractions and the urge to push.

    C. **CORRECT:** Crowning is bulging of the perineum and the appearance of the fetal head.

    D. Crowning occurs with an increase in rectal pressure as the fetal head descends onto the perineum.

    Ⓝ *NCLEX® Connection: Health Promotion and Maintenance, Ante/Intra/Postpartum and Newborn Care*

2. A. The urge to have a bowel movement indicates fetal descent and complete dilation. Assisting the client to the bathroom is not an appropriate action in view of the impending delivery.

    B. **CORRECT:** The urge to have a bowel movement indicates fetal descent and complete dilation. Preparing for an imminent delivery is appropriate.

    C. The nurse cleanses the perineal area to remove fecal matter that can be expelled due to the descent of the fetus. The nurse does not prepare to remove an impaction.

    D. Deep cleansing breaths are encouraged between contractions. The client will be encouraged to push because the sensation of a bowel movement indicates complete dilation and fetal descent.

    Ⓝ *NCLEX® Connection: Health Promotion and Maintenance, Ante/Intra/Postpartum and Newborn Care*

3. A. **CORRECT:** The umbilical cord lengthens as the placenta is being expulsed.

    B. A sudden gush of clear amniotic fluid occurs when membranes rupture.

    C. Softening of the lower uterine segment is not an indication of placental separation.

    D. **CORRECT:** A gush of dark blood from the introitus is an indication of placental separation.

    E. **CORRECT:** The uterus contracts firmly with placental separation.

    Ⓝ *NCLEX® Connection: Health Promotion and Maintenance, Ante/Intra/Postpartum and Newborn Care*

4. A. Active vaginal bleeding is not an indication of ruptured membranes. Therefore, the nurse should not anticipate cord prolapse.

    B. A test for ferning is performed if there is suspected amniotic fluid and there is no indication of ruptured membranes.

    C. Station is monitored by vaginal examination, which should not be performed if there is vaginal bleeding, which can be related to placenta previa or abruptio placentae.

    D. **CORRECT:** Vaginal examinations should not be performed until placenta previa or abruptio placentae has been ruled out as the cause of vaginal bleeding.

    Ⓝ *NCLEX® Connection: Physiological Adaptation, Unexpected Response to Therapies*

5. A. A full bladder does not place the fetus at risk for trauma.

    B. Urinary stasis, which occurs due to long periods between voiding, increases the risk for bladder infections.

    C. The urethra can be traumatized by frequent pelvic exams.

    D. **CORRECT:** A distended bladder reduces pelvic space, impedes fetal descent, and places the bladder at risk for trauma during the labor process.

    Ⓝ *NCLEX® Connection: Health Promotion and Maintenance, Ante/Intra/Postpartum and Newborn Care*

PRACTICE Answer

Using the ATI Active Learning Template: Basic Concept

UNDERLYING PRINCIPLES: The focus of care in the fourth stage is to maintain uterine tone and to prevent hemorrhage.

NURSING INTERVENTIONS

- Assess vital signs, fundus, and lochia every 15 min for the first hour, then according to facility protocol.
- Massage the uterus.
- Encourage voiding to prevent bladder distention.
- Promote parental-newborn bonding.

Ⓝ *NCLEX® Connection: Health Promotion and Maintenance, Ante/Intra/Postpartum and Newborn Care*

CHAPTER 15 Therapeutic Procedures to Assist with Labor and Delivery

In this chapter, the various therapeutic procedures to assist with labor and delivery will be discussed.

The therapeutic procedures that will be reviewed include external cephalic version, Bishop score, cervical ripening, induction of labor, augmentation of labor, amniotomy, amnioinfusion, vacuum-assisted delivery, forceps-assisted delivery, episiotomy, cesarean birth, and vaginal birth after cesarean birth.

External cephalic version

External cephalic version is an ultrasound-guided hands-on procedure to externally manipulate the fetus into a cephalic lie done at 36 to 37 weeks gestation in a hospital setting. There is a high risk of placental abruption, umbilical cord compression, and emergent cesarean birth with this procedure. Contraindications to performing a version include uterine anomalies, previous cesarean birth, cephalopelvic disproportion, placenta previa, multifetal gestation, and oligohydramnios.

INDICATIONS

POTENTIAL DIAGNOSES: A malpositioned fetus in a breech or transverse position after 36 weeks of gestation.

CONSIDERATIONS

PREPARATION OF THE CLIENT
- Obtain an informed consent form.
- The provider will perform ultrasound screening prior to the procedure to evaluate fetal position, locate the umbilical cord, assess placental placement to rule out placenta previa, determine the amount of amniotic fluid, determine fetal age, assess for the presence of anomalies, evaluate pelvic adequacy for delivery, and/or guide the direction of the fetus during the procedure.
- Perform a nonstress test to evaluate fetal well-being.
- Ensure that Rho(D) immune globulin was administered at 28 weeks of gestation if the mother is Rh-negative.
- Administer IV fluid and tocolytics to relax uterus to permit easier manipulation.

ONGOING CARE
- Continuously monitor FHR patterns to assess for bradycardia and variable decelerations during the version and for 1 hr following the procedure.
- Monitor vital signs.
- Assess for hypotension to determine whether vena cava compression is occurring. Qs
- Monitor for client report of pain.
- Rh-negative clients require a Kleihauer–Betke test to detect for the presence and amount of fetal blood in the maternal circulation because a version can cause fetomaternal bleeding. If more than 15 mL fetal blood is present, Rho(D) immune globulin must be administered to suppress the maternal immune response to fetal Rh-positive blood.

INTERVENTIONS
- Monitor uterine activity, contraction frequency, duration, and intensity.
- Monitor for rupture of membranes.
- Monitor for bleeding until maternal condition is stable.
- Monitor for a decrease in fetal activity.

Bishop score

- A Bishop score is used to determine maternal readiness for labor by evaluating whether the cervix is favorable by rating the following.
  - Cervical dilation
  - Cervical effacement
  - Cervical consistency (firm, medium, or soft)
  - Cervical position (posterior, midposition, or anterior)
  - Station of presenting part
- The five factors are assigned a numerical value of 0 to 3, and the total score is calculated.

INDICATIONS

POTENTIAL DIAGNOSES: Any condition in which augmentation or induction of labor is indicated.

CLIENT READINESS: A Bishop score for a client at 39 weeks of gestation should be greater than 8 for a multiparous client and greater than 10 for a nulliparous client as an indicator of readiness for labor induction.

Cervical ripening

Cervical ripening by various methods increases cervical readiness for labor through promotion of cervical softening, dilation, and effacement.
- Cervical ripening can eliminate the need for oxytocin administration to induce labor, lower the dosage of oxytocin needed and promote a more successful induction.
- Administration of a low-dose infusion of oxytocin is used for cervical priming.

MECHANICAL AND PHYSICAL METHODS

- A balloon catheter is inserted into the intracervical canal to dilate the cervix.
- Membrane stripping and an amniotomy may be performed.
- Hygroscopic dilators may be inserted to absorb fluid from surrounding tissues and then enlarge. Fresh dilators may be inserted if further dilation is required.
  - Laminaria tents are made from desiccated seaweed.
  - Synthetic dilators contain magnesium sulfate

CHEMICAL AGENTS based on prostaglandins are used to soften and thin the cervix. They can be in the form of oral medication or vaginal suppositories/gels.
  - Misoprostol: prostaglandin E_1
  - Dinoprostone: prostaglandin E_2

INDICATIONS

POTENTIAL DIAGNOSES: Any condition in which augmentation or induction of labor is indicated

CLIENT PRESENTATION
- Failure of the cervix to dilate and efface
- Failure of labor to progress

CONSIDERATIONS

NURSING ACTIONS
Ongoing care includes the nurse assessing for
- Urinary retention
- Rupture of membranes
- Uterine tenderness or pain
- Contractions
- Vaginal bleeding
- Fetal distress

INTERVENTIONS
- Obtain the client's informed consent form.
- Obtain baseline data on fetal and maternal well-being.
- Assist the client to void prior to the procedure.
- Document the number of dilators and/or sponges inserted during the procedure.
- The client should remain in a side-lying position.
- Assist with augmentation or induction of labor as prescribed.
- The nurse should monitor FHR and uterine activity after administration of cervical-ripening agents.
- The nurse should notify the provider if uterine hyperstimulation or fetal distress is noted.
- Monitor the client for potential side effects such as nausea, vomiting, diarrhea, fever, and uterine tachysystole.
- The nurse should proceed with caution in clients who have glaucoma, asthma, and cardiovascular or renal disorders.

COMPLICATIONS

Hyperstimulation

NURSING ACTIONS: Administer subcutaneous injection of terbutaline

Fetal distress

NURSING ACTIONS
- Apply O_2 via face mask at 10 L/min.
- Position the client on her left side.
- Increase rate of IV fluid administration.
- Notify the provider.

Induction of labor

Induction of labor is the deliberate initiation of uterine contractions to stimulate labor before spontaneous onset to bring about the birth by chemical or mechanical means.

METHODS
- Mechanical or chemical approaches
- Administration of IV oxytocin
- Nipple stimulation to trigger the release of endogenous oxytocin

INDICATIONS

Any condition in which augmentation or induction of labor is indicated. Elective induction for nonmedical indications must meet the criteria of at least 39 weeks of gestation and a Bishop score of greater than 8 for a multiparous client and greater than 10 for a nulliparous. Elective inductions that do not meet recommended criteria can result in increased risk for infection, premature delivery, longer labor, and need for cesarean birth.

CLIENT PRESENTATION
- Postterm pregnancy (greater than 42 weeks of gestation)
- Dystocia (prolonged, difficult labor) due to inadequate uterine contractions.
- Prolonged rupture of membranes predisposes the client and fetus to risk of infection.
- Maternal medical complications
  - Rh-isoimmunization
  - Diabetes mellitus
  - Pulmonary disease
  - Gestational hypertension
- Fetal demise
- Chorioamnionitis

CONSIDERATIONS

CLIENT PREPARATION

- Prepare the client for cervical ripening.
  - Obtain the client's informed consent form.
  - If cervical-ripening agents are used, baseline data on fetal and maternal well-being should be obtained.
  - The nurse may initiate oxytocin 6 to 12 hr after administration of the prostaglandin.
  - The nurse should monitor FHR and uterine activity after administration of cervical-ripening agents.
  - The nurse should notify the provider if uterine hyperstimulation or fetal distress is noted.
- Prepare the client for an amniotomy or amniotic membrane stripping.
- Prepare of the client for oxytocin.
  - Prior to the administration of oxytocin, it is essential that the nurse confirm that the fetus is engaged in the birth canal at a minimum of station 0.
  - Use the infusion port closest to the client for administration. Oxytocin should be connected "piggyback" to the main IV line and administered via an infusion pump.
  - An intrauterine pressure catheter (IUPC) may be used to monitor frequency, duration, and intensity of contractions.
  - When oxytocin is administered, assessments include maternal blood pressure, pulse, and respirations every 30 to 60 min and with every change in dose.
  - Monitor FHR and contraction pattern every 15 min and with every change in dose.
  - Assess fluid intake and urinary output.
  - A Bishop score rating should be obtained prior to starting any labor induction protocol.

ONGOING CARE

- Assist with or perform administration of labor induction agents as prescribed.
  - Increase oxytocin as prescribed until desired contraction pattern is obtained and then maintain the dose if there is
    - Contraction frequency of 2 to 3 min
    - Contraction duration of 60 to 90 seconds
    - Contraction intensity of 40 to 90 mm Hg on IUPC
    - Uterine resting tone of 10 to 15 mm Hg on IUPC
    - Cervical dilation of 1 cm/hr
    - Reassuring FHR between 110 to 160/min
- Discontinue oxytocin if uterine hyperstimulation occurs. Clinical findings of uterine hyperstimulation include the following. Qs
  - Contraction frequency more often than every 2 min
  - Contraction duration longer than 90 seconds
  - Contraction intensity that results in pressures greater than 90 mm Hg as shown by IUPC
  - Uterine resting tone greater than 20 mm Hg between contractions
  - No relaxation of uterus between contractions

COMPLICATIONS

Nonreassuring FHR

- Abnormal baseline less than 110 or greater than 160/min
- Loss of variability
- Late or prolonged decelerations

NURSING ACTIONS

- Notify the provider.
- Position the client in a side-lying position to increase uteroplacental perfusion.
- Keep the IV line open and increase the rate of IV fluid administration to 200 mL/hr unless contraindicated.
- Administer O_2 by a face mask at 8 to 10 L/min as prescribed.
- Administer the tocolytic terbutaline 0.25 mg subcutaneously as prescribed to diminish uterine activity.
- Monitor FHR and patterns in conjunction with uterine activity.
- Document responses to interventions.
- If unable to restore reassuring FHR, prepare for an emergency cesarean birth.

Augmentation of labor

Augmentation of labor is the stimulation of hypotonic contractions once labor has spontaneously begun, but progress is inadequate.

Some providers favor active management of labor to establish effective labor with the aggressive use of oxytocin or rupture of membranes.

RISK FACTORS REQUIRING AUGMENTATION OF LABOR: Administration procedures, nursing assessments and interventions, and possible procedure complications are the same for labor induction.

Amniotomy

- An amniotomy is the artificial rupture of the amniotic membranes (AROM) by the provider using an Amnihook or other sharp instrument.
- Labor typically begins within 12 hr after the membranes rupture and can decrease the duration of labor by up to 2 hr.
- The client is at an increased risk for cord prolapse or infection.

INDICATIONS

- Labor progression is too slow and augmentation or induction of labor is indicated.
- An amnioinfusion is indicated for cord compression.

CONSIDERATIONS

ONGOING CARE
- Ensure that the presenting part of the fetus is engaged prior to an amniotomy to prevent cord prolapse.
- Monitor FHR prior to and immediately following AROM to assess for cord prolapse as evidenced by variable or late decelerations.
- Assess and document characteristics of amniotic fluid including color, odor, and consistency.

INTERVENTIONS
- Document the time of rupture.
- Obtain temperature every 2 hr.
- Provide comfort measures, e.g. frequently change pads, perineal cleansing

Amnioinfusion

An amnioinfusion of normal saline or lactated Ringer's is instilled into the amniotic cavity through a transcervical catheter introduced into the uterus to supplement the amount of amniotic fluid. The instillation reduces the severity of variable decelerations caused by cord compression.

INDICATIONS

POTENTIAL DIAGNOSES
- Oligohydramnios (scant amount or absence of amniotic fluid) caused by any of the following
  - Uteroplacental insufficiency
  - Premature rupture of membranes
  - Postmaturity of the fetus
- Fetal cord compression secondary to postmaturity of fetus (macrosomic, large body), which places the fetus at risk for variable deceleration from cord compression

CONSIDERATIONS

INTERVENTIONS
- Assist with the amniotomy if membranes have not already ruptured. Membranes must have ruptured to perform an amnioinfusion.
- Warm fluid using a blood warmer prior to infusion.
- Perform nursing measures to maintain comfort and dryness because the infused fluid will leak continuously.
- Monitor the client to prevent uterine overdistention and increased uterine tone, which can initiate, accelerate, or intensify uterine contractions and cause nonreassuring FHR changes.
- Continually assess intensity and frequency of uterine contractions.
- Continually monitor FHR.
- Monitor fluid output from vagina to prevent uterine overdistention.

Vacuum-assisted delivery

A vacuum-assisted birth involves the use of a cuplike suction device that is attached to the fetal head. Traction is applied during contractions to assist in the descent and birth of the head, after which, the vacuum cup is released and removed preceding delivery of the fetal body.

Follow recommendations by the manufacturer for product use to ensure safety.

CONDITIONS FOR USE
- Vertex presentation
- Absence of cephalopelvic disproportion
- Ruptured membranes

ASSOCIATED RISKS
- Scalp lacerations
- Subdural hematoma of the neonate
- Cephalohematoma
- Maternal lacerations to the cervix, vagina, or perineum

INDICATIONS

- Maternal exhaustion and ineffective pushing efforts
- Fetal distress during second stage of labor
- Generally not used to assist birth before 34 weeks gestation

CONSIDERATIONS

PREPARATION OF THE CLIENT
- Provide the client and her partner with support and education regarding the procedure.
- Assist the client into the lithotomy position to allow for sufficient traction of the vacuum cup when it is applied to the fetal head.
- Assess and record FHR before and during vacuum assistance.
- Assess for bladder distention, and catheterize if necessary.

ONGOING CARE: Prepare for a forceps-assisted birth if a vacuum-assisted birth is not successful.

INTERVENTIONS
- Alert postpartum care providers that vacuum assistance was used.
- Observe the neonate for lacerations, cephalohematomas, or subdural hematomas after delivery.
- Check the neonate for caput succedaneum. Caput succedaneum is swelling of the scalp in a newborn that usually disappears within 3 to 5 days.

Forceps-assisted birth

A forceps-assisted birth consists of using an instrument with two curved spoon-like blades to assist in the delivery of the fetal head. Traction is applied during contractions.

INDICATIONS

CLIENT PRESENTATION
- Prolonged second stage of labor and need to shorten duration (e.g., maternal exhaustion)
- Fetal distress during labor
- Abnormal presentation or a breech position requiring delivery of the head
- Arrest of rotation

CONSIDERATIONS

PREPARATION OF THE CLIENT
- Explain the procedure to the client and her partner.
- Assist the client into the lithotomy position.
- Assess to ensure that the client's bladder is empty, and catheterize if necessary.
- Assess to ensure that the fetus is engaged and that membranes have ruptured.

ONGOING CARE: Assist with the procedure as necessary.

INTERVENTIONS
- Assess and record FHR before, during, and after forceps assistance.
  - Compression of the cord between the fetal head and forceps will cause a decrease in the FHR.
  - If a FHR decrease occurs, the forceps are removed and reapplied.
- Observe the neonate for bruising and abrasions at the site of forceps application after birth.
- Check the client for any possible injuries after birth.
  - Vaginal or cervical lacerations indicated by bleeding in spite of contracted uterus
  - Urine retention resulting from bladder or urethral injuries
  - Hematoma formation in the pelvic soft tissues resulting from blood vessel damage
- Report to the postpartum nursing caregivers that forceps or vacuum-assisted delivery methods were used.

COMPLICATIONS

- Lacerations of the cervix
- Lacerations of the vagina and perineum
- Injury to the bladder
- Facial nerve palsy of the neonate
- Facial bruising on the neonate

Episiotomy

An episiotomy is an incision made into the perineum to enlarge the vaginal opening to facilitate birth and minimize soft tissue damage.

INDICATIONS

- Shorten the second stage of labor
- Facilitate forceps-assisted or vacuum-assisted delivery
- Prevent cerebral hemorrhage in a fragile preterm fetus
- Facilitate birth of a macrosomic (large) infant

CONSIDERATIONS

The site and direction of the incision designates the type of episiotomy.
- A **median (midline) episiotomy** extends from the vaginal outlet toward the rectum, and is the most commonly used.
  - Effective
  - Easily repaired
  - Generally least painful
  - Associated with a higher incidence of third- and fourth-degree lacerations
- A **mediolateral episiotomy** extends from the vaginal outlet posterolateral, either to the left or right of the midline, and is used when posterior extension is likely.
  - Third-degree laceration can occur.
  - Blood loss is greater, and the repair is more difficult and painful.
  - Local anesthetic is administered to the perineum prior to the incision.

ONGOING CARE: Encourage alternate labor positions to reduce pressure on the perineum and promote perineal stretching to reduce the necessity for an episiotomy.

Cesarean birth

- A cesarean birth is the delivery of the fetus through a transabdominal incision of the uterus to preserve the life or health of the client and fetus when there is evidence of complications.
- Incisions are made horizontally into the lower segment of the uterus.

INDICATIONS

POTENTIAL DIAGNOSES
- Malpresentation, particularly breech presentation
- Cephalopelvic disproportion
- Nonreassuring fetal heart tones
- Placental abnormalities
- Placenta previa
- Abruptio placentae
- High-risk pregnancy
  - Positive HIV status
  - Hypertensive disorders such as preeclampsia and eclampsia
  - Diabetes mellitus
  - Active genital herpes lesions
- Previous cesarean birth
- Dystocia
- Multiple gestations
- Umbilical cord prolapse

CONSIDERATIONS

PREPROCEDURE

NURSING ACTIONS
- Assess and record FHR and vital signs.
- Assist with obtaining an ultrasound to determine whether a cesarean birth is indicated.
- Position the client in a supine position with a wedge under one hip to prevent compression of the vena cava.
- Insert an indwelling urinary catheter.
- Obtain informed consent from the client.
- Apply a sequential compression device.
- Administer preoperative medications as prescribed.
- Prepare the surgical site.
- Insert an IV catheter, and initiate administration of IV fluids as prescribed.
- Determine whether the client has had nothing by mouth since midnight before the procedure. If the client has, notify the anesthesiologist.
- Ensure that preoperative diagnostic tests are complete, including an Rh-factor test.

CLIENT EDUCATION
- Explain the procedure to the client and her partner.
- Provide emotional support.

INTRAPROCEDURE

- Assist in positioning the client on the operating table.
- Continue to monitor FHR.
- Continue to monitor vital signs, IV fluids, and urinary output.
- Conduct instrument and sponge counts per protocol.

POSTPROCEDURE

- Monitor for evidence of infection and excessive bleeding at the incision site.
- Assess the uterine fundus for firmness or tenderness.
- Assess the lochia for amount and characteristics.

> A tender uterus and foul-smelling lochia can indicate endometritis.

- Assess for productive cough or chills, which could be a manifestation of pneumonia.
- Assess for indications of thrombophlebitis, which include tenderness, pain, and heat on palpation.
- Monitor I&O.
- Monitor vital signs per protocol.
- Provide pain relief and antiemetics as prescribed.
- Encourage the client to turn, cough, and deep breathe to prevent pulmonary complications.
- Encourage splinting of the incision with pillows.
- Encourage ambulation to prevent thrombus formation.
- Assess the client for burning and pain on urination, which could be suggestive of a urinary tract infection.

COMPLICATIONS

MATERNAL
- Aspiration
- Amniotic fluid pulmonary embolism
- Wound infection
- Wound dehiscence
- Severe abdominal pain
- Thrombophlebitis
- Hemorrhage
- Urinary tract infection
- Injuries to the bladder or bowel
- Anesthesia associated complications

FETAL
- Premature birth of fetus if gestational age is inaccurate
- Fetal injuries during surgery

Vaginal birth after cesarean (VBAC)

A vaginal birth after cesarean birth is when the client delivers vaginally after having had a previous cesarean birth.

INDICATIONS

CLIENT PRESENTATION: Selection criteria for VBAC
- No other uterine scars or history of previous rupture
- One or two previous low transverse cesarean births
- Clinically adequate pelvis
- Providers immediately available throughout active labor capable of monitoring labor and performing an emergency cesarean birth if necessary
- No current contraindications
  - Large for gestational age newborn
  - Malpresentation
  - Cephalopelvic disproportion
  - Previous classical vertical uterine incision

CONSIDERATIONS

PREPROCEDURE

NURSING ACTIONS: Review medical records for evidence of a previous low-segment transverse cesarean incision.

CLIENT EDUCATION: Explain the procedure to the client and her partner.

INTRAPROCEDURE

- Assess and record FHR during the labor.
- Assess and record contraction patterns for strength, duration, and frequency of contractions.
- Assess for evidence of uterine rupture.
- Promote relaxation and breathing techniques during labor.
- Provide analgesia as prescribed and requested.

POSTPROCEDURE

Nursing interventions for a vaginal delivery after a cesarean birth are the same as for a vaginal delivery.

PRACTICE Active Learning Scenario

A nurse is planning care for a client who experienced a cesarean birth. What should the nurse include in the plan of care? Use the ATI Active Learning Template: Therapeutic Procedure to complete this item.

DESCRIPTION OF PROCEDURE

INDICATIONS: Describe at least four.

NURSING INTERVENTIONS: Describe four that are preprocedure.

POTENTIAL COMPLICATIONS: Describe two that are maternal and two that are fetal.

Application Exercises

1. A nurse is caring for a client who is at 42 weeks of gestation and is admitted to the labor and delivery unit. During an ultrasound, it is noted that the fetus is large for gestational age. The nurse reviews the prescription from the provider to begin an amnioinfusion. Which of the following conditions should the nurse plan to prepare an amnioinfusion? (Select all that apply.)
   - A. Oligohydramnios
   - B. Hydramnios
   - C. Fetal cord compression
   - D. Hydration
   - E. Fetal immaturity

2. A nurse is caring for a client who has been in labor for 12 hr, and her membranes are intact. The provider has decided to perform an amniotomy in an effort to facilitate the progress of labor. The nurse performs a vaginal examination to ensure which of the following prior to the performance of the amniotomy?
   - A. Fetal engagement
   - B. Fetal lie
   - C. Fetal attitude
   - D. Fetal position

3. A nurse is caring for client who had no prenatal care, is Rh-negative, and will undergo an external version at 37 weeks of gestation. Which of the following medication should the nurse plan to administer prior to the version?
   - A. Prostaglandin gel
   - B. Magnesium sulfate
   - C. Rho(D) immune globulin
   - D. Oxytocin

4. A nurse is caring for a client who is receiving oxytocin for induction of labor and has an intrauterine pressure catheter (IUPC) placed to monitor uterine contractions. For which of the following contraction patterns should the nurse discontinue the infusion of oxytocin?
   - A. Frequency of every 2 min
   - B. Duration of 90 to 120 seconds
   - C. Intensity of 60 to 90 mm Hg
   - D. Resting tone of 15 mm Hg

5. A nurse educator in the labor and delivery unit is reviewing the use of chemical agents to promote cervical ripening with a group of newly hired nurses. Which of the following statements by a nurse indicates understanding of the teaching?
   - A. "They are administered in an oral form."
   - B. "They act by absorbing fluid from tissues."
   - C. "They promote dilation of the os."
   - D. "They include an amniotomy."

Application Exercises Key

1. A. **CORRECT:** Oligohydramnios is an indication for an amnioinfusion because inadequate amniotic fluid can contribute to intrauterine growth restriction of the fetus, restrict fetal movement, and cause fetal distress during labor.

   B. Hydramnios is excessive amniotic fluid.

   C. **CORRECT:** Oligohydramnios results in fetal cord compression, which decreases fetal oxygenation. Amnioinfusion prevents cord compression.

   D. Amnioinfusion does not increase hydration. IV fluids or oral intake would provide hydration.

   E. Fetal immaturity is not a reason for performing an amnioinfusion.

   Ⓝ *NCLEX® Connection: Physiological Adaptation, Unexpected Response to Therapies*

2. A. **CORRECT:** Prior to the performance of an amniotomy, the amniotic membranes should have ruptured. It is also imperative that the fetus is engaged at 0 station and at the level of the maternal ischial spines to prevent prolapse of the umbilical cord.

   B. Fetal lie pertains to the axis of the maternal spine in relation to the fetal spine and is determined by Leopold maneuvers.

   C. Fetal attitude is the relationship of the fetal extremities and chin to the fetal torso. It is determined by Leopold maneuvers.

   D. Fetal position refers to the direction of a reference point in the fetal presenting part to the maternal pelvis. It is not a criterion when performing an amniotomy.

   Ⓝ *NCLEX® Connection: Health Promotion and Maintenance, Ante/Intra/Postpartum and Newborn Care*

3. A. Prostaglandin gel is a cervical ripening agent and is not administered prior to an external version.

   B. Magnesium sulfate is a tocolytic, which may be administered prior to the version. But because the client had no prenatal care and is Rh-negative, there is another medication the nurse should anticipate administering.

   C. **CORRECT:** Rho(D) immune globulin is administered to an Rh-negative client at 28 weeks of gestation. Because this client had no prenatal care, it should be given prior to the version to prevent isoimmunization.

   D. Oxytocin is administered to increase contraction frequency, intensity and duration. It is not administered prior to an external version.

   Ⓝ *NCLEX® Connection: Pharmacological and Parenteral Therapies, Medication Administration*

4. A. This contraction pattern does not require discontinuing the infusion of oxytocin.

   B. **CORRECT:** Oxytocin is discontinued if uterine hyperstimulation occurs with contraction duration longer than 90 seconds.

   C. This contraction pattern does not require discontinuing the infusion of oxytocin.

   D. This contraction pattern does not require discontinuing the infusion of oxytocin.

   Ⓝ *NCLEX® Connection: Pharmacological and Parenteral Therapies, Medication Administration*

5. A. **CORRECT:** Chemical agents that promote cervical ripening include medications administered in oral form.

   B. Hygroscopic sponges, which are a mechanical method to promote cervical ripening, act by absorbing fluid from surrounding tissues to enlarge the cervical opening.

   C. Mechanical and physical methods promote cervical ripening by dilation.

   D. An amniotomy is a mechanical method to promote cervical ripening.

   Ⓝ *NCLEX® Connection: Pharmacological and Parenteral Therapies, Medication Administration*

PRACTICE Answer

Using the ATI Active Learning Template: Therapeutic Procedure

DESCRIPTION OF PROCEDURE: Delivery of the fetus through a transabdominal incision of the uterus to preserve the life or health of the client and fetus when there is evidence of complications; incisions are made horizontally into the lower uterine segment.

INDICATIONS
- Malpresentation, breech
- Cephalopelvic disproportion
- Fetal distress
- Placenta previa
- Abruptio placentae
- HIV-positive status
- Dystocia
- Multiple gestations
- Umbilical cord prolapse
- Preeclampsia
- Eclampsia
- Active herpes lesions
- Previous cesarean birth

NURSING INTERVENTIONS
- Assess and record FHR, vital signs.
- Assist with ultrasound.
- Position client in a supine position with a wedge under one hip.
- Insert an indwelling urinary catheter.
- Administer preoperative medications as prescribed.
- Prepare the surgical site.
- Insert an IV catheter, and administer IV fluids as prescribed.
- Obtain signed informed consent form.
- Determine client's NPO status.
- Verify preoperative testing results.
- Provide emotional support.

POTENTIAL COMPLICATIONS
Maternal
- Aspiration
- Amniotic fluid pulmonary embolism
- Wound infection
- Wound dehiscence
- Severe abdominal pain
- Thrombophlebitis
- Hemorrhage
- Urinary tract infection
- Injury to bladder or bowel
- Anesthesia-associated complications
Fetal
- Premature birth
- Fetal injury during surgery

Ⓝ *NCLEX® Connection: Reduction of Risk Potential, Therapeutic Procedures*

CHAPTER 16 ## Complications Related to the Labor Process

Complications occurring during the labor process are emergent and require immediate intervention in order to improve maternal fetal outcomes. This chapter explores prolapsed umbilical cord, meconium-stained amniotic fluid, fetal distress, dystocia (dysfunctional labor), precipitous labor, uterine rupture, and anaphylactoid syndrome of pregnancy (amniotic fluid embolism).

Prolapsed umbilical cord

A prolapsed umbilical cord occurs when the umbilical cord is displaced, preceding the presenting part of the fetus, or protruding through the cervix. This results in cord compression and compromised fetal circulation.

ASSESSMENT

RISK FACTORS

- Rupture of amniotic membranes
- Abnormal fetal presentation (any presentation other than vertex [occiput as presenting part])
- Transverse lie: Presenting part is not engaged, which leaves room for the cord to descend.
- Small-for-gestational-age fetus
- Unusually long umbilical cord
- Multifetal pregnancy
- Unengaged presenting part
- Hydramnios or polyhydramnios

EXPECTED FINDINGS

Client reports that she feels something coming through her vagina.

PHYSICAL ASSESSMENT FINDINGS
- Visualization or palpation of the umbilical cord protruding from the introitus
- FHR monitoring shows variable or prolonged deceleration
- Excessive fetal activity followed by cessation of movement; suggestive of severe fetal hypoxia

PATIENT-CENTERED CARE

NURSING CARE

- Call for assistance immediately.
- Notify the provider.
- Use a sterile-gloved hand, insert two fingers into the vagina, and apply finger pressure on either side of the cord to the fetal presenting part to elevate it off of the cord. Qs
- Reposition the client in a knee-chest, Trendelenburg, or a side-lying position with a rolled towel under the client's right or left hip to relieve pressure on the cord. QEBP
- Apply a warm, sterile, saline-soaked towel to the visible cord to prevent drying and to maintain blood flow.
- Provide continuous electronic monitoring of FHR for variable decelerations, which indicate fetal asphyxia and hypoxia.
- Administer oxygen at 8 to 10 L/min via a face mask to improve fetal oxygenation.
- Initiate IV access, and administer IV fluid bolus.
- Prepare for an immediate vaginal birth if cervix is fully dilated or cesarean section if it is not.
- Inform and educate the client and her partner about the interventions.

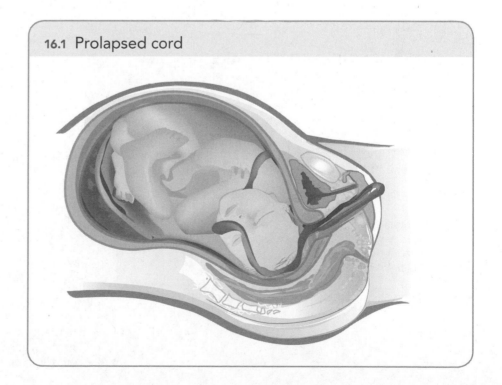

16.1 Prolapsed cord

Meconium-stained amniotic fluid

- Meconium passage in the amniotic fluid during the antepartum period prior to the start of labor is typically not associated with an unfavorable fetal outcome.
- The fetus has had an episode of loss of sphincter control, allowing meconium to pass into amniotic fluid.

ASSESSMENT

RISK FACTORS

- There is an increased incidence for meconium in the amniotic fluid after 38 weeks of gestation due to fetal maturity of normal physiological functions.
- Umbilical cord compression results in fetal hypoxia that stimulates the vagal nerve in mature fetuses.
- Hypoxia stimulates the vagal nerve, which induces peristalsis of the fetal gastrointestinal tract and relaxation of the anal sphincter.

EXPECTED FINDINGS

PHYSICAL ASSESSMENT FINDINGS
- Amniotic fluid can vary in color: black to greenish, yellow, or brown, though meconium–stained amniotic fluid is often green. Consistency can be thin or thick.
- Criteria for evaluation of meconium–stained amniotic fluid
  - Often present in breech presentation, and might not indicate fetal hypoxia
  - Present with no changes in FHR
  - Stained fluid accompanied by variable or late decelerations in FHR (ominous sign)

DIAGNOSTIC PROCEDURES

Electronic fetal monitoring

PATIENT-CENTERED CARE

NURSING CARE

- Document color and consistency of stained amniotic fluid.
- Notify neonatal resuscitation team to be present at birth.
- Gather equipment needed for neonatal resuscitation.
- Follow designated suction protocol.
  - Assess neonate's respiratory efforts, muscle tone, and heart rate.
  - Suction mouth and nose using bulb syringe if respiratory efforts strong, muscle tone good, and heart rate greater than 100/min.
  - Suction below the vocal cords using an endotracheal tube before spontaneous breaths occur if respirations are depressed, muscle tone decreased, and heart rate less than 100/min.

Fetal distress

Fetal distress is present when
- The FHR is below 110/min or above 160/min.
- The FHR shows decreased or no variability.
- There is fetal hyperactivity or no fetal activity.

ASSESSMENT

EXPECTED FINDINGS: Nonreassuring FHR pattern with decreased or no variability

DIAGNOSTIC PROCEDURES
- Monitor uterine contractions.
- Monitor FHR.
- Monitor findings of ultrasound and any other prescribed diagnostics.

RISK FACTORS
- Fetal anomalies
- Uterine anomalies
- Complications of labor and birth

PATIENT-CENTERED CARE

NURSING CARE

- Monitor vital signs and FHR.
- Position the client in a left side–lying reclining position with legs elevated.
- Administer 8 to 10 L/min of oxygen via a face mask.
- Discontinue oxytocin if being administered.
- Increase IV fluid rate to treat hypotension if indicated.
- Prepare the client for an emergency cesarean birth.

Dystocia (dysfunctional labor)

- Dystocia, or dysfunctional labor, is a difficult or abnormal labor related to the five P's of labor (passenger, passageway, powers, position, and psychologic response).
- Atypical uterine contraction patterns prevent the normal process of labor and its progression. Contractions can be hypotonic (weak, inefficient, or completely absent) or hypertonic (excessively frequent, uncoordinated, and of strong intensity with inadequate uterine relaxation) with failure to efface and dilate the cervix.

ASSESSMENT

RISK FACTORS

- Short stature, overweight status
- Age greater than 40 years
- Uterine abnormalities
- Pelvic soft tissue obstructions or pelvic contracture
- Cephalopelvic disproportion (fetal head is larger than maternal pelvis)
- Congenital anomalies
- Fetal macrosomia

- Fetal malpresentation, malposition
- Multifetal pregnancy
- Hypertonic or hypotonic uterus
- Maternal fatigue, fear, or dehydration
- Inappropriate timing of anesthesia or analgesics

EXPECTED FINDINGS

PHYSICAL ASSESSMENT FINDINGS
- Lack of progress in dilatation, effacement, or fetal descent during labor.
  - A **hypotonic uterus** is easily indentable, even at peak of contractions.
  - A **hypertonic uterus** cannot be indented, even between contractions.
- Client is ineffective in pushing with no voluntary urge to bear down.
  - Persistent occiput posterior presentation is when the fetal occiput is directed toward the posterior maternal pelvis rather than the anterior pelvis.
  - Persistent occiput posterior position prolongs labor and the client reports greater back pain as the fetus presses against the maternal sacrum.

DIAGNOSTIC AND THERAPEUTIC PROCEDURES

- Ultrasound
- Amniotomy or stripping of membranes if not ruptured
- Oxytocin infusion
- Vacuum-assisted birth
- Cesarean birth

PATIENT-CENTERED CARE

NURSING CARE

Dysfunctional labor

- Assist with application of fetal scalp electrode and/or intrauterine pressure catheter.
- Assist with amniotomy (artificial rupture of membranes).
- Encourage client to engage in regular voiding to empty her bladder.
- Encourage position changes to aid in fetal descent or to open up the pelvic outlet. Assist the client to a position on her hands and knees to help the fetus to rotate from a posterior to anterior position.
- Encourage ambulation to enhance the progression of labor.
- Encourage hydrotherapy and other relaxation techniques to aid in the progression of labor.
- Apply counterpressure using fist or heel of hand to sacral area to alleviate discomfort.
- Assist the client into a beneficial position for pushing and coach her about how to bear down with contractions.
- Prepare for a possible forceps-assisted, vacuum-assisted, or cesarean birth.
- Continue monitoring FHR in response to labor.

Hypertonic contractions

- Maintain hydration.
- Promote rest and relaxation, and provide comfort measures between contractions.
- Place the client in a lateral position, and provide oxygen by mask.

MEDICATIONS

Administer analgesics if prescribed (for rest from hypertonic contractions).

Oxytocin

THERAPEUTIC INTENT: Used to augment labor and strengthen uterine contractions

NURSING CONSIDERATIONS: Administer if prescribed to augment labor. Oxytocin is not administered for hypertonic contractions.

Precipitous labor

Precipitous labor is defined as labor that lasts 3 hr or less from the onset of contractions to the time of delivery.

ASSESSMENT

RISK FACTORS

Hypertonic uterine dysfunction
- Nonproductive, uncoordinated, painful, uterine contractions during labor that are too frequent and too long in duration and do not allow for relaxation of the uterine muscle between contractions (uterine tetany).
- Hypertonic contractions do not contribute to the progression of labor (cervical effacement, dilation, and fetal descent).
- Hypertonic contractions can result in uteroplacental insufficiency leading to fetal hypoxia.

Oxytocin stimulation
- Administered to augment or induce labor by increasing intensity and duration of contractions.
- Oxytocin stimulation can lead to hypertonic uterine contractions.

Multiparous client: Can move through the stages of labor more rapidly.

EXPECTED FINDINGS

DURING LABOR
- Low backache
- Abdominal pressure and cramping
- Increased or bloody vaginal discharge
- Palpable uterine contractions
- Progress of cervical dilation and effacement
- Diarrhea
- Fetal presentation, station, and position
- Status of amniotic membranes (membranes can be intact or ruptured)

PHYSICAL ASSESSMENT FINDINGS (POSTBIRTH)
- Assess maternal perineal area for indications of trauma or lacerations.
- Assess neonate's color and for indications of hypoxia.
- Assess for indications of trauma to presenting part of neonate, especially on cephalic presentation.

PATIENT-CENTERED CARE

NURSING CARE

- Do not leave the client unattended.
  - Provide reassurance and emotional support to help the client remain calm.
  - Prepare for emergency delivery of the neonate.
- Encourage the client to pant with an open mouth between contractions to control the urge to push.
- Encourage the client to maintain a side-lying position to optimize uteroplacental perfusion and fetal oxygenation. Q EBP
- Prepare for rupturing of membranes upon crowning (fetal head visible at perineum) if not already ruptured.
- Do not attempt to stop delivery.
- Control rapid delivery by applying light pressure to the perineal area and fetal head, gently pressing upward toward the vagina. This eases the rapid expulsion of the fetus and prevents cerebral damage to the newborn and perineal lacerations to the client.
  - Deliver the fetus between contractions assuring the cord is not around the fetal neck.
  - If the cord is around the fetal neck, attempt to gently slip it over the head. If not possible, clamp the cord with two clamps and cut between the clamps.
- Suction mucus from the fetal mouth and nose with a bulb syringe when the head appears.
- Next, deliver the anterior shoulder located under the maternal symphysis pubis: next, the posterior shoulder; and then allow the rest of the fetal body to slip out.
- Assess for complications of precipitous labor.
  - MATERNAL
    - Cervical, vaginal, or perineal lacerations
    - Resultant tissue trauma secondary to rapid birth
    - Uterine rupture
    - Amniotic fluid embolism
    - Postpartum hemorrhage
  - FETAL
    - Fetal hypoxia due to hypertonic contractions or umbilical cord around fetal neck
    - Fetal intracranial hemorrhage due to head trauma from rapid birth

Uterine rupture

- Complete rupture involves the uterine wall, peritoneal cavity, and/or broad ligament. Internal bleeding is present.
- Incomplete rupture occurs with dehiscence at the site of a prior scar (cesarean birth, surgical intervention). Internal bleeding might not be present.
- This is a rare but life-threatening obstetric injury.

ASSESSMENT

RISK FACTORS

- Congenital uterine abnormality
- Uterine trauma due to accident or surgery (previous multiple cesarean births)
- Overdistention of the uterus from a fetus who is large for gestational age, a multifetal gestation, or polyhydramnios
- Hyperstimulation of the uterus, either spontaneous or from oxytocin administration
- External or internal fetal version done to correct malposition of the fetus
- Forceps-assisted birth
- Multigravida clients

EXPECTED FINDINGS

- Client reports sensation of "ripping," "tearing," or sharp pain.
- Client reports abdominal pain, uterine tenderness.

PHYSICAL ASSESSMENT FINDINGS
- Nonreassuring FHR with indications of distress (bradycardia, variable and late decelerations, and absent or minimal variability)
- Change in uterine shape and fetal parts palpable
- Cessation of contractions and loss of fetal station
- Manifestations of hypovolemic shock: tachypnea, hypotension, pallor, and cool, clammy skin

PATIENT-CENTERED CARE

NURSING CARE

- Administer IV fluids.
- Administer oxygen.
- Administer blood product transfusions if prescribed.
- Prepare the client for an immediate cesarean birth, which can involve a laparotomy and/or hysterectomy.
- Inform the client and her partner about the treatment.

Anaphylactoid syndrome of pregnancy (amniotic fluid embolism)

- An amniotic fluid embolism occurs when there is a rupture in the amniotic sac or maternal uterine veins accompanied by high intrauterine pressure that causes infiltration of the amniotic fluid into the maternal circulation. The amniotic fluid then travels to and obstructs pulmonary vessels and causes respiratory distress and circulatory collapse. It can occur during labor, birth, or within 30 min following birth.
- Meconium-stained amniotic fluid or fluid containing particulate matter can cause devastating maternal damage because it readily clogs the pulmonary veins completely.
- Serious coagulation problems, such as disseminated intravascular coagulopathy (DIC), can occur.

ASSESSMENT

RISK FACTORS

- Multiparity and advanced maternal age
- Placenta previa or abruption
- Preeclampsia
- Eclampsia
- Oxytocin administration
- Diabetes mellitus
- Cesarean birth
- Forceps-assisted birth
- Uterine rupture
- Cervical laceration
- Meconium-stained amniotic fluid

EXPECTED FINDINGS

Report of sudden chest pain and/or sudden shortness of breath

PHYSICAL ASSESSMENT FINDINGS

- **Indications of respiratory distress**
  - Restlessness
  - Cyanosis
  - Dyspnea
  - Pulmonary edema
  - Respiratory arrest
- **Indications of coagulation failure**
  - Bleeding from incisions and venipuncture sites
  - Petechiae and ecchymosis
  - Uterine atony
- **Indications of circulatory collapse**
  - Tachycardia
  - Hypotension
  - Shock
  - Cardiac arrest

PATIENT-CENTERED CARE

NURSING CARE

- Administer oxygen via a mask at 8 to 10 L/min.
- Assist with intubation and mechanical ventilation as indicated.
- Perform cardiopulmonary resuscitation if necessary.
- Administer IV fluids.
- Position the client on her side with her pelvis tilted at a 30° angle to displace the uterus.
- Administer blood products as prescribed to correct coagulation failure.
- Insert an indwelling urinary catheter, and measure hourly urine output.
- Monitor maternal and fetal status.
- Prepare the client for an emergency cesarean birth if the fetus is not yet delivered.

Application Exercises

1. A nurse is caring for a client who is in labor and experiencing incomplete uterine relaxation between hypertonic contractions. The nurse should identify that this contraction pattern increases the risk for which of the following complications?

   A. Prolonged labor

   B. Reduced fetal oxygen supply

   C. Delayed cervical dilation

   D. Increased maternal stress

2. A nurse is caring for a client who is in active labor and reports severe back pain. During assessment, the fetus is noted to be in the occiput posterior position. Which of the following maternal positions should the nurse suggest to the client to facilitate normal labor progress?

   A. Hands and knees

   B. Lithotomy

   C. Trendelenburg

   D. Supine with a rolled towel under one hip

3. A nurse is caring for a client who is admitted to the labor and delivery unit. With the use of Leopold maneuvers, it is noted that the fetus is in a breech presentation. For which of the following possible complications should the nurse observe?

   A. Precipitous labor

   B. Premature rupture of membranes

   C. Postmaturity syndrome

   D. Prolapsed umbilical cord

4. A nurse is caring for a client who is at 42 weeks of gestation and in active labor. Which of the following findings is the fetus is at risk for developing?

   A. Intrauterine growth restriction

   B. Hyperglycemia

   C. Meconium aspiration

   D. Polyhydramnios

5. A nurse is caring for a client in active labor. When last examined 2 hr ago, the client's cervix was 3 cm dilated, 100% effaced, membranes intact, and the fetus was at a -2 station. The client suddenly states "My water broke." The monitor reveals a FHR of 80 to 85/min, and the nurse performs a vaginal examination, noticing clear fluid and a pulsing loop of umbilical cord in the client's vagina. Which of the following actions should the nurse perform first?

   A. Place the client in the Trendelenburg position.

   B. Apply pressure to the presenting part with her fingers.

   C. Administer oxygen at 10 L/min via a face mask.

   D. Call for assistance.

PRACTICE Active Learning Scenario

A nurse is caring for a client and observes meconium-stained amniotic fluid upon rupture of the client's membranes. What actions should the nurse take? Use the ATI Active Learning Template: System Disorder to complete this item.

EXPECTED FINDINGS: Describe at least two observations the nurse should make.

RISK FACTORS: Describe two.

NURSING CARE: Describe three actions the nurse should take.

Application Exercises Key

1. A. Precipitous labor, not prolonged labor, is often the result of hypertonic contractions and inadequate uterine relaxation between contractions.

   B. **CORRECT:** Inadequate uterine relaxation results in reduced oxygen supply to the fetus.

   C. Hypertonic contractions and inadequate relaxation of the uterus between contractions does not delay cervical dilation.

   D. A contraction pattern of hypertonic contractions and inadequate relaxation between contractions will increase maternal distress, but this is not an adverse effect.

   Ⓝ *NCLEX® Connection: Health Promotion and Maintenance, Ante/Intra/Postpartum and Newborn Care*

2. A. **CORRECT:** Having the client assume a position on her hands and knees can help the fetus rotate from a posterior to an anterior position.

   B. The lithotomy position is when the client lies on her back with her knees elevated and does not facilitate labor progression.

   C. The Trendelenburg position requires the client to lie on her back and does not assist in the rotation of the fetus.

   D. The supine position with a rolled towel under one hip can assist in preventing vena cava syndrome but does not assist in the rotation of the fetus.

   Ⓝ *NCLEX® Connection: Health Promotion and Maintenance, Ante/Intra/Postpartum and Newborn Care*

3. A. Breech presentation would most likely cause dystocia (prolonged, difficult labor) rather than a precipitous labor.

   B. Breech presentation has no effect on rupture of the membranes.

   C. Breech presentation is not associated with postmaturity syndrome.

   D. **CORRECT:** A prolapsed umbilical cord is a potential complication for a fetus in a breech presentation.

   Ⓝ *NCLEX® Connection: Health Promotion and Maintenance, Ante/Intra/Postpartum and Newborn Care*

4. A. Intrauterine growth restriction occurs earlier in the pregnancy and not at this point.

   B. A postterm neonate is at risk for hypoglycemia, not hyperglycemia.

   C. **CORRECT:** Postterm neonates are at risk for aspiration of meconium.

   D. Postterm pregnancies result in oligohydramnios, not polyhydramnios.

   Ⓝ *NCLEX® Connection: Health Promotion and Maintenance, Health Screening*

5. A. The nurse should place the client in the Trendelenburg position. However, evidence-based practice indicates that another action/assessment is the priority.

   B. The nurse should apply pressure to the presenting part with her fingers. However, evidence-based practice indicates that another action/assessment is the priority.

   C. The nurse should administer oxygen at 10 L/min via a face mask. However, evidence-based practice indicates that another action/assessment is the priority.

   D. **CORRECT:** According to evidenced-based practice, the nurse should first call for assistance.

   Ⓝ *NCLEX® Connection: Physiological Adaptation, Medical Emergencies*

PRACTICE Answer

Using ATI Active Learning Template: System Disorder

EXPECTED FINDINGS
- Color and consistency
- FHR pattern (presence of decelerations)

RISK FACTORS
- 38 weeks or later in gestation
- Episodes of fetal hypoxia due to cord compression

NURSING CARE
- Document color and consistency of amniotic fluid.
- Notify neonatal resuscitation team to be present at birth.
- Gather equipment needed for neonatal resuscitation and make available.
- Follow designated suction protocol.
  - Assess neonate's respiratory efforts, muscle tone, and heart rate.
  - If respiratory efforts are strong, muscle tone good, and heart rate greater than 100/min, suction mouth and nose using bulb syringe.
  - If respirations are depressed, muscle tone decreased, and heart rate less than 100/min, suction below the vocal cords using an endotracheal tube before spontaneous breaths occur.

Ⓝ *NCLEX® Connection: Physiological Adaptation, Medical Emergencies*

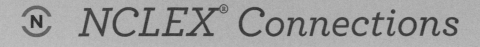

When reviewing the following chapters, keep in mind the relevant topics and tasks of the NCLEX outline, in particular:

Client Needs: Health Promotion and Maintenance

ANTE/INTRA/POSTPARTUM AND NEWBORN CARE: Provide post-partum care and education.

DEVELOPMENTAL STAGES AND TRANSITIONS: Assist client to cope with life transitions.

HEALTH PROMOTION/DISEASE PREVENTION: Provide information about health promotion and maintenance recommendations.

Client Needs: Pharmacological and Parenteral Therapies

ADVERSE EFFECTS/CONTRAINDICATIONS/SIDE EFFECTS/ INTERACTIONS: Provide information to the client on common side effects/adverse effects/potential interactions of medications and inform the client when to notify the primary health care provider.

EXPECTED ACTIONS/OUTCOMES: Evaluate client response to medication.

MEDICATION ADMINISTRATION: Review pertinent data prior to medication administration.

Client Needs: Reduction of Risk Potential

CHANGES/ABNORMALITIES IN VITAL SIGNS: Assess and respond to changes in client vital signs.

LABORATORY VALUES: Educate client about the purpose and procedure of prescribed laboratory tests.

POTENTIAL FOR COMPLICATIONS FROM SURGICAL PROCEDURES AND HEALTH ALTERATIONS: Apply knowledge of pathophysiology to monitoring for complications.

UNIT 3   POSTPARTUM NURSING CARE
SECTION: ROUTINE POSTPARTUM CARE

CHAPTER 17 *Postpartum Physiological Adaptations*

It is important for a nurse to provide comfort measures for the client during the fourth stage of labor. This maternal recovery period starts with delivery of the placenta and includes at least the first 2 hr after birth. Also during this stage, parent-newborn bonding should begin to occur.

The main goal during the immediate postpartum period is to prevent postpartum hemorrhage. Other goals include assisting in a client's recovery, identifying deviations in the expected recovery process, providing comfort measures and pharmacological pain relief, providing client education about newborn and self-care, and providing baby-friendly activities to promote infant/family bonding.

PHYSICAL CHANGES

The postpartum period, also known as the puerperium, includes physiological and psychological adjustments. This period is the interval between birth and the return of the reproductive organs to their normal nonpregnant state. Although traditionally this has been considered to last 6 weeks, this timeframe varies among women.

- Physiological maternal changes consist of uterine involution; lochia flow; cervical involution; decrease in vaginal distention; alteration in ovarian function and menstruation; and cardiovascular, urinary tract, breast, and gastrointestinal tract changes.
- The greatest risks during the postpartum period are hemorrhage, shock, and infection.
- Oxytocin, a hormone released from the pituitary gland, coordinates and strengthens uterine contractions.
  - Breastfeeding stimulates the release of endogenous oxytocin from the pituitary gland.
  - Exogenous oxytocin can be administered postpartum to improve the quality of the uterine contractions. A firm and contracted uterus prevents excessive bleeding and hemorrhage.
  - Uncomfortable uterine cramping is referred to as afterpains.

- After delivery of the placenta, hormones (estrogen, progesterone, and placental enzyme insulinase) decrease, thus resulting in decreased blood glucose, estrogen, and progesterone levels.
  - Decreased estrogen is associated with breast engorgement, diaphoresis (profuse perspiration), and diuresis (increased formation and excretion of urine) of excess extracellular fluid accumulated during pregnancy.
  - Decreased estrogen diminishes vaginal lubrication. Local dryness and intercourse discomfort can persist until ovarian function returns and menstruation resumes.
  - Decreased progesterone results in an increase in muscle tone throughout the body.
  - Decreased placental enzyme insulinase results in reversal of the diabetogenic effects of pregnancy, which lowers blood glucose levels immediately in the puerperium.
- Lactating and nonlactating women differ in the timing of the first ovulation and the resumption of menstruation.
  - In lactating women, the serum prolactin levels remain elevated and suppress ovulation.
    - The return of ovulation is influenced by breastfeeding frequency, the length of each feeding, and the use of supplementation.
    - The infant's suck is also believed to affect prolactin levels.
    - Length of time to the first postpartum ovulation is approximately 6 months.
  - In nonlactating women, prolactin declines and reaches the prepregnant level by the third week postpartum.
    - Ovulation occurs 27 to 75 days after birth.
    - Menses resume by 4 to 6 weeks postpartum.

ASSESSMENT

Postpartum assessments immediately following delivery include monitoring vital signs, uterine firmness and its location in relation to the umbilicus, uterine position in relation to the midline of the abdomen, and amount of vaginal bleeding.

- American Academy of Pediatrics and American Congress of Obstetricians and Gynecologists recommends that blood pressure and pulse be assessed at least every 15 min for the first 2 hr after birth. Temperature should be assessed every 4 hr for the first 8 hr after birth and then at least every 8 hr.

A focused postpartum physical assessment should include assessing the client's
- **B: Breasts**
- **U: Uterus** (fundal height, uterine placement, and consistency)
- **B: Bowel** and GI function
- **B: Bladder** function
- **L: Lochia** (color, odor, consistency, and amount [COCA])
- **E: Episiotomy** (edema, ecchymosis, approximation)
- Vital signs, to include pain assessment
- Teaching needs

LABORATORY TESTS

Can include CBC with monitoring of Hgb, Hct, and WBC and platelet counts.

DIAGNOSTIC AND THERAPEUTIC PROCEDURES

RH-NEGATIVE MOTHERS

- **Rho(D) immune globulin** is administered within 72 hr to women who are Rh-negative and gave birth to infants who are Rh-positive to prevent sensitization in future pregnancies. Q͏s
- The **Kleihauer–Betke test** determines the amount of fetal blood in maternal circulation if a large fetomaternal transfusion is suspected. If 15 mL or more of fetal blood is detected, the mother should receive an increased Rho(D) immune globulin dose.

Thermoregulation

Postpartum chill, which occurs in the first 2 hr puerperium, is an uncontrollable shaking chill immediately following birth. Postpartum chill is possibly related to a nervous system response, vasomotor changes, a shift in fluids, and/or the work of labor. This is a normal occurrence unless accompanied by an elevated temperature.

- Provide warm blankets and fluids.
- Assure client that these chills are a self-limiting, common occurrence that will last only a short while.

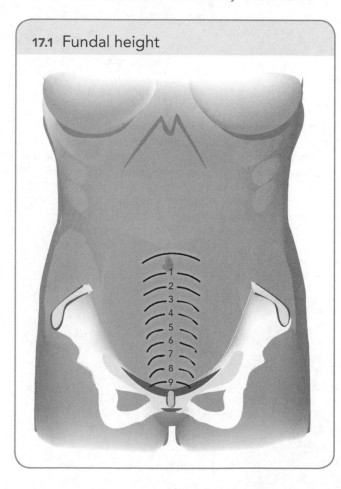

17.1 Fundal height

Fundus

Physical changes of the uterus include involution of the uterus. Involution occurs with contractions of the uterine smooth muscle, whereby the uterus returns to its prepregnant state. The uterus also rapidly decreases in size from approximately 1 kg (2.2 lb) to 60 to 80 g at 6 weeks with the fundal height steadily descending into the pelvis approximately one fingerbreadth (1 cm) per day. **(17.1)**

- Immediately after delivery, the fundus should be firm, midline with the umbilicus, and approximately at the level of the umbilicus. At 12 hr postpartum, the fundus may be palpated at 1 cm above the umbilicus.
- Every 24 hr, the fundus should descend approximately 1 to 2 cm. It should be halfway between the symphysis pubis and the umbilicus by the sixth postpartum day.
- After 2 weeks, the uterus should lie within the true pelvis and should not be palpable.

ASSESSMENT

The nurse should assess the fundal height, uterine placement, and uterine consistency at least every 8 hr after the recovery period has ended.

- Explain the procedure to the client.
- Apply clean gloves and a lower perineal pad, and observe lochia flow as the fundus is palpated.
- Cup one hand just above the symphysis pubis to support the lower segment of the uterus, and with the other hand, palpate the abdomen to locate the fundus.
- Document the fundal height, location, and uterine consistency.
  - Determine the fundal height by placing fingers on the abdomen and measuring how many fingerbreadths (centimeters) fit between the fundus and the umbilicus above, below, or at the umbilical level.
  - Determine whether the fundus is midline in the pelvis or displaced laterally (caused by a full bladder).
  - Determine whether the fundus is firm or boggy. If the fundus is boggy (not firm), lightly massage the fundus in a circular motion. Q͏EBP

PATIENT-CENTERED CARE

- Administer oxytocics intramuscularly or IV after the placenta is delivered to promote uterine contractions and to prevent hemorrhage.
  - Oxytocics include oxytocin, methylergonovine, and carboprost. Misoprostol, a prostaglandin, also may be administered.
- Monitor for adverse effects of medications.
  - Oxytocin and misoprostol can cause hypotension.
  - Methylergonovine, ergonovine, and carboprost can cause hypertension.
- Encourage early breastfeeding for a client who is lactating. This will stimulate the production of natural oxytocin and prevent hemorrhage.
- Encourage emptying of the bladder every 2 to 3 hr to prevent possible uterine displacement and atony.

Lochia

Lochia is post-birth uterine discharge that contains blood, mucus, and uterine tissue.

Three stages of lochia

Lochia rubra: Bright red color, bloody consistency, fleshy odor, can contain small clots, transient flow increases during breastfeeding and upon rising. Lasts 1 to 3 days after delivery.

Lochia serosa: Pinkish brown color and serosanguineous consistency. Lasts from approximately day 4 to day 10 after delivery.

Lochia alba: Yellowish white creamy color, fleshy odor. Lasts from approximately day 11 up to 4 to 8 weeks postpartum.

ASSESSMENT

- Lochia amount is assessed by the quantity of saturation on the perineal pad as being
  - Scant: less than 2.5 cm
  - Light: 2.5 to 10 cm
  - Moderate: more than 10 cm
  - Heavy: one pad saturated within 2 hr
  - Excessive blood loss: one pad saturated in 15 min or less, or pooling of blood under buttocks **(17.2)** Qs
- Assess the lochia flow for normal color, amount, and consistency.
  - Lochia typically trickles from the vaginal opening but flows more steadily during uterine contractions.
  - Assess for pooled lochia on the pad under the client, which she might not feel. Massaging the uterus or ambulation can result in a gush of lochia with the expression of clots and dark blood that has pooled in the vagina, but should soon decrease back to a trickle of bright red lochia when in the early puerperium.

PATIENT-CENTERED CARE

Nursing interventions for abnormal lochia include notifying the provider and performing prescribed interventions based on the cause of the abnormality.

Manifestations of abnormal lochia
- Excessive spurting of bright red blood from the vagina, possibly indicating a cervical or vaginal tear
- Numerous large clots and excessive blood loss (saturation of one pad in 15 min or less), which can indicate hemorrhage
- Foul odor, which is suggestive of infection
- Persistent lochia rubra in the early postpartum period beyond day 3, which can indicate retained placental fragments
- Continued flow of lochia serosa or alba beyond the normal length of time can indicate endometritis, especially if it is accompanied by fever, pain, or abdominal tenderness.

Cervix, vagina, and perineum

PHYSICAL CHANGES
- The cervix is soft directly after birth and can be edematous, bruised, and have small lacerations. Within 2 to 3 days postpartum, it shortens, regains its form, and becomes firm, with the os gradually closing. Lacerations can delay the production of estrogen-influenced cervical mucus and are a predisposing factor to infection.
- The vagina, which has distended, gradually returns to its prepregnancy size with the reappearance of rugae and a thickening of the vaginal mucosa. However, muscle tone is never restored completely.
- The soft tissues of the perineum can be erythematous and edematous, especially in areas of an episiotomy or lacerations. Hematomas or hemorrhoids can be present. Pelvic floor muscles can be overstretched and weak.

ASSESSMENT

Assess for cervical, vaginal, and perineal healing.
- Observe the perineum for erythema, edema, and hematoma.
- Assess episiotomy and lacerations for approximation, drainage, quantity, and quality. A bright red trickle of blood from the episiotomy site in the early postpartum period is a normal finding.

PATIENT-CENTERED CARE

Perineal tenderness, laceration, and episiotomy
- Promote measures to help soften the client's stools.
- Educate the client about proper cleansing to prevent infection.
  - The client should wash her hands thoroughly before and after voiding.
  - The client should use a squeeze bottle filled with warm water or antiseptic solution after each voiding to cleanse the perineal area.
  - The client should clean her perineal area from front to back (urethra to anus).
  - The client should blot dry, not wipe.
  - The client should sparingly use a topical application of antiseptic cream or spray.
  - The client's perineal pad should be changed from front to back after voiding or defecating.

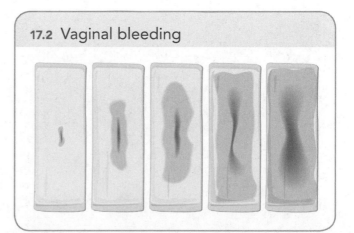

17.2 Vaginal bleeding

- Promote comfort measures.
  - Apply ice packs to the perineum for the first 24 to 48 hr to reduce edema and provide anesthetic effect.
  - Encourage sitz baths at a temperature of 38° to 40° C (100° to 104° F) or cooler at least twice a day. Ⓠ EBP

17.3 Breastfeeding positions

Football hold

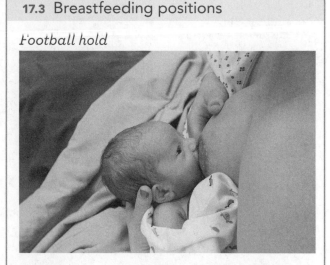

Cradle

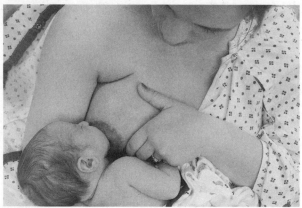

Modified cradle

The mother positions the baby as in the cradle position shown above, but reverses the function of each arm.

Side-lying

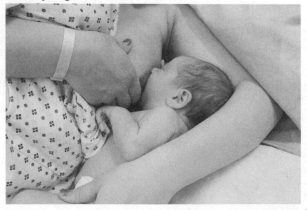

  - Administer analgesia, such as nonopioids (acetaminophen), nonsteroidal anti-inflammatories (ibuprofen), and opioids (codeine, hydrocodone) for pain and discomfort.
  - Opioid analgesia may be administered via a patient-controlled analgesia (PCA) pump after cesarean birth. Continuous epidural infusions may also be used for pain control after cesarean birth.
  - Apply topical anesthetics (benzocaine spray) to the client's perineal area as needed or witch hazel compresses to the rectal area for hemorrhoids.

Breasts

Physical changes of the breasts include the secretion of colostrum, which occurs during pregnancy and 2 to 3 days immediately after birth. Milk is produced 3 to 5 days after the delivery of the newborn.

ASSESSMENT

The nurse should assess the client's breasts as well as her ability to assist the newborn with latching on if breastfeeding.

- Colostrum (early milk) transitions to mature milk by about 72 to 96 hr after birth and is referred to as the milk coming in.
- Engorgement of the breast tissue as a result of lymphatic circulation, milk production, and temporary vein congestion.
- Redness and tenderness of the breast.
- Cracked nipples and indications of mastitis (infection in a milk duct of the breast with concurrent flu-like manifestations).
- Ascertain that the newborn who is breastfeeding has latched on correctly to prevent sore nipples.
- Ineffective newborn feeding patterns related to maternal dehydration, maternal discomfort, newborn positioning, or difficulty with the newborn latching onto the breast.

PATIENT-CENTERED CARE

- Encourage early demand breastfeeding for the client who is lactating, which will also stimulate the production of natural oxytocin and help prevent uterine hemorrhage.
- Assist the client into a comfortable position, and have her try various positions during breastfeeding. The four traditional positions for breastfeeding are football hold (under the arm), cradle, across the lap (modified cradle), and side-lying. Explain how varying positions can prevent nipple soreness. **(17.3)**
- Teach the client the importance of proper latch techniques (the newborn takes in part of the areola and nipple, not just the tip of the nipple) to prevent nipple soreness.
- Inform the client that breastfeeding causes the release of oxytocin, which stimulates uterine contractions. This is a normal occurrence and beneficial to uterine tone.

Cardiovascular system and fluid and hematologic status

PHYSICAL CHANGES

In the cardiovascular system during the postpartum period

- The cardiovascular system undergoes a decrease in blood volume during the postpartum period related to
  - Blood loss during childbirth (average blood loss is 300 to 500 mL (10% of blood volume) in an uncomplicated vaginal delivery and 500 to 1,000 mL (15% to 30% of blood volume) for a cesarean birth).
  - Diaphoresis and diuresis of the excess fluid accumulated during the last part of the pregnancy. Loss occurs within the first 2 to 3 days post-delivery.
- Hypovolemic shock does not usually occur in response to the normal blood loss of labor and birth because of the expanded blood volume of pregnancy and the readjustment in the maternal vasculature, which occurs in response to the following.
  - Elimination of the placenta, diverting 500 mL of blood into the maternal systemic circulation
  - Rapid reduction in the size of the uterus, putting more blood into the maternal systemic circulation

In blood values, coagulation factors, and fibrinogen levels during the puerperium

- Hematocrit levels drop moderately for 3 to 4 days then begin to increase and reach nonpregnant levels by 8 weeks postpartum. During the first 4 to 7 days after birth, WBC values between 20,000 and 25,000mm^3 are common.
- Coagulation factors and fibrinogen levels increase during pregnancy and remain elevated for 2 to 3 weeks postpartum. Hypercoagulability predisposes the postpartum client to thrombus formation and thromboembolism.

VITAL SIGN CHANGES

- Blood pressure is usually unchanged with an uncomplicated pregnancy but may have an insignificant, slight transient increase.
- Possible orthostatic hypotension within the first 48 hr postpartum can occur immediately after standing up with feelings of faintness or dizziness resulting from splanchnic (viscera/internal organs) engorgement that can occur after birth.
- Elevation of pulse, stroke volume, and cardiac output for the first hour postpartum occurs and then gradually decreases to a prepregnant state baseline by 8 to 10 weeks.
- Elevation of temperature to 38° C (100.4° F) resulting from dehydration after labor during the first 24 hr can occur, but should return to normal after 24 hr postpartum.

ASSESSMENT

- Assess for cardiovascular and vital sign changes and monitor blood component changes.
- Inspect the legs for redness, swelling, and warmth, which are additional indications of venous thrombosis.

PATIENT-CENTERED CARE

Nursing interventions for alterations in findings include notifying the provider and performing prescribed interventions based on the cause of the alteration.

- Encourage early ambulation to prevent venous stasis and thrombosis.
- Apply antiembolism stockings to the lower extremities if the client is at high risk for developing venous stasis and thrombosis. Remove the stockings as soon as the client is ambulating.
- Administer medications as prescribed.

Gastrointestinal system and bowel function

PHYSICAL CHANGES IN THE GASTROINTESTINAL SYSTEM

- Increased appetite following delivery
- Constipation with bowel evacuation delayed until 2 to 3 days after birth
- Hemorrhoids

ASSESSMENT

The nurse should assess the gastrointestinal system including bowel function.

- Assess for reports of hunger. Expect the client to have a good appetite.
- Assess for bowel sounds and the return of normal bowel function. Spontaneous bowel movement might not occur for 2 to 3 days after delivery secondary to decreased intestinal muscle tone during labor and puerperium and prelabor diarrhea and dehydration. The client can also anticipate discomfort with defecation because of perineal tenderness, episiotomy, lacerations, or hemorrhoids.
- Assess the rectal area for varicosities (hemorrhoids).
- Operative vaginal birth (forceps-and vacuum-assisted) and anal sphincter lacerations increase the risk of temporary postpartum anal incontinence that usually resolves within 6 months.

PATIENT-CENTERED CARE

- Encourage the client to take measures to soften her stools and promote bowel function (early ambulation, increased fluids, and high-fiber food sources).
- Administer stool softeners (docusate sodium) to prevent constipation.
- Enemas and suppositories are contraindicated for clients who have third- or fourth-degree perineal lacerations. Qs

Urinary system and bladder function

The urinary system can show evidence of the following.
- Urinary retention secondary to loss of bladder elasticity and tone and/or loss of bladder sensation resulting from trauma, medications, or anesthesia. A distended bladder as a result of urinary retention can cause uterine atony and displacement to one side, usually to the right. The ability of the uterus to contract is also lessened.
- Postpartal diuresis with increased urinary output begins within 12 hr of delivery.

ASSESSMENT

Assess the urinary system and bladder function.
- Assess the client's ability to void every 2 to 3 hr (perineal/urethral edema may cause pain and difficulty in voiding during the first 24 to 48 hr).
- Assess bladder elimination pattern (client should be voiding every 2 to 3 hr). Excessive urine diuresis (more than 3,000 mL/day) is normal within the first 2 to 3 days after delivery.
- Assess for evidence of a distended bladder.
  - Fundal height above the umbilicus or baseline level
  - Fundus displaced from the midline over to the side
  - Bladder bulges above the symphysis pubis
  - Excessive lochia
  - Tenderness over the bladder area
- Frequent voiding of less than 150 mL of urine is indicative of urinary retention with overflow.

PATIENT-CENTERED CARE

- Encourage the client to empty her bladder frequently (every 2 to 3 hr) to prevent possible displacement of the uterus and atony.
- Measure the client's first few voidings after delivery to assess for bladder emptying.
- Encourage the client to increase her oral fluid intake to replace fluids lost at delivery and to prevent or correct dehydration.
- Catheterize if necessary for bladder distention if the client is unable to void to ensure complete emptying of the bladder and allow uterine involution.

Musculoskeletal system

Physical changes of the musculoskeletal system involve a reversal of the musculoskeletal adaptations that occurred during pregnancy. By 6 to 8 weeks after birth:
- The joints return to their prepregnant state and are completely restabilized. The feet, however, can remain permanently increased in size.
- Muscle tone begins to be restored throughout the body with the removal of progesterone's effect following delivery of the placenta. The rectus abdominis muscles of the abdomen and the pubococcygeus muscle tone are restored following placental expulsion and return to the prepregnant state about 6 weeks postpartum.

ASSESSMENT

- Assess the musculoskeletal system for changes.
- Assess the abdominal wall for diastasis recti (separation of the rectus muscle) from 2 to 4 cm. It usually resolves within 6 weeks.

PATIENT-CENTERED CARE

- Teach the client postpartum strengthening exercises, advising her to start with simple exercises, and then gradually progressing to more strenuous ones.
- Instruct clients who have had a cesarean birth to postpone abdominal exercises until about 4 weeks after delivery, or follow recommendations of her provider.
- Advise the client on good body mechanics and proper posture.

Immune system

Review the status of the following.

Rubella: A client who has a titer of less than 1:8 is administered a subcutaneous injection of rubella vaccine or a measles, mumps, and rubella (MMR) vaccine during the postpartum period to protect a subsequent fetus from malformations. The client should not get pregnant for 1 month following the immunization. Qs

Hepatitis B: Newborns born to infected mothers should receive the hepatitis B vaccine and the hepatitis B immune globulin within 12 hr of birth.

Rh: All Rh-negative mothers who have newborns who are Rh-positive must be given Rho(D) immune globulin administered IM within 72 hr of the newborn being born to suppress antibody formation in the mother.
- Test the client who receives both the rubella vaccine and Rho(D) immune globulin after 3 months to determine whether immunity to rubella has been developed. QEBP

Varicella: If the client has no immunity, varicella vaccine is administered before discharge. The client should not get pregnant for 1 month following the immunization. A second dose of vaccine is given at 4 to 8 weeks.

Tetanus–diphtheria–acellular pertussis vaccine: The vaccine is recommended for women who have not previously received it. Administer prior to discharge or as soon as possible in the postpartum period.

Comfort level

ASSESSMENTS AND INTERVENTIONS
- Assess pain related to episiotomy, lacerations, incisions, afterpains, and sore nipples.
- Assess location, type, and quality of the pain to guide nursing interventions and client education.
- Administer pain medications as prescribed.

Application Exercises

1. A nurse is performing a fundal assessment for a client who is 2 days postpartum and observes the perineal pad for lochia. She notes the pad to be saturated approximately 12 cm with lochia that is bright red and contains small clots. Which of the following findings should the nurse document?

    A. Moderate lochia rubra

    B. Excessive blood loss

    C. Light lochia rubra

    D. Scant lochia serosa

2. During ambulation to the bathroom, a postpartum client experiences a gush of dark red blood that soon stops. On assessment, a nurse finds the uterus to be firm, midline, and at the level of the umbilicus. Which of the following findings should the nurse interpret this data as being?

    A. Evidence of a possible vaginal hematoma

    B. An indication of a cervical or perineal laceration

    C. A normal postural discharge of lochia

    D. Abnormally excessive lochia rubra flow

3. A nurse is completing postpartum discharge teaching to a client who had no immunity to varicella and was given varicella vaccine. Which of the following statements by the client indicates understanding of the teaching?

    A. "I will need to use contraception for 3 months before considering pregnancy."

    B. "I need a second vaccination at my postpartum visit."

    C. "I was given the vaccine because my baby is O-positive."

    D. "I will be tested in 3 months to see if I have developed immunity."

4. A nurse is assessing a postpartum client for fundal height, location, and consistency. The fundus is noted to be displaced laterally to the right, and there is uterine atony. The nurse should identify which of the following conditions as the cause of the uterine atony?

    A. Poor involution

    B. Urinary retention

    C. Hemorrhage

    D. Infection

5. A nurse is caring for a client who is 1 hr postpartum following a vaginal birth and experiencing uncontrollable shaking. The nurse should understand that the shaking is due to which of the following factors? (Select all that apply.)

    A. Change in body fluids

    B. Metabolic effort of labor

    C. Diaphoresis

    D. Decrease in body temperature

    E. Decrease in prolactin levels

PRACTICE Active Learning Scenario

A nurse on the postpartum unit is leading a discussion with a group of clients about perineal care after delivery. What education should the nurse include in the discussion? Use the ATI Active Learning Template: Basic Concept to complete this item.

UNDERLYING PRINCIPLES: Describe three concepts that are the basis for perineal hygiene.

NURSING INTERVENTIONS
- Describe four actions the client should take to prevent infection.
- Describe four actions the nurse can take to promote client comfort.

Application Exercises Key

1. A. **CORRECT:** The client has moderate lochia rubra containing small clots, which is an expected finding for the second day postpartum.

   B. Excessive blood loss is saturation of a perineal pad in 15 min or less or pooling of blood under the client's buttocks.

   C. Light lochia rubra is a perineal pad that is saturated less than 10 cm with lochia.

   D. Scant lochia serosa (less than 2.5 cm on perineal pad) is pinkish brown in color and serosanguineous in consistency. It occurs on day 4 to 12 following delivery.

   Ⓝ *NCLEX® Connection: Health Promotion and Maintenance, Ante/Intra/Postpartum and Newborn Care*

2. A. A client who has a vaginal hematoma is expected to report excessive pain or vaginal pressure.

   B. Excessive spurting of bright red blood from the vagina indicates a possible cervical or perineal laceration.

   C. **CORRECT:** Lochia typically trickles from the vaginal opening but flows more steadily during uterine contractions. Massaging the uterus or ambulation can result in a gush of lochia with the expression of clots and dark blood that has been pooled in the vagina, but it should soon decrease back to a trickle of bright red lochia in the early puerperium.

   D. Excessive blood loss consists of one pad saturated in 15 min or less or the pooling of blood under the buttocks, which is not affected by the client's postural changes.

   Ⓝ *NCLEX® Connection: Health Promotion and Maintenance, Ante/Intra/Postpartum and Newborn Care*

3. A. A client is instructed to not get pregnant for 1 month following administration of varicella vaccine.

   B. **CORRECT:** A second varicella immunization is needed at 4 to 8 weeks following delivery by clients who had no history of immunity.

   C. Rho(D) immune globulin is administered to a Rh-negative mother who has an Rh-positive newborn.

   D. A client requires testing for immunity at 3 months following administration of rubella vaccine and Rho(D) immune globulin.

   Ⓝ *NCLEX® Connection: Pharmacological and Parenteral Therapies, Medication Administration*

4. A. Poor involution is the result of uterine atony and does not cause it.

   B. **CORRECT:** Urinary retention can result in a distention of the bladder. A distended bladder can cause uterine atony and lateral displacement from the midline, usually to the right.

   C. Hemorrhage is the result of uterine atony and does not cause it.

   D. Infection does not cause uterine displacement or atony and would be characterized by foul-smelling vaginal discharge and elevated temperature.

   Ⓝ *NCLEX® Connection: Health Promotion and Maintenance, Ante/Intra/Postpartum and Newborn Care*

5. A. **CORRECT:** A shift in body fluids during the first 2 hr puerperium can cause a postpartum chill.

   B. **CORRECT:** The work of labor can cause a postpartum chill during the first 2 hr puerperium.

   C. Diaphoresis is the mechanism by which the excess fluid of pregnancy is removed from the body. It usually occurs within the first 2 to 3 days following delivery.

   D. An increase in body temperature is associated with a postpartum chill, but it is not the cause of it.

   E. Changes in prolactin levels affect ovulation and menses and are not the cause of a postpartum chill.

   Ⓝ *NCLEX® Connection: Health Promotion and Maintenance, Ante/Intra/Postpartum and Newborn Care*

PRACTICE Answer

Using the ATI Active Learning Template: Basic Concept

UNDERLYING PRINCIPLES
- Promote stool softening.
- Promote comfort.

NURSING INTERVENTIONS
- Prevent infection.
  - Wash hands thoroughly before and after voiding.
  - Use a squeeze bottle with warm water or antiseptic solution after each voiding.
  - Clean the perineal area from front to back.
  - Blot dry; do not wipe.
  - Use topical application of antiseptic cream or spray sparingly.
  - Change perineal pad from front to back after voiding and defecating.
- Promote comfort.
  - Apply ice packs to the perineum for 24 to 48 hr.
  - Encourage sitz baths at least twice a day.
  - Administer analgesics.
  - Administer PCA pump after cesarean birth.
  - Apply topical anesthetics to perineal area or witch hazel compresses to the rectal area.

Ⓝ *NCLEX® Connection: Health Promotion and Maintenance, Ante/Intra/Postpartum and Newborn Care*

UNIT 3   POSTPARTUM NURSING CARE
SECTION: ROUTINE POSTPARTUM CARE

CHAPTER 18 *Baby-Friendly Care*

Bonding and integration of an infant into the family structure should start during pregnancy, and continue into the fourth stage of labor and throughout hospitalization.

Assessment of bonding and integration of an infant into the family structure requires that a nurse understand the normal postpartum psychological changes the client undergoes in the attainment of the maternal role and the recognition of deviations. Baby-friendly care can be promoted by delaying nursing procedures during the first hour after birth and through the first attempt of the client to breastfeed to allow for immediate parent-infant contact.

A client's emotional and physical condition (unwanted pregnancy, adolescent pregnancy, history of depression, difficult pregnancy and birth) and the newborn's physical condition (prematurity, congenital anomalies) after birth can affect the family's bonding process. Culture, age, and socioeconomic level are factors that can influence the bonding process. Bonding can be delayed secondary to maternal or neonatal factors.

PSYCHOSOCIAL AND MATERNAL ADAPTATION

Psychosocial adaptation and maternal adjustment begin during pregnancy as the client goes through commitment, attachment, and preparation for the birth of the newborn.
- During the first 2 to 6 weeks after birth, the client goes through a period of acquaintance with her newborn, as well as physical restoration. During this time she also focuses on competently caring for her newborn.
- Finally, the act of achieving maternal identity is accomplished around 4 months following birth.
- These stages can overlap, and are variable based on maternal, infant, and the environmental factors.

PHASES OF MATERNAL ROLE ATTAINMENT

Dependent: taking-in phase
- First 24 to 48 hr
- Focus on meeting personal needs
- Rely on others for assistance
- Excited, talkative
- Need to review birth experience with others

Dependent-independent: taking-hold phase
- Begins on day 2 or 3
- Lasts 10 days to several weeks
- Focus on baby care and improving caregiving competency
- Want to take charge but need acceptance from others
- Want to learn and practice
- Dealing with physical and emotional discomforts, can experience "baby blues"

Interdependent: letting-go phase
- Focus on family as a unit
- Resumption of role (intimate partner, individual)

ASSESSMENT

Nursing assessments include noting the client's condition after birth, observing the maternal adaptation process, assessing maternal emotional readiness to care for the infant, and assessing how comfortable the client appears in providing infant care.
- Assess for behaviors that facilitate and indicate mother-infant bonding.
  - Considers the infant a family member
  - Holds the infant face-to-face (en face position), maintaining eye contact
  - Assigns meaning to the infant's behavior and views this positively
  - Identifies the infant's unique characteristics and relates them to those of other family members.
  - Names the infant, indicating bonding is occurring
  - Touches the infant and maintains close physical proximity and contact
  - Provides physical care for the infant, such as feeding and diapering
  - Responds to the infant's cries
  - Smiles at, talks to, and sings to the infant
- Assess for behaviors that impair and indicate a lack of mother-infant bonding.
  - Apathy when the infant cries
  - Disgust when the infant voids, stools, or spits up
  - Expresses disappointment in the infant
  - Turns away from the infant
  - Does not seek close physical proximity to the infant
  - Does not talk about the infant's unique features
  - Handles the infant roughly
  - Ignores the infant entirely
  - Does not include the infant in the family context
  - Perceives infant behavior as uncooperative
- Assess for manifestations of mood swings, conflict about maternal role, or personal insecurity.
  - Feelings of being "down"
  - Feelings of inadequacy
  - Feelings of anxiety related to ineffective breastfeeding
  - Emotional lability with frequent crying
  - Flat affect and being withdrawn
  - Feeling unable to care for the infant

NURSING CONSIDERATIONS

- Facilitate the bonding process by placing the infant skin-to-skin or in the en face position with the client immediately after birth.
- Promote rooming-in as a quiet and private environment that enhances the family bonding process.
- Promote early initiation of breastfeeding, and encourage the client to recognize infant readiness cues. Offer assistance as needed.
- Teaching the client about infant care facilitates bonding as the client's confidence improves.
- Encourage parents to bond with the infant through cuddling, bathing, feeding, diapering, and inspection.
- Provide frequent praise, support, and reassurance to the client as she moves toward independence in caring for her infant and adjusting to her maternal role.
- Encourage parents to express feelings, fears, and anxieties about caring for the infant.

PATERNAL ADAPTATION

Paternal adaptation takes place as the father develops a parent-infant bond.

- The father has skin-to-skin contact, holds the infant, and maintains eye-to-eye contact with the infant.
- The father observes the infant for features similar to his own to validate his claim of the infant.
- The father talks, sings, and reads to the infant.

TRANSITION

Paternal transition to fatherhood consists of a predictable three-stage process during the first few weeks of transition.

Expectations and intentions: The father desires to be deeply and emotionally connected with the infant.

Confronting reality: The father discovers that his expectations might not be met. Commonly expressed emotions include feeling sad, frustrated, and jealous. He embraces the need to be actively involved in parenting.

Creating the role of the involved father: The father decides to become actively involved in the care of the infant.

Reaping rewards: Rewards include infant smiles and a sense of completeness and meaning.

ASSESSMENT

Nursing assessment of paternal adaptation includes observing for the characteristics of father-infant bonding.

NURSING ACTIONS

- Provide education about infant care when the father is present, and encourage the father to take a hands-on approach.
- Assist the father in his transition to fatherhood by providing guidance and involving him as a full partner rather than just a helper.
- Encourage couples to verbalize concerns and expectations related to infant care.

SIBLING ADAPTATION

The addition of an infant into the family unit affects everyone in the family, including siblings who can experience a temporary separation from parents. Siblings become aware of changes in the parents' behavior because the infant requires much more of parents' time.

ASSESSMENT

Nursing assessment of sibling adaptation to the infant includes the following.

- Assess for positive responses from the sibling.
  - Interest and concern for the infant
  - Increased independence
- Assess for adverse responses from the sibling.
  - Signs of sibling rivalry and jealousy
  - Regression in toileting and sleep habits
  - Aggression toward the infant
  - Increased attention-seeking behaviors and whining

NURSING ACTIONS

- Take the sibling on a tour of the obstetric unit.
- Encourage the parents to do the following.
  - Let the sibling be one of the first to see the infant.
  - Provide a gift from the infant to give the sibling.
  - Arrange for one parent to spend time with the sibling while the other parent is caring for the infant.
  - Allow older siblings to help in providing care for the infant.
  - Provide preschool-aged siblings with a doll to care for.

COMPLICATIONS

Impaired parenting can include the following.

- Emotional detachment and inability to care for the infant, thus placing the infant at risk for neglect and failure to thrive.
- Failure to bond with the infant increases the risk of physical and/or emotional abuse.

NURSING ACTIONS

- Emphasize verbal and nonverbal communication skills between the client, caregivers, and the infant.
- Provide continued assessment of the client's parenting abilities, as well as any other caregivers for the infant.
- Encourage continued support of grandparents and other family members.
- Provide home visits and group sessions for discussion regarding infant care and parenting problems.
- Give the client and caregivers information about social networks that provide a support system where they can seek assistance.
- Involve outreach programs concerned with self-care, parent-child interactions, child injuries, and failure to thrive.
- Notify programs that provide prompt and effective community interventions to prevent more serious problems from occurring.

Application Exercises

1. A nurse concludes that the father of an infant is not showing positive signs of parent-infant bonding. He appears very anxious and nervous when the infant's mother asks him to bring her the infant. Which of the following actions should the nurse use to promote father-infant bonding?

   A. Hand the father the infant, and suggest that he change the diaper.

   B. Ask the father why he is so anxious and nervous.

   C. Tell the father that he will grow accustomed to the infant.

   D. Provide education about infant care when the father is present.

2. A client in the early postpartum period is very excited and talkative. She is repeatedly telling the nurse every detail of her labor and birth. Because the client will not stop talking, the nurse is having difficulty completing the postpartum assessments. Which of the following action should the nurse take?

   A. Come back later when the client is more cooperative.

   B. Give the client time to express her feelings.

   C. Tell the client she needs to be quiet so the assessment can be completed.

   D. Redirect the client's focus so that she will become quiet.

3. A nurse is caring for a client who is 1 day postpartum. The nurse is assessing for maternal adaptation and mother-infant bonding. Which of the following behaviors by the client indicates a need for the nurse to intervene? (Select all that apply.)

   A. Demonstrates apathy when the infant cries

   B. Touches the infant and maintains close physical proximity

   C. Views the infant's behavior as uncooperative during diaper changing

   D. Identifies and relates infant's characteristics to those of family members

   E. Interprets the infant's behavior as meaningful and a way of expressing needs

4. A nurse is caring for a client who is 2 days postpartum. The client states, "My 4-year old son was toilet trained and now he is frequently wetting himself." Which of the following statements should the nurse provide to the client?

   A. "Your son was probably not ready for toilet training and should wear training pants."

   B. "Your son is showing an adverse sibling response."

   C. "Your son may need counseling."

   D. "You should try sending your son to preschool to resolve the behavior."

5. A nurse in the delivery room is planning to promote maternal-infant bonding for a client who just delivered. Which of the following is the priority action by the nurse?

   A. Encourage the parents to touch and explore the neonate's features.

   B. Limit noise and interruption in the delivery room.

   C. Place the neonate at the client's breast.

   D. Position the neonate skin-to-skin on the client's chest.

PRACTICE Active Learning Scenario

A nurse is leading a parenting class on paternal adaptation for expectant women and their partners. What concepts on paternal adaptation should the nurse include in the presentation? Use ATI Active Learning Template: Basic Concept to complete this item.

RELATED CONTENT: Describe three ways the father develops a parent-infant bond.

UNDERLYING PRINCIPLES
• Describe three stages of paternal transition to parenthood.
• Describe three stages of the development of the father-infant bond.

NURSING INTERVENTIONS: Describe three actions to assist in the father-infant bonding process.

Application Exercises Key

1. A. It is not helpful to push the father into infant care activities without first providing education.

   B. This is a nontherapeutic statement and presumes the nurse knows what the father is feeling.

   C. This is a nontherapeutic statement and offers the nurse's opinion.

   D. **CORRECT:** Nursing interventions to promote paternal bonding include providing education about infant care and encouraging the father to take a hands-on approach.

   Ⓝ *NCLEX® Connection: Psychosocial Integrity, Family Dynamics*

2. A. The nurse should continue her activities while encouraging the client to talk.

   B. **CORRECT:** The nurse should recognize that the client in is the taking-in phase, which begins immediately following birth and lasts a few hours to a couple of days.

   C. It is not necessary for the client to stop talking while the nurse completes the needed assessments.

   D. The client is in the taking-in phase, which includes talking about the birth experience. The client should be encouraged.

   Ⓝ *NCLEX® Connection: Psychosocial Integrity, Therapeutic Communication*

3. A. **CORRECT:** This behavior demonstrates a lack of interest in the infant and impaired maternal-infant bonding.

   B. Touching the infant and maintaining close proximity are signs of effective maternal-infant bonding.

   C. **CORRECT:** A client's view of her infant as being uncooperative during diaper changing is a sign of impaired maternal-infant bonding.

   D. Endowing the infant with family characteristics indicates effective maternal-infant bonding.

   E. Recognizing the infant's behavior as meaningful and a way to express needs is an indication of effective maternal-infant bonding.

   Ⓝ *NCLEX® Connection: Psychosocial Integrity, Family Dynamics*

4. A. This is not an appropriate intervention by the nurse because it overlooks the child's emotional response to a new family member.

   B. **CORRECT:** Adverse responses by a sibling to a new infant can include regression in toileting habits.

   C. Recommending that the child receive counseling is not an appropriate nursing intervention for a child who is demonstrating an adverse sibling response.

   D. Recommending that the child be sent to preschool is not an appropriate nursing intervention for a child who is demonstrating an adverse sibling response.

   Ⓝ *NCLEX® Connection: Psychosocial Integrity, Therapeutic Communication*

5. A. This is an appropriate action, but another intervention is the priority.

   B. This is an appropriate action, but another intervention is the priority.

   C. This is an appropriate action, but another intervention is the priority.

   D. **CORRECT:** Placing the neonate in the en face position on the client's chest immediately after birth is the priority nursing intervention to promote maternal-infant bonding.

   Ⓝ *NCLEX® Connection: Psychosocial Integrity, Family Dynamics*

PRACTICE Answer

Using the ATI Active Learning Template: Basic Concept

RELATED CONTENT
- Development of parent-infant bond
- Touching, holding, skin-to-skin contact, and maintaining eye-to-eye contact
- Recognizing personal features in the infant, and validating his claim to the infant
- Talking, reading, singing, and verbally interacting with the infant

UNDERLYING PRINCIPLES

Stages of paternal transition to parenthood
- Expectations: Having preconceived ideas about fatherhood
- Reality: Recognizing expectations might not be met, facing these feelings, and then embracing the need to become actively involved in parenting
- Transition to mastery: Taking an active role in parenting

Development of the father-infant bond
- Making a commitment and assuming responsibility for parenting
- Becoming connected and having feelings of attachment to the infant
- Modifying lifestyle to make room to care for the infant

NURSING INTERVENTIONS
- Provide education about infant care when the father is present.
- Encourage the father to take a hands-on role in care when present.
- Provide guidance.
- Involve the father as a full partner, not a helper, in the parenting process.
- Encourage the couple to verbalize concerns and expectations about infant care.

Ⓝ *NCLEX® Connection: Psychosocial Integrity, Family Dynamics*

CHAPTER 19 *Client Education and Discharge Teaching*

Discharge teaching is an important aspect of postpartum care. It is important for a client to be able to perform self-care and recognize effects that suggest possible complications prior to discharge.

Discharge planning should be initiated at admission with time spent during the hospitalization on providing client education regarding postpartum self-care.

A nurse should use a variety of teaching strategies to promote learning. Return demonstrations are important to ensure that adequate learning has taken place.

ASSESSING A CLIENT'S KNOWLEDGE OF POSTPARTUM CARE

- Inquire about the client's current knowledge regarding self-care.
- Assess the client's home support system and who will be there to assist. Include support persons in the educational process.
- Determine the client's readiness for learning and her ability to verbalize or demonstrate the information she has been given.

NURSING INTERVENTIONS FOR POSTPARTUM CARE

SELF-CARE

Provide client teaching on self-care.

Perineal care

- Cleanse the perineal area from front to back with warm water after each voiding and bowel movement.
- Blot perineal area from front to back.
- Remove and apply perineal pads from front to back.

Breast care

CLIENTS WHO ARE LACTATING

- Place the newborn skin-to-skin as soon as possible following birth and initiate breastfeeding within the first 1 to 2 hr after birth unless contraindicated.
- Wear a well-fitting, supportive bra continuously for the duration of lactation.
- Emphasize the importance of hand hygiene prior to breastfeeding to prevent infection.
- To relieve breast engorgement, have the client completely empty her breasts at each feeding. Allow the infant to nurse on demand, which would be about 8 to 12 times in 24-hr period. Massaging the breasts during feeding can help with emptying. Allow the infant to feed until the breast softens. If the second breast does not soften after the infant's feeding, the breast can be emptied with a breast pump. Alternate breasts with each feeding.
- For breast engorgement, apply cool compresses after feedings and apply warm compresses, or take a warm shower prior to breastfeeding. These actions will increase milk flow and promote the letdown reflex.
- For flat or inverted nipples, suggest that the client roll the nipples between her fingers just before breastfeeding to help them become more erect and make it easier for the infant to latch on. Use a breast shield between feedings.
- For sore nipples, the client should apply a small amount of breast milk to her nipple and allow it to air dry after breastfeeding.
- Have the client apply breast creams as prescribed and wear breast shields in her bra to soften her nipples if they are irritated and cracked.
- Promote adequate fluid intake to replace fluid lost from breastfeeding as well as to provide an adequate amount of milk for the infant.

NONLACTATING CLIENTS

- Wear a well-fitting, supportive bra continuously for the first 72 hr.
- Suppression of lactation is necessary for clients who are not breastfeeding. Avoid breast stimulation and running warm water over the breasts for prolonged periods until no longer lactating.
- For breast engorgement, which can occur on the third or fifth postpartum day, apply cold compresses 15 min on and 45 min off. Fresh, cold cabbage leaves can be placed inside the bra. Mild analgesics or anti-inflammatory medication can be taken for pain and discomfort of breast engorgement.

Rest/sleep

Plan at least one daily rest period; rest when the infant naps.

Activity

- Do not perform housework requiring heavy lifting for at least 3 weeks. Do not lift anything heavier than the infant.
- Avoid sitting for prolonged periods of time with legs crossed (to prevent thrombophlebitis).
- Limit stair climbing for the first few weeks postpartum.
- Clients who have had a cesarean birth should wait until the 4- to 6-week follow-up visit before performing strenuous exercise, heavy lifting, or excessive stair climbing.
- Instruct not to drive for the first 2 weeks postpartum, or while taking opioids for pain control.

Nutrition

- Teach the importance of eating a nutritious diet including all food groups. Encourage a diet high in protein, which will aid in tissue repair. The client should also consume 2 to 3 L of fluid each day from food and beverage sources.
- Encourage nonlactating clients to consume 1,800 to 2,200 kcal/day.
- Instruct the lactating client to increase her caloric intake and to include calcium-enriched foods in her diet.
  - The Institute of Medicine recommends an increase of 330 calories/day for the first 6 months of lactation.
  - The American Academy of Pediatrics recommends that clients who are lactating add an additional 450 to 500 calories/day to their prepregnancy diet.

Postpartum exercises

- Regain pelvic floor muscle control by performing Kegel exercises. The same muscles are used when starting and stopping the flow of urine. Have the client relax and contract the pelvic floor muscles 10 times 8 times a day.
- Teach how to perform pelvic tilt exercises to strengthen back muscles and relieve strain on the lower back. These exercises involve alternately arching and straightening the back.

Sexual intercourse

- Avoid sexual intercourse until the episiotomy/laceration is healed and vaginal discharge has turned white (lochia alba). This usually takes 2 to 4 weeks or until the client is seen by the provider. Over-the-counter lubricants might be needed during the first 6 weeks to 6 months.
- Physiological reactions to sexual activity can be slower and less intense for the first 3 months following birth.

Contraception

- Discuss the use of contraception upon resumption of sexual activity and inform the client that pregnancy can occur while breastfeeding even though menses has not returned.
- Clients who are lactating should be advised that oral contraceptives should not be taken until milk production is well established (usually 4 weeks).
- Menses for nonlactating clients might not resume until around 4 to 10 weeks. However, ovulation can occur as early as 1 month after delivery.
- Menses for lactating clients might not resume for 3 months or until cessation of breastfeeding.

INDICATIONS OF POTENTIAL COMPLICATIONS

- Provide client education on indications of potential complications to report to the provider.
  - **Chills or fever** greater than 38° C (100.4° F) for 2 or more days.
  - **Change in vaginal discharge** with increased amount, large clots, change to a previous lochia color, such as bright red bleeding, and a foul odor. Qs
    - NORMAL LOCHIAL FLOW PATTERNS
      - Rubra: Dark red vaginal drainage for 1 to 3 days.
      - Serosa: Brownish red or pink vaginal drainage from days 3 to 10.
      - Alba: Yellowish white vaginal discharge after day 10 to 6 weeks.
  - **Episiotomy, laceration, or incisional pain**, that does not resolve with analgesics, foul-smelling drainage, redness, and/or edema.
  - **Pain or tenderness in the abdominal or pelvic areas** that does not resolve with analgesics.
  - **Breast(s) with localized areas of pain and tenderness** with firmness, heat, and swelling, and/or nipples with cracks, redness, bruising, blisters, or fissures.
  - **Calves with localized pain, tenderness, redness, and swelling**. A lower extremity with either areas of redness and warmth or coolness and paleness.
  - **Urination with burning, pain, frequency, urgency**; urine that is cloudy or has blood.
- **Postpartum depression** is when the client feels apathy toward the infant, cannot provide self- or infant-care, or has feelings that she might hurt herself or her infant.
- The client should be discharged with an appointment set for a postpartum follow-up visit or a number to call and schedule an appointment. Following a vaginal delivery, the follow-up visit should take place in 4 to 6 weeks; following a cesarean birth, the visit should take place in 2 weeks.
- Date and time of the follow-up appointment should be written and discussed in the discharge instructions.

Application Exercises

1. A nurse is conducting a home visit for a client who is 1 week postpartum and breastfeeding. The client reports breast engorgement. Which of the following recommendations should the nurse make?

   A. "Apply cold compresses between feedings."

   B. "Take a warm shower right after feedings."

   C. "Apply breast milk to the nipples and allow them to air dry."

   D. "Use the various infant positions for feedings."

2. A nurse is providing discharge instructions for a client. At 4 weeks postpartum, the client should contact her provider for which of the following client findings?

   A. Scant, nonodorous white vaginal discharge

   B. Uterine cramping during breastfeeding

   C. Sore nipple with cracks and fissures

   D. Decreased response with sexual activity

3. A nurse is providing discharge teaching for a nonlactating client. Which of the following instructions should the nurse include in the teaching?

   A. "Wear a supportive bra continuously for the first 72 hours."

   B. "Pump your breast every 4 hours to relieve discomfort."

   C. "Use breast shells throughout the day to decrease milk supply."

   D. "Apply warm compresses until milk suppression occurs."

4. A nurse is providing discharge instructions to a postpartum client following a cesarean birth. The client reports leaking urine every time she sneezes or coughs. Which of the following interventions should the nurse suggest?

   A. Sit-ups

   B. Pelvic tilt exercises

   C. Kegel exercises

   D. Abdominal crunches

5. A nurse is providing care to four clients on the postpartum unit. Which of the following clients is at greatest risk for developing a postpartum infection?

   A. A client who has an episiotomy that is erythematous and has extended into a third-degree laceration

   B. A client who does not wash her hands between perineal care and breastfeeding

   C. A client who is not breastfeeding and is using measures to suppress lactation

   D. A client who has a cesarean incision that is well-approximated with no drainage

---

PRACTICE Active Learning Scenario

A nurse is reviewing discharge teaching with a client who is not breastfeeding. What information should the nurse include in the teaching? Use the ATI Active Learning Template: Basic Concept to complete this item.

UNDERLYING PRINCIPLES

- Nutrition: Describe the nutrition and fluid plan the client should use.
- Resumption of sexual intercourse: Describe appropriate actions by the client.
- Indications of complications to report to the provider: List two that the client should report.

Application Exercises Key

1. A. **CORRECT:** Cold compresses applied to the breasts after the feedings can help with breast engorgement.

   B. Taking a warm shower prior to feedings, not immediately after, can assist with the letdown reflex and milk flow.

   C. Applying breast milk to the nipples and air drying is recommended for the client who has sore nipples, but it has no effect on breast engorgement.

   D. Using the various positions for feedings helps to prevent nipple soreness but has no effect on breast engorgement.

   Ⓝ *NCLEX® Connection: Health Promotion and Maintenance, Ante/Intra/Postpartum and Newborn Care*

2. A. Lochia alba, a white vaginal discharge, is normal from the 11th day postpartum to approximately 6 weeks following birth.

   B. Oxytocin, which is released with breastfeeding, causes the uterus to contract and can cause discomfort.

   C. **CORRECT:** A sore nipple that has cracks and fissures is an indication of mastitis.

   D. Physiological reactions to sexual activity can be slower and less intense for the first 3 months following birth.

   Ⓝ *NCLEX® Connection: Health Promotion and Maintenance, Ante/Intra/Postpartum and Newborn Care*

3. A. **CORRECT:** The nurse should instruct the client to wear a well-fitting support bra continuously for the first 72 hr.

   B. The nurse should not recommend using a breast pump for the nonlactating client.

   C. The nurse should recommend using a breast shell for clients who have flat or inverted nipples.

   D. The nurse should instruct the nonlactating client to avoid application of warm compresses. Cold compresses can be applied to relieve discomfort.

   Ⓝ *NCLEX® Connection: Health Promotion and Maintenance, Ante/Intra/Postpartum and Newborn Care*

4. A. Sit-ups should not be performed until after the postpartum follow-up appointment.

   B. Pelvic tilt exercises consist of the alternate arching and straightening of the back to strengthen the back muscles and relieve back discomfort.

   C. **CORRECT:** Kegel exercises consist of the voluntary contraction and relaxation of the pubococcygeus muscle to strengthen the pelvic muscles, which will assist the client in decreasing urinary stress incontinence that occurs with sneezing and coughing.

   D. Abdominal crunches should not be performed until after the postpartum follow-up appointment.

   Ⓝ *NCLEX® Connection: Health Promotion and Maintenance, Ante/Intra/Postpartum and Newborn Care*

5. A. An episiotomy with a laceration is at risk for an infection, but there is a client who is at greater risk for a postpartum infection.

   B. **CORRECT:** The client who does not wash her hands between perineal care and breastfeeding is at an increased risk for developing mastitis. Therefore, she is most at risk for developing a postpartum infection.

   C. A client who is suppressing lactation (increases the risk of milk stasis) is at risk for an infection, but there is a client who is at greater risk for a postpartum infection.

   D. A client who has an abdominal incision is at risk for an infection, but there is a client who is at greater risk for a postpartum infection.

   Ⓝ *NCLEX® Connection: Physiological Adaptation, Illness Management*

PRACTICE Answer

Using the ATI Active Learning Template: Basic Concept

UNDERLYING PRINCIPLES

Nutrition
- Eat a diet that includes all food groups and higher protein content.
- Consume 2 to 3 L of fluid daily from food and beverage sources.
- Encourage an intake of 1,800 to 2,200 kcal/day.

Sexual intercourse
- Avoid sexual intercourse until episiotomy/laceration is healed and vaginal discharge is lochia alba (2 to 4 weeks).
- Over-the-counter lubricants might be needed.
- Physiological reactions to sexual activity can be slower and less intense.

Indications of complications
- Chills or fever greater than 38° C (100.4° F) for 2 or more days.
- Change in vaginal discharge with increased amount, large clots, change to previous lochia color, foul odor.
- Episiotomy, laceration, or incisional pain that does not resolve with analgesics; foul-smelling drainage; redness; and/or edema.
- Pain or tenderness in the abdominal or pelvic area that does not resolve with analgesics.

- Breasts with localized areas of pain and tenderness with firmness, heat, and swelling and/or nipples with cracks or fissures.
- Calves with localized pain and tenderness, redness, and swelling. Lower extremity with either areas of redness and warmth, or coolness and paleness.
- Urination with burning, pain, frequency, urgency; urine that is cloudy or bloody.

Ⓝ *NCLEX® Connection: Health Promotion and Maintenance, Ante/Intra/Postpartum and Newborn Care*

CHAPTER 20 *Postpartum Disorders*

Postpartum disorders are unexpected events or occurrences that can happen during the postpartum period. It is imperative for a nurse to have a thorough understanding of each disorder and initiate appropriate nursing interventions to achieve positive outcomes.

Postpartum disorders reviewed in this chapter include superficial and deep-vein thrombosis, pulmonary embolus, coagulopathies (idiopathic thrombocytopenic purpura and disseminated intravascular coagulation), postpartum hemorrhage, uterine atony, subinvolution of the uterus, inversion of the uterus, retained placenta, lacerations, and hematomas.

Deep-vein thrombosis

- Thrombophlebitis refers to a thrombus that is associated with inflammation.
- Thrombophlebitis of the lower extremities can be of superficial or deep veins, which are most often of the femoral, saphenous, or popliteal veins. The postpartum client is at greatest risk for a deep-vein thrombosis (DVT) that can lead to a pulmonary embolism.

ASSESSMENT

RISK FACTORS

- Pregnancy
- Cesarean birth (doubles the risk)
- Operative vaginal birth
- Pulmonary embolism or varicosities
- Immobility
- Obesity
- Smoking
- Multiparity
- Age greater than 35 years
- History of thromboembolism
- Diabetes mellitus

EXPECTED FINDINGS

Leg pain and tenderness

PHYSICAL ASSESSMENT FINDINGS

- Unilateral area of swelling, warmth, and redness
- Hardened vein over the thrombosis
- Calf tenderness

DIAGNOSTIC PROCEDURES

NONINVASIVE

- Doppler ultrasound scanning
- Computed tomography
- Magnetic resonance imaging

PATIENT-CENTERED CARE

NURSING CARE

PREVENTION OF THROMBOPHLEBITIS
Provide the client with education and encouragement pertaining to measures for prevention of DVT.
- Maintain sequential compression device until ambulation established.
- If bed rest is prolonged longer than 8 hr, perform active and passive range of motion to promote circulation in the legs if warranted.
- Initiate early and frequent ambulation postpartum.
- Avoid prolonged periods of standing, sitting, or immobility.
- Have the client elevate her legs when sitting.
- Tell the client to avoid crossing her legs, which will reduce the circulation and exacerbate venous stasis.
- Maintain fluid intake of 2 to 3 L each day from food and beverage sources to prevent dehydration, which causes circulation to be sluggish.
- Tell the client to discontinue smoking.
- Measure the lower extremities for fitted elastic thromboembolic hose to lower extremities.

MANAGEMENT OF THROMBOPHLEBITIS
- Encourage rest.
- Facilitate bed rest and elevation of the client's extremity above the level of her heart. (Avoid using a knee gatch or pillow under knees.)
- Administer intermittent or continuous warm moist compresses.
- Do **NOT** massage the affected limb to prevent thrombus from dislodging and becoming an embolus.
- Measure the client's leg circumferences.
- Provide thigh-high antiembolism stockings for the client at high risk for venous insufficiency.
- Administer analgesics (nonsteroidal anti-inflammatory agents).
- Administer anticoagulants for DVT.

MEDICATIONS

Heparin

CLASSIFICATION: Anticoagulant

THERAPEUTIC INTENT: Given IV to prevent formation of other clots and to prevent enlargement of the existing clot.

NURSING CONSIDERATIONS
- Initially, IV heparin is administered by continuous infusion for 3 to 5 days with doses adjusted according to coagulation studies. Protamine sulfate, the heparin antidote, should be readily available to counteract the development of heparin-induced antiplatelet antibodies.
- Monitor aPTT (1.5 to 2.5 times the control level of 30 to 40 seconds).

CLIENT EDUCATION: Instruct the client to report bleeding from the gums or nose, increased vaginal bleeding, blood in the urine, and frequent bruising.

Warfarin

CLASSIFICATION: Anticoagulant

THERAPEUTIC INTENT: Used for treatment of clots. It is administered orally and is continued by the client for approximately 3 months.

NURSING CONSIDERATIONS
- Phytonadione, the warfarin antidote, should be readily available for prolonged clotting times.
- Monitor PT (1.5 to 2.5 times the control level of 11 to 12.5 seconds) and INR of 2 to 3.

CLIENT EDUCATION
- Instruct the client to watch for bleeding from the gums or nose, increased vaginal bleeding, blood in the urine, and frequent bruising. Qs
- Instruct the client to use birth control to avoid pregnancy due to the teratogenic effects of warfarin. Oral contraceptives are contraindicated because of the increased risk for thrombosis.

CLIENT EDUCATION

PRECAUTIONS WHILE RECEIVING ANTICOAGULANTS QEBP
- Instruct the client to avoid taking aspirin or ibuprofen (increases bleeding tendencies).
- Instruct the client to use an electric razor for shaving.
- Instruct the client to avoid alcohol use (inhibits warfarin).
- Instruct the client to brush teeth gently using a soft toothbrush.
- Instruct the client to avoid rubbing or massaging legs.
- Instruct the client to avoid periods of prolonged sitting or crossing legs.

Pulmonary embolus

- An embolus occurs when fragments or an entire clot dislodges and moves into circulation.
- A pulmonary embolism is a complication of DVT that occurs if the embolus moves into the pulmonary artery or one of its branches and lodges in a lung, occluding the vessel and obstructing blood flow to the lungs.
- Acute pulmonary embolus is an emergent situation.

ASSESSMENT

RISK FACTORS

Risk factors are the same as those for DVT.

EXPECTED FINDINGS

- Apprehension
- Pleuritic chest pain
- Dyspnea
- Tachypnea
- Hemoptysis
- Heart murmurs
- Peripheral edema
- Distended neck veins
- Elevated temperature
- Hypotension
- Hypoxia

DIAGNOSTIC AND THERAPEUTIC PROCEDURES

- Ventilation/perfusion lung scan
- Chest radiographic study
- Radioisotope lung scan
- Pulmonary angiogram
- Embolectomy to surgically remove the embolus

PATIENT-CENTERED CARE

NURSING CARE

- Place the client in a semi-Fowler's position with the head of the bed elevated to facilitate breathing.
- Administer oxygen by mask.

MEDICATIONS

- Medications prescribed include the medications listed under DVT.
- Thrombolytic therapy to break up blood clots may be prescribed.
  - **Alteplase**, **streptokinase**: Similar side effects and contraindications as anticoagulants.

Coagulopathies

- **Idiopathic thrombocytopenic purpura (ITP)** is a coagulopathy that is an autoimmune disorder in which the life span of platelets is decreased by antiplatelet antibodies. This can result in severe hemorrhage following a cesarean birth or lacerations.
- **Disseminated intravascular coagulation (DIC)** is a coagulopathy in which clotting and anticlotting mechanisms occur at the same time. The client is at risk for both internal and external bleeding, as well as damage to organs resulting from ischemia caused by microclots.
- Coagulopathies are suspected when the usual measures to stimulate uterine contractions fail to stop vaginal bleeding.

ASSESSMENT

RISK FACTORS

ITP: genetic in origin

DIC: can occur secondary to other complications to include the following
- Abruptio placentae, most common cause
- Amniotic fluid embolism
- Missed abortion
- Fetal death in utero (fetus has died but is retained in the uterus for at least 6 weeks)
- Severe preeclampsia or eclampsia (gestational hypertension), HELLP syndrome
- Septicemia
- Cardiopulmonary arrest
- Hemorrhage
- Hydatidiform mole

EXPECTED FINDINGS

PHYSICAL ASSESSMENT FINDINGS
- Unusual spontaneous bleeding from the gums and nose (epistaxis)
- Oozing, trickling, or flow of blood from incision, lacerations, or episiotomy
- Petechiae and ecchymoses
- Excessive bleeding from venipuncture, injection sites, or slight traumas
- Hematuria
- Gastrointestinal bleeding
- Tachycardia, hypotension, and diaphoresis
- Oliguria

LABORATORY TESTS

- CBC with differential
- Blood typing and crossmatch

CLOTTING FACTORS
- Platelet levels (thrombocytopenia): decreased
- Fibrinogen levels: decreased
- PT: prolonged
- Fibrin split product levels: increased
- D-dimer test (specific fibrin degradation fragment): increased

PATIENT-CENTERED CARE

NURSING CARE

- Assess skin, venipuncture, injection sites, lacerations, and episiotomy for bleeding.
- Monitor vital signs and hemodynamic status.
- Monitor urinary output, usually by insertion of an indwelling urinary catheter.
- Transfuse platelets.
- Assist in preparing the client for a splenectomy if ITP does not respond to medical management and provide postsurgical care.

DIC: Focus is on assessing for and correcting the underlying cause (removal of dead fetus or placental abruption, treatment of infection, preeclampsia, or eclampsia).
- Administer fluid volume replacement, which can include blood and blood products.
- Administer pharmacological interventions, including antibiotics, vasoactive medications, and uterotonic agents.
- Administer supplemental oxygen.
- Provide protection from injury.

THERAPEUTIC PROCEDURES

- Correction of the underlying cause
- Volume expansion, blood products, and clotting factors
- Optimize oxygen
- Splenectomy: may be performed by the provider if ITP does not respond to medical management
- Surgical intervention (hysterectomy) for DIC: performed by the provider as indicated

Postpartum hemorrhage

Postpartum hemorrhage is considered to occur if the client loses more than 500 mL blood after a vaginal birth or more than 1,000 mL blood after a cesarean birth. Two complications that can occur following postpartum hemorrhage include hypovolemic shock and anemia.

ASSESSMENT

RISK FACTORS

- Uterine atony
- Overdistended uterus
- Previous history of uterine atony
- Prolonged labor, oxytocin-induced labor
- High parity
- Ruptured uterus
- Complications during pregnancy (e.g., placenta previa, abruptio placentae)
- Precipitous delivery
- Administration of magnesium sulfate therapy during labor
- Lacerations and hematomas
- Inversion of uterus
- Subinvolution of the uterus
- Retained placental fragments
- Coagulopathies (DIC)

EXPECTED FINDINGS

Increase or change in lochial pattern (return to previous stage, large clots)

PHYSICAL ASSESSMENT FINDINGS
- Uterine atony (hypotonic or boggy)
- Blood clots larger than a quarter
- Perineal pad saturation in 15 min or less
- Constant oozing, trickling, or frank flow of bright red blood from the vagina
- Tachycardia and hypotension
- Skin pale, cool, and clammy with loss of turgor and pale mucous membranes
- Oliguria

LABORATORY TESTS

- Hgb and Hct
- Coagulation profile (PT)
- Blood type and crossmatch

PATIENT-CENTERED CARE

NURSING CARE

- Firmly massage the uterine fundus.
- Monitor vital signs.
- Assess for source of bleeding.
  - Assess fundus for height, firmness, and position. If uterus is boggy, massage fundus to increase muscle contraction.
  - Assess lochia for color, quantity, and clots.
  - Assess for clinical findings of bleeding from lacerations, episiotomy site, or hematomas.
- Assess bladder for distention. Insert an indwelling urinary catheter to assess kidney function and obtain an accurate measurement of urinary output.
- Maintain or initiate IV fluids to replace fluid volume loss with IV isotonic solutions, such as lactated Ringer's or 0.9% sodium chloride; colloid volume expanders, such as albumin; and blood products (packed RBCs and fresh frozen plasma).
- Provide oxygen at 2 to 3 L/min per nasal cannula, and monitor oxygen saturation.
- Elevate the client's legs to a 20° to 30° angle to increase venous return.

MEDICATIONS

Oxytocin

CLASSIFICATION: Uterine stimulant

THERAPEUTIC INTENT: Promotes uterine contractions

NURSING CONSIDERATIONS
- Assess uterine tone and vaginal bleeding.
- Monitor for adverse reactions of water intoxication, such as lightheadedness, nausea, vomiting, headache, and malaise. These reactions can progress to cerebral edema with seizures, coma, and death.

Methylergonovine

CLASSIFICATION: Uterine stimulant

THERAPEUTIC INTENT: Controls postpartum hemorrhage

NURSING CONSIDERATIONS
- Assess uterine tone and vaginal bleeding. Do not administer to clients who have hypertension.
- Monitor for adverse reactions, including hypertension, nausea, vomiting, and headache.

Misoprostol

CLASSIFICATION: Uterine stimulant

THERAPEUTIC INTENT: Controls postpartum hemorrhage.

NURSING CONSIDERATIONS: Assess uterine tone and vaginal bleeding.

Carboprost tromethamine

CLASSIFICATION: Uterine stimulant

THERAPEUTIC INTENT: Controls postpartum hemorrhage

NURSING CONSIDERATIONS
- Assess uterine tone and vaginal bleeding.
- Monitor for adverse reactions, including fever, chills, headache, nausea, vomiting, and diarrhea.

CLIENT EDUCATION

Instruct the client to limit physical activity to conserve strength, to increase iron and protein intake to promote the rebuilding of RBC volume, and to take iron with vitamin C to enhance absorption.

Uterine atony

Uterine atony results from the inability of the uterine muscle to contract adequately after birth. This can lead to postpartum hemorrhage.

ASSESSMENT

RISK FACTORS

- Retained placental fragments
- Prolonged labor
- Oxytocin induction or augmentation of labor
- Overdistention of the uterine muscle (multiparity, multiple gestations, polyhydramnios [hydramnios], macrosomic fetus)
- Precipitous labor
- Magnesium sulfate administration as a tocolytic
- Anesthesia and analgesia administration
- Trauma during labor and birth from operative delivery (forceps- or vacuum-assisted birth, cesarean birth)

EXPECTED FINDINGS

Increased vaginal bleeding

PHYSICAL ASSESSMENT FINDINGS
- Uterus that is larger than normal and boggy with possible lateral displacement on palpation
- Prolonged lochial discharge
- Irregular or excessive bleeding
- Tachycardia and hypotension
- Skin that is pale, cool, and clammy with loss of turgor and pale mucous membranes

DIAGNOSTIC PROCEDURES

- Bimanual compression or manual exploration of the uterine cavity for retained placental fragments by the provider
- Surgical management, such as a hysterectomy

PATIENT-CENTERED CARE

NURSING CARE

- Ensure that the urinary bladder is empty.
- Monitor the following.
  - Fundal height, consistency, and location
  - Lochia for quantity, color, and consistency
- Perform fundal massage if indicated.
  - If the uterus becomes firm, continue assessing hemodynamic status.
  - If uterine atony persists, anticipate surgical intervention, such as a hysterectomy.
- Express clots that can have accumulated in the uterus, but only after the uterus is firmly contracted. It is critical not to express clots prior to the uterus becoming firmly contracted because pushing on an uncontracted uterus can invert the uterus and result in extensive hemorrhage. Qᴇʙᴘ
- Monitor vital signs.
- Maintain or initiate IV fluids.
- Provide oxygen at 2 to 3 L/min per nasal cannula.

MEDICATIONS

As noted for postpartum hemorrhage

CLIENT EDUCATION

Instruct the client to limit physical activity to conserve strength and to increase iron and protein intake to promote the rebuilding of RBC volume.

Subinvolution of the uterus

Subinvolution is when the uterus remains enlarged with continued lochial discharge and can result in postpartum hemorrhage.

ASSESSMENT

RISK FACTORS

- Pelvic infection and endometritis
- Retained placental fragments not completely expelled from the uterus

EXPECTED FINDINGS

- Prolonged vaginal bleeding
- Irregular or excessive vaginal bleeding

PHYSICAL ASSESSMENT FINDINGS
- Uterus that is enlarged and higher than normal in the abdomen relative to the umbilicus
- Boggy uterus
- Prolonged lochia discharge with irregular or excessive bleeding

LABORATORY TESTS

Blood, intracervical, and intrauterine bacterial cultures to check for evidence of infection and endometritis

DIAGNOSTIC PROCEDURES

Dilation and curettage (D&C) is performed by the provider to remove retained placental fragments if indicated.

PATIENT-CENTERED CARE

NURSING CARE

- Monitor fundal position and consistency.
- Monitor lochia for color, amount, consistency, and odor.
- Monitor vital signs.
- Encourage the client to use activities that can enhance uterine involution.
  - Breastfeeding
  - Early and frequent ambulation
  - Frequent voiding
- D&C can be necessary to remove retained placental fragments.

MEDICATIONS

Oxytocin, methylergonovine

CLASSIFICATION: Uterine stimulant

THERAPEUTIC INTENT: To promote uterine contractions and expel the retained fragments of placenta.

NURSING CONSIDERATIONS
- Assess uterine tone and vaginal bleeding.
- Monitor for adverse reactions of water intoxication, such as lightheadedness, nausea, vomiting, headache, and malaise, which can progress to cerebral edema with seizures, coma, and death. Qs

Antibiotic therapy may be prescribed to prevent or treat infection.

Inversion of the uterus

Inversion of the uterus is the turning inside out of the uterus and can be partial or complete. Uterine inversion is an emergency situation that can result in postpartum hemorrhage and requires immediate intervention.

ASSESSMENT

RISK FACTORS

- Retained placenta
- Uterine atony
- Vigorous fundal pressure
- Abnormally adherent placental tissue
- Fundal implantation of the placenta
- Excessive traction applied to the umbilical cord
- Short umbilical cord
- Prolonged labor

EXPECTED FINDINGS

Pain in lower abdomen

PHYSICAL ASSESSMENT FINDINGS
- Vaginal bleeding: hemorrhage
  - Complete inversion as evidenced by a large, red, rounded mass that protrudes 20 to 30 cm outside the introitus
  - Partial inversion as evidenced by the palpation of a smooth mass through the dilated cervix
- Dizziness
- Low blood pressure, increased pulse (shock)
- Pallor

DIAGNOSTIC PROCEDURES

Manual replacement of the uterus into the uterine cavity and repositioning of the uterus by the provider

PATIENT-CENTERED CARE

NURSING CARE

- Assess for an inverted uterus.
  - Visualize the introitus.
  - Perform a pelvic exam.
  - Maintain IV fluids.
  - Administer oxygen.
- Stop oxytocin if it is being administered at the time uterine inversion occurred.
- Avoid excessive traction on the umbilical cord.
- Anticipate surgery if nonsurgical interventions and management are unsuccessful.

MEDICATIONS

Terbutaline

CLASSIFICATION: Tocolytic

THERAPEUTIC INTENT: To relax the uterus prior to the provider's attempt at replacement of the uterus into the uterine cavity and uterus repositioning

NURSING CONSIDERATIONS
Following replacement of the uterus into the uterine cavity
- Closely observe the client's response to treatment and assess for stabilization of hemodynamic status.
- Avoid aggressive fundal massage.
- Administer oxytocics as prescribed.
- Administer broad-spectrum antibiotics for infection prophylaxis.

CLIENT EDUCATION: Inform the client that a cesarean birth will be needed for subsequent pregnancies.

Retained placenta

The placenta or fragments of the placenta remain in the uterus and prevents the uterus from contracting, which can lead to uterine atony or subinvolution.

ASSESSMENT

RISK FACTORS

- Partial separation of a normal placenta
- Entrapment of a partially or completely separated placenta by a constricting ring of the uterus
- Excessive traction on the umbilical cord prior to complete separation of the placenta
- Placental tissue that is abnormally adherent to the uterine wall
- Preterm births between 20 and 24 weeks of gestation

EXPECTED FINDINGS

PHYSICAL ASSESSMENT FINDINGS
- Uterine atony, subinvolution, or inversion
- Excessive bleeding or blood clots larger than a quarter
- Return of lochia rubra once lochia has progressed to serosa alba
- Malodorous lochia or vaginal discharge
- Elevated temperature

LABORATORY TESTS

Hgb and Hct

DIAGNOSTIC PROCEDURES

- Manual separation and removal of the placenta is done by the provider.
- D&C if oxytocics are ineffective in expelling the placental fragments.

PATIENT-CENTERED CARE

NURSING CARE

- Monitor the uterus for fundal height, consistency, and position.
- Monitor lochia for color, amount, consistency, and odor.
- Monitor vital signs.
- Maintain or initiate IV fluids.
- Provide oxygen at 2 to 3 L/min per nasal cannula.
- Anticipate surgical interventions, such as a D&C or hysterectomy, if postpartum bleeding is present and continues.

MEDICATIONS

Oxytocin

To expel retained fragments of the placenta

CLASSIFICATION: Uterine stimulant

THERAPEUTIC INTENT: Promotes uterine contractions and expel the retained fragments of placenta.

NURSING CONSIDERATIONS
- Assess uterine tone and vaginal bleeding.
- Monitor for adverse reactions of water intoxication, such as lightheadedness, nausea, vomiting, headache, and malaise, which can progress to cerebral edema with seizures, coma, and death.

Terbutaline

CLASSIFICATION: Tocolytic

THERAPEUTIC INTENT: Relaxes the uterus prior to D&C if placental expulsion with oxytocics is unsuccessful.

CLIENT EDUCATION

Instruct the client to limit physical activity to conserve strength, and to increase iron and protein intake to promote the rebuilding of RBC volume.

Lacerations and hematomas

- Lacerations that occur during labor and birth consist of the tearing of soft tissues in the birth canal and adjacent structures including the cervical, vaginal, vulvar, perineal, and/or rectal areas.
- An episiotomy can extend and become a third- or fourth-degree laceration.
- A hematoma is a collection of 250 to 500 mL of clotted blood within tissues that can appear as a bulging bluish mass. Hematomas can occur in the pelvic region or higher in the vagina or broad ligament.
- Pain, rather than noticeable bleeding, is the distinguishable clinical finding of hematomas.
- The client is at risk for hemorrhage or infection due to a laceration or hematoma.

ASSESSMENT

RISK FACTORS

- Operative vaginal birth (forceps-assisted, vacuum assisted birth)
- Precipitous birth
- Cephalopelvic disproportion
- Size (macrosomic infant) and abnormal presentation or position of the fetus
- Prolonged pressure of the fetal head on the vaginal mucosa
- Previous scarring of the birth canal from infection, injury, or operation
- Clients who are nulliparous are at a greater risk for injury due to firmer and less resistant tissue.
- Women who have light skin, especially those with reddish hair, have less distensible tissue than women who are dark skin.

EXPECTED FINDINGS

Laceration
- Sensation of oozing or trickling of blood
- Excessive rubra lochia (with or without clots)

Hematoma
- Pain
- Pressure sensation in rectum (urge to defecate) or vagina
- Difficulty voiding

PHYSICAL ASSESSMENT FINDINGS
- **Laceration**
  - Vaginal bleeding even though the uterus is firm and contracted
  - Continuous slow trickle of bright red blood from vagina, laceration, episiotomy
- **Hematoma:** Bulging, bluish mass or area of red-purple discoloration on vulva, perineum, or rectum

PATIENT-CENTERED CARE

NURSING CARE

- Assess pain.
- Visually or manually inspect the vulva, perineum, and rectum for lacerations and/or hematomas.
- Assess an episiotomy for extension into a third- or fourth-degree laceration.
- Evaluate lochia.
- Continue to assess vital signs and hemodynamic status.
- Attempt to identify the source of the bleeding.
- Assist the provider with repair procedures.
- Use ice packs to treat small hematomas.
- Administer pain medication.
- Encourage sitz baths and frequent perineal hygiene.

THERAPEUTIC PROCEDURES

- Repair and suturing of the episiotomy or lacerations is done by the provider.
- Ligation of the bleeding vessel or surgical incision for evacuation of the clotted blood from the hematoma is done by the provider.

Application Exercises

1. A nurse is caring for a client who is postpartum. The nurse should identify which of the following findings as an early indicator of hypovolemia caused by hemorrhage?

   A. Increasing pulse and decreasing blood pressure

   B. Dizziness and increasing respiratory rate

   C. Cool, clammy skin, and pale mucous membranes

   D. Altered mental status and level of consciousness

2. A nurse educator on the postpartum unit is reviewing risk factors for postpartum hemorrhage with a group of nurses. Which of the following factors should the nurse include in the teaching? (Select all that apply.)

   A. Precipitous delivery

   B. Obesity

   C. Inversion of the uterus

   D. Oligohydramnios

   E. Retained placental fragments

3. A nurse on the postpartum unit is performing a physical assessment of a client who is being admitted with a suspected deep-vein thrombosis (DVT). Which of the following clinical findings should the nurse expect? (Select all that apply.)

   A. Calf tenderness to palpation

   B. Mottling of the affected extremity

   C. Elevated temperature

   D. Area of warmth

   E. Report of nausea

4. A nurse on the postpartum unit is planning care for a client who has thrombophlebitis. Which of the following nursing interventions should the nurse include in the plan of care?

   A. Apply cold compresses to the affected extremity.

   B. Massage the affected extremity.

   C. Allow the client to ambulate.

   D. Measure leg circumferences.

5. A nurse is caring for a client who has disseminated intravascular coagulation (DIC). Which of the following antepartum complications should the nurse understand is a risk factor for this condition?

   A. Preeclampsia

   B. Thrombophlebitis

   C. Placenta previa

   D. Hyperemesis gravidarum

PRACTICE Active Learning Scenario

A nurse is planning care for a client who has a deep-vein thrombosis (DVT). What interventions should the nurse include in the plan of care? Use the ATI Active Learning Template: System Disorder to complete this item.

ALTERATION IN HEALTH (DIAGNOSIS): Describe the disease process and location.

RISK FACTORS: Describe four risk factors for the disorder.

CLIENT EDUCATION: Describe four teaching points for prevention of a DVT.

MEDICATIONS: Describe two medications and their related laboratory tests.

Application Exercises Key

1. A. **CORRECT:** A rising pulse rate and decreasing blood pressure are often the first indications of inadequate blood volume.

   B. Dizziness and increased respiratory rate are findings that occur in hypovolemia, but they are not the earliest indicators.

   C. Skin that is cool, clammy, and pale, along with pale mucous membranes, are changes that occur in the physical status of a client who has decreased blood volume, but they are not the first indicators of inadequate blood volume.

   D. Altered mental status and changes in level of consciousness are late manifestations of decreased blood volume, which leads to hypoxia and low oxygen saturation.

   (N) *NCLEX® Connection: Physiological Adaptation, Alterations in Body Systems*

2. A. **CORRECT:** Rapid, precipitous delivery is a risk factor for postpartum hemorrhage.

   B. Obesity is not a risk factor for postpartum hemorrhage.

   C. **CORRECT:** Inversion of the uterus in a risk factor for postpartum hemorrhage.

   D. Oligohydramnios does not place a client at risk for postpartum hemorrhage.

   E. **CORRECT:** Retained placental fragments is a risk factor for postpartum hemorrhage.

   (N) *NCLEX® Connection: Reduction of Risk Potential, Potential for Complications from Surgical Procedures and Health Alterations*

3. A. **CORRECT:** A client report of calf tenderness to palpation is an expected finding in a client who has a DVT.

   B. Mottling of the affected extremity is not an expected finding in a client who has a DVT.

   C. **CORRECT:** Elevated temperature is an expected finding in a client who has a DVT.

   D. **CORRECT:** An area of warmth over the thrombus is an expected finding in a client who has a DVT.

   E. A report of nausea is not an expected finding in a client who has a DVT.

   (N) *NCLEX® Connection: Health Promotion and Maintenance, Ante/Intra/Postpartum and Newborn Care*

4. A. The nurse should plan to apply warm compresses to the affected extremity.

   B. The nurse should not massage the affected extremity. This action can result in dislodgement of the clot.

   C. The client should be encouraged to rest with the affected extremity elevated.

   D. **CORRECT:** The nurse should plan to measure the circumference of the leg to assess for changes in the client's condition.

   (N) *NCLEX® Connection: Physiological Adaptation, Unexpected Response to Therapies*

5. A. **CORRECT:** DIC can occur secondary in a client who has preeclampsia.

   B. Thrombophlebitis is not a risk factor for DIC.

   C. Placenta previa is not a risk factor for DIC.

   D. Hyperemesis gravidarum is not a risk factor for DIC.

   (N) *NCLEX® Connection: Physiological Adaptation, Hemodynamics*

PRACTICE Answer

Using the ATI Active Learning Template: System Disorder

ALTERATION IN HEALTH (DIAGNOSIS): DVT refers to a thrombus that is associated with inflammation. It can occur in a superficial or deep vein (femoral, saphenous, or popliteal).

RISK FACTORS
- Pregnancy
- Immobility
- Obesity
- Smoking
- Cesarean birth
- Multiparity
- Older than 35 years of age
- History of previous thromboembolism
- Diabetes mellitus

CLIENT EDUCATION
- Wear antiembolic stockings until ambulation established.
- Perform active range of motion when on bed rest for longer than 8 hr.
- Initiate early and frequent postpartum ambulation.
- Avoid prolonged periods of standing, sitting, or immobility.
- Elevate the legs when sitting.
- Avoid crossing legs.
- Maintain 2 to 3 L of daily fluid intake from food and beverage sources.
- Discontinue smoking

MEDICATIONS
- Heparin: aPTT
- Warfarin: PT and INR

(N) *NCLEX® Connection: Physiological Adaptation, Alterations in Body Systems*

UNIT 3   POSTPARTUM NURSING CARE
SECTION: COMPLICATIONS OF THE POSTPARTUM PERIOD

CHAPTER 21

Postpartum Infections

Postpartum infections are complications that can occur up to 28 days following childbirth, or a spontaneous or induced abortion. Fever of 38° C (100.4° F) or higher for 2 consecutive days during the first 10 days of the postpartum period is indicative of a postpartum infection and requires further investigation. The infection can be present in the bladder, uterus, wound, or breast of a postpartum client. The major complication of puerperal infection is septicemia.

Uterine infection, wound infection, mastitis, and a urinary tract infection are examples of postpartum infections. Early identification and prompt treatment are necessary to promote positive outcomes.

Infections (endometritis, mastitis, and wound infections)

Uterine infection is also referred to as **endometritis**.
- Endometritis is an infection of the uterine lining or endometrium. It is the most frequently occurring puerperal infection.
- Endometritis usually begins on the second to fifth postpartum day, generally starting as a localized infection at the placental attachment site and spreading to include the entire uterine endometrium.

Sites of **wound infections** include cesarean incisions, episiotomies, lacerations, and any trauma wounds present in the birth canal following labor and birth.

Mastitis is an infection of the breast involving the interlobular connective tissue and is usually unilateral. Mastitis can progress to an abscess if untreated.
- It occurs most commonly in mothers breastfeeding for the first time and well after the establishment of milk flow, which is usually 6 weeks after delivery.
- *Staphylococcus aureus* is usually the infecting organism.

ASSESSMENT

RISK FACTORS

The immediate postpartum period following birth is a time of increased risk for all women for micro-organisms entering the reproductive tract and migrating into the blood and other parts of the body, which can result in life-threatening septicemia.
- Urinary tract infection, mastitis, pneumonia, or history of previous venous thrombus
- History of diabetes mellitus, immunosuppression, anemia, or malnutrition
- History of alcohol or drug use disorder
- Cervical dilation that provides the uterus with exposure to the external environment through the vagina
- Well-supplied exposed blood vessels
- Wounds from lacerations, incisions, or hematomas
- Alkalinity of amniotic fluid, blood, and lochia during pregnancy and the early postpartum period, decreasing the acidity of the vaginal secretions
- Cesarean birth
- Prolonged rupture of membranes
- Retained placental fragments and manual extraction of the placenta
- Chorioamnionitis
- Internal fetal/uterine pressure monitoring
- Multiple vaginal examinations after rupture of membranes
- Prolonged labor
- Postpartum hemorrhage
- Operative vaginal birth
- Epidural analgesia/anesthesia
- Hematomas
- Episiotomy or lacerations

Mastitis

- Milk stasis from a blocked duct
- Nipple trauma and cracked or fissured nipples
- Poor breastfeeding technique with improper latching of the infant onto the breast, which can lead to sore and cracked nipples
- Decrease in breastfeeding frequency due to supplementation with bottle feeding
- Poor hygiene and inadequate handwashing when handling perineal pads and touching the breasts

EXPECTED FINDINGS

Puerperal infections
- Flu-like clinical findings, such as body aches, chills, fever, and malaise
- Anorexia and nausea

Endometritis
- Pelvic pain
- Chills
- Fatigue
- Loss of appetite

Mastitis
- Painful or tender localized hard mass and reddened area, usually on one breast
- Chills
- Fatigue

PHYSICAL ASSESSMENT FINDINGS
- **Puerperal infections**
  - Elevated temperature of at least 38° C (100.4° F) for 2 or more consecutive days
  - Tachycardia
- **Endometritis**
  - Uterine tenderness and enlargement
  - Dark, profuse lochia
  - Lochia that is either malodorous or purulent
  - Temperature greater than 38° C (100.4° F), typically on the third to fourth postpartum day
  - Tachycardia
- **Wound infection**
  - Wound warmth, erythema, tenderness, pain, edema, seropurulent drainage, and wound dehiscence (separation of wound or incision edges) or evisceration (protrusion of internal contents through the separated wound edges)
  - Temperature greater than 38° C (100.4° F) for 2 or more consecutive days
- **Mastitis:** Axillary adenopathy in the affected side (enlarged tender axillary lymph nodes) with an area of inflammation that can be red, swollen, warm, and tender

LABORATORY TESTS

- Blood, intracervical, or intrauterine bacterial cultures to reveal the offending organism
- WBC count: leukocytosis
- RBC sedimentation rate: distinctly increased
- RBC count: anemia

PATIENT-CENTERED CARE

NURSING CARE

- Obtain frequent vital signs.
- Assess pain.
- Assess fundal height, position, and consistency.
- Observe lochia for color, quantity, and consistency.
- Inspect incisions, episiotomy, and lacerations.
- Inspect breasts.

Puerperal infections

- Use aseptic technique for appropriate procedures; perform proper hand hygiene; and don gloves for labor, birth, and postpartum care.
- Provide client education about preventative measures to include thorough handwashing and good perineal hygiene.
- Maintain or initiate IV access.
- Administer IV broad-spectrum antibiotic therapy (penicillins or cephalosporins).
- Provide comfort measures, such as warm blankets or cool compresses, depending on findings.
- Educate the client about signs of worsening conditions to report and the importance of adherence to the treatment plan with the completion of a full course of antibiotics.
- Encourage a diet high in protein to promote tissue healing.

Endometritis

- Collect vaginal and blood cultures.
- Administer IV antibiotics.
- Administer analgesics.
- Teach the client hand hygiene techniques.
- Encourage the client to maintain interaction with her infant to facilitate bonding.

Wound infection

- Perform wound care.
- Administer IV antibiotics.
- Provide or encourage comfort measures, such as sitz baths, perineal care, and warm or cold compresses.
- Teach the client good hand hygiene techniques (changing perineal pads from front to back, performing thorough hand hygiene prior to and after perineal care).

Mastitis

Provide the client with education regarding breast hygiene to prevent and manage mastitis.
- Instruct the client to thoroughly wash hands prior to breastfeeding.
- Instruct the client to maintain cleanliness of breasts with frequent changes of breast pads.
- Encourage the client to allow nipples to air-dry.
- Teach the client proper infant positioning and latching-on techniques, including both the nipple and the areola. The client should release the infant's grasp on the nipple prior to removing the infant from the breast.
- Instruct the client about completely emptying her breasts with each feeding to prevent milk stasis, which provides a medium for bacterial growth.
- Encourage the client to use ice packs or warm packs on affected breasts for discomfort.
- Instruct the client to continue breastfeeding frequently (at least every 2 to 4 hr), especially on the affected side.
- Instruct the client to manually express breast milk or use a breast pump if breastfeeding is too painful.
- Instruct the client to begin breastfeeding from the unaffected breast first to initiate the letdown reflex in the affected breast that is distended or tender.
- Encourage rest, analgesics, and fluid intake of at least 3,000 mL per day.
- Encourage the client to wear a well-fitting bra for support.
- Tell the client to report redness and fever.
- Administer antibiotics, and teach the client the importance of completing the entire course of antibiotics as prescribed.

MEDICATIONS

For endometritis

Clindamycin

Cephalosporins, penicillins, and gentamicin

CLASSIFICATION: Antibiotic

THERAPEUTIC INTENT: Treatment of bacterial infections

CLIENT EDUCATION
- Educate the client to take all the medication as prescribed.
- Tell the client to notify the provider of the development of watery, bloody diarrhea.
- Tell the client to notify the provider if the client is breastfeeding.

THERAPEUTIC PROCEDURES

The provider might need to open and drain the wound or perform wound debridement if indicated.

Urinary tract infection

- Urinary tract infections (UTIs) are a common postpartum infection secondary to bladder trauma incurred during the delivery or a break in aseptic technique during bladder catheterization.
- A potential complication of a UTI is the progression to pyelonephritis with permanent kidney damage leading to kidney failure.

ASSESSMENT

RISK FACTORS

- Postpartal hypotonic bladder or urethra (urinary stasis and retention)
- Epidural anesthesia
- Urinary bladder catheterization
- Frequent pelvic examinations
- Genital tract injuries
- History of UTIs
- Cesarean birth

EXPECTED FINDINGS

- Reports of urgency, frequency, dysuria, and discomfort in the pelvic area
- Fever
- Chills
- Malaise

PHYSICAL ASSESSMENT FINDINGS
- Change in vital signs, elevated temperature
- Urine (cloudy, blood-tinged, malodorous, sediment visible)
- Urinary retention
- Pain in the suprapubic area
- Pain at the costovertebral angle (pyelonephritis)

DIAGNOSTIC PROCEDURES

Urinalysis for WBCs, RBCs, protein, bacteria

PATIENT-CENTERED CARE

NURSING CARE

- Obtain a random or clean-catch urine sample.
- Administer antibiotics, and teach the client the importance of completing the entire course of antibiotics as prescribed.
- Acetaminophen is taken to reduce discomfort and pain associated with a urinary tract infection.
- Teach the client proper perineal hygiene, such as wiping from front to back.
- Encourage the client to increase her fluid intake to 3,000 mL/day to dilute the bacteria and flush her bladder.
- Recommend that the client drink cranberry and prune juice to promote urine acidification, which inhibits bacterial multiplication. Q EBP

Application Exercises

1. A nurse on the postpartum unit is caring for four clients. Which of the following clients should the nurse recognize as the greatest risk for development of a postpartum infection?
   - A. A client who experienced a precipitous labor less than 3 hr in duration
   - B. A client who had premature rupture of membranes and prolonged labor
   - C. A client who delivered a large for gestational age infant
   - D. A client who had a boggy uterus that was not well-contracted

2. A nurse is teaching a client who is breastfeeding and has mastitis. Which of the following responses should the nurse make?
   - A. "Limit the amount of time the infant nurses on each breast."
   - B. "Nurse the infant only on the unaffected breast until resolved."
   - C. "Completely empty each breast at each feeding or use a pump."
   - D. "Wear a tight-fitting bra until lactation has ceased."

3. A nurse is reviewing discharge teaching with a client who has a urinary tract infection. Which of the following statements by the client indicates understanding of the teaching? (Select all that apply.)
   - A. "I will perform peri care and apply a perineal pad in a back-to-front direction."
   - B. "I will drink cranberry and prune juices to make my urine more acidic."
   - C. "I will drink large amounts of fluids to flush the bacteria from my urinary tract."
   - D. "I will go back to breastfeeding after I have finished taking the antibiotic."
   - E. "I will take Tylenol for any discomfort."

4. A nurse is caring for a client who has mastitis. Which of the following is the typical causative agent of mastitis?
   - A. *Staphylococcus aureus*
   - B. *Chlamydia trachomatis*
   - C. *Klebsiella pneumonia*
   - D. *Clostridium perfringens*

5. A nurse is discussing risks factors for urinary tract infections with a newly licensed nurse. Which of the following conditions should the nurse include in the teaching? (Select all that apply).
   - A. Epidural anesthesia
   - B. Urinary bladder catheterization
   - C. Frequent pelvic examinations
   - D. History of UTIs
   - E. Vaginal birth

PRACTICE Active Learning Scenario

A nurse educator is reviewing care of a client who has endometritis with a group of newly hired nurses. What information should the nurse educator include in the teaching? Use the ATI Active Learning Template: System Disorder to complete this item.

ALTERATION IN HEALTH (DIAGNOSIS)

EXPECTED FINDINGS: Describe at least six.

NURSING CARE: Describe at least three nursing interventions.

Application Exercises Key

1. A. A precipitous labor places the client at risk for trauma and lacerations during delivery, but there is another client who is at greater risk for postpartum infection.

    B. **CORRECT:** Premature rupture of membranes with prolonged labor poses the greatest risk for developing a postpartum infection because the birth canal was open, allowing pathogens to enter.

    C. Delivery of a large infant places the client at risk for a postpartum infection, but there is another client who is at greater risk.

    D. A boggy uterus that did not remain well-contracted places the client at risk for a postpartum infection, but there is another client who is at greater risk.

    Ⓝ *NCLEX® Connection: Physiological Adaptation, Alterations in Body Systems*

2. A. Frequent, on-demand breastfeeding should be encouraged to promote milk flow.

    B. The client should be instructed to continue breastfeeding, especially on the affected side.

    C. **CORRECT:** Instruct the client to completely empty each breast at each feeding to prevent milk stasis, which provides a medium for bacterial growth.

    D. The client should wear a well-fitting bra, not one that is too tight or a binder.

    Ⓝ *NCLEX® Connection: Physiological Adaptation, Illness Management*

3. A. Perineal cleansing and pad application should be done front to back, not back to front.

    B. **CORRECT:** Acidification of urine inhibits bacterial multiplication.

    C. **CORRECT:** Increased fluid intake can help to flush the bacteria from the urinary tract.

    D. Breastfeeding does not have to be delayed until the course of antibiotics is completed.

    E. **CORRECT:** Acetaminophen is taken to reduce discomfort and pain associated with a urinary tract infection.

    Ⓝ *NCLEX® Connection: Physiological Adaptation, Illness Management*

4. A. **CORRECT:** *Staphylococcus aureus, Escherichia coli*, and streptococcus are usually the infecting agents that enter the breast due to sore or cracked nipples, which results in mastitis.

    B. *Chlamydia trachomatis* is an STI but not the causative agent of mastitis.

    C. *Klebsiella pneumonia* is a causative agent of pneumonia.

    D. *Clostridium perfringens* can cause wound infections but is not a causative agent of mastitis.

    Ⓝ *NCLEX® Connection: Physiological Adaptation, Illness Management*

5. A. **CORRECT:** Epidural anesthesia is a risk factor for a UTI.

    B. **CORRECT:** Urinary bladder catheterization is a risk factor for a UTI.

    C. **CORRECT:** A history of frequent pelvic examinations is a risk factor for a UTI.

    D. **CORRECT:** A history of UTIs is a risk factor for developing UTIs.

    B. Cesarean birth places a client at risk for development of a UTI.

    Ⓝ *NCLEX® Connection: Physiological Adaptation, Illness Management*

PRACTICE Answer

Using the ATI Active Learning Template: System Disorder

ALTERATION IN HEALTH (DIAGNOSIS): Endometritis is an infection of the uterine lining or endometrium. It usually begins on the second to fifth postpartum day as a localized infection at the placental attachment site and spreads to include the entire endometrium. It is the most frequently occurring puerperal infection.

EXPECTED FINDINGS
- Uterine tenderness and enlargement
- Dark, profuse lochia
- Malodorous or purulent lochia
- Temperature greater than 38° C (100.4° F) on the third or fourth postpartum day
- Tachycardia
- Pelvic pain
- Chills
- Fatigue, loss of appetite

NURSING CARE
- Collect vaginal and blood cultures.
- Administer IV antibiotics.
- Administer analgesics.
- Teach client hand hygiene techniques.
- Encourage client interaction with her infant to facilitate bonding.

Ⓝ *NCLEX® Connection: Physiological Adaptation, Illness Management*

CHAPTER 22 *Postpartum Depression*

Postpartum blues can occur in approximately 50% to 85% of women during the first few days after birth and generally continues for up to 10 days. It is characterized by tearfulness, insomnia, lack of appetite, and a feeling of letdown. A mother can experience an intense fear, anxiety, anger, and inability to cope with the slightest problems and become despondent. Postpartum blues typically resolves in 10 days without intervention.

Postpartum depression occurs within 6 months of delivery and is characterized by persistent feelings of sadness and intense mood swings. It occurs in 10% to 15% of new mothers and usually does not resolve without intervention. It is similar to nonpostpartum mood disorders.

Postpartum psychosis develops within the first 2 to 3 weeks of the postpartum period. Clients who have a history of bipolar disorder are at a higher risk. Clinical findings are **severe** and can include confusion, disorientation, hallucinations, delusions, obsessive behaviors, and paranoia. The client might attempt to harm herself or her infant.

A nurse should monitor clients for suicidal or delusional thoughts. The nurse should monitor infants for failure to thrive secondary to an inability of the mother to provide care.

ASSESSMENT

RISK FACTORS

- Hormonal changes with a rapid decline in estrogen and progesterone levels
- Postpartum physical discomfort or pain
- Individual socioeconomic factors
- Decreased social support system
- Anxiety about assuming new role as a mother
- Unplanned or unwanted pregnancy
- History of previous depressive disorder
- Low self-esteem
- History of intimate partner abuse

EXPECTED FINDINGS

Postpartum blues

- Feelings of sadness
- Lack of appetite
- Sleep pattern disturbances
- Feeling of inadequacies
- Crying easily for no apparent reason
- Restlessness, insomnia, fatigue
- Headache
- Anxiety, anger, sadness

PHYSICAL ASSESSMENT FINDINGS: Crying

Postpartum depression

- Feelings of guilt and inadequacies
- Irritability
- Anxiety
- Fatigue persisting beyond a reasonable amount of time
- Feeling of loss
- Lack of appetite
- Persistent feelings of sadness
- Intense mood swings
- Sleep pattern disturbances

PHYSICAL ASSESSMENT FINDINGS
- Crying
- Weight loss
- Flat affect
- Irritability
- Rejection of the infant
- Severe anxiety and panic attack

Postpartum psychosis

- Pronounced sadness
- Disorientation
- Confusion
- Paranoia

PHYSICAL ASSESSMENT FINDINGS: Behaviors indicating hallucinations or delusional thoughts of self-harm or harming the infant

PATIENT-CENTERED CARE

NURSING CARE

- Monitor interactions between the client and her infant. Encourage bonding activities.
- Monitor the client's mood and affect.
- Reinforce that feeling down in the postpartum period is normal and self-limiting. Encourage the client to notify her provider if the condition persists.
- Encourage the client to communicate feelings, validate and address personal conflicts, and reinforce personal power and autonomy.
- Reinforce the importance of compliance with any prescribed medication regimen.
- Contact a community resource to schedule a follow-up visit after discharge for clients who are at high risk for postpartum depression.
- Ask the client if she has thoughts of self-harm, suicide, or harming her infant. Provide for the safety of the infant and client as the priority of care.

MEDICATIONS

- **Antidepressants** may be prescribed by the provider if indicated.
- **Antipsychotics** and **mood stabilizers** may be prescribed for clients who have postpartum psychosis.

CLIENT EDUCATION

CARE AFTER DISCHARGE

- Advise the client to get plenty of rest and to nap when the infant sleeps.
- Reinforce the importance of the client taking time out for herself.
- Schedule a follow-up visit prior to the traditional postpartum visit for clients who are at risk for developing postpartum depression.
- Provide information about community resources such as La Leche League or community mental health centers.
- Encourage the client to seek counseling, and make referrals to social agencies as indicated.

Application Exercises

1. A nurse is assessing a postpartum client who is exhibiting tearfulness, insomnia, lack of appetite, and a feeling of letdown. Which of the following conditions are associated with these clinical findings?

   A. Postpartum fatigue

   B. Postpartum psychosis

   C. Letting-go phase

   D. Postpartum blues

2. A nurse is caring for a postpartum client who delivered her third infant 2 days ago. The nurse recognizes that which of the following findings are suggestive of postpartum depression? (Select all that apply.)

   A. Fatigue

   B. Insomnia

   C. Euphoria

   D. Flat affect

   E. Delusions

3. A nurse is assessing a client who has postpartum depression. The nurse should expect which of the following findings? (Select all that apply.)

   A. Paranoia that her infant will be harmed

   B. Concerns about lack of income to pay bills

   C. Anxiety about assuming a new role as a mother

   D. Rapid decline in estrogen and progesterone

   E. Feeling of inadequacy with the new role as a mother

4. A nurse is caring for a client who has postpartum psychosis. Which of the following actions is the nurse's priority?

   A. Reinforce the need to take antipsychotics as prescribed.

   B. Ask the client if she has thoughts of harming herself or her infant.

   C. Monitor the infant for indications of failure to thrive.

   D. Review the client's medical record for a history of bipolar disorder.

PRACTICE Active Learning Scenario

A nurse manager is reviewing the facility's protocol for the care of a client who has postpartum depression. What information should the nurse manager include in the protocol? Use the ATI Active Learning Template: System Disorder to complete this item.

ALTERATION IN HEALTH (DIAGNOSIS)

MEDICATIONS

NURSING CARE: Describe four nursing interventions.

CLIENT EDUCATION: Describe two teaching points for the client.

Application Exercises Key

1. A. Postpartum fatigue results from the work of labor. It is normally self-limiting.

   B. The client who has postpartum psychosis will exhibit pronounced feelings of sadness, confusion, disorientation, hallucinations, delusions, and paranoia, and might attempt to harm herself or her infant.

   C. The letting-go phase is the phase in which the client assumes her position at home and her new maternal role, focusing on the forward movement of the family unit.

   D. **CORRECT:** Postpartum blues are characterized by tearfulness, insomnia, lack of appetite, and feeling let-down.

   Ⓝ *NCLEX® Connection: Health Promotion and Maintenance, Ante/Intra/Postpartum and Newborn Care*

2. A. **CORRECT:** Fatigue is a finding suggestive of postpartum depression.

   B. **CORRECT:** Insomnia is a finding suggestive of postpartum depression.

   C. Persistent sadness, rather than euphoria, is associated with postpartum depression.

   D. **CORRECT:** A flat affect is a finding suggestive of postpartum depression.

   E. Delusions are a finding suggestive of postpartum psychosis .

   Ⓝ *NCLEX® Connection: Health Promotion and Maintenance, Health Screening*

3. A. Paranoia is a finding associated with postpartum psychosis.

   B. **CORRECT:** Feelings of financial inadequacy to provide for family is a finding associated with postpartum depression.

   C. **CORRECT:** Anxiety about assuming a new role as a mother is a finding associated with postpartum depression.

   D. **CORRECT:** The rapid decline in estrogen and progesterone is a finding associated with postpartum depression.

   E. **CORRECT:** Feeling of inadequacies with the new role as a mother is a finding associated with postpartum depression.

   Ⓝ *NCLEX® Connection: Health Promotion and Maintenance, Ante/Intra/Postpartum und Newborn Care*

4. A. The nurse should reinforce the need to take antipsychotics as prescribed to manage the manifestations of postpartum psychosis; however, there is another action that is the nurse's priority.

   B. **CORRECT:** The nurse should identify that the greatest risk to the client and her infant is self-harm or harm directed toward the infant. Therefore, the priority action the nurse should take is to directly ask the client if she has thoughts of self-harm, suicide, or harming the infant.

   C. The nurse should monitor the infant for indications of failure to thrive as the client who has postpartum psychosis might be unable to provide care for the infant; however, there is another action that is the nurse's priority.

   D. The nurse should review the client's medical record for a history of bipolar disorder as this is associated with an increased risk for postpartum psychosis; however, there is another action that is the nurse's priority.

   Ⓝ *NCLEX® Connection: Health Promotion and Maintenance, Health Screening*

PRACTICE Answer

Using the ATI Active Learning Template: System Disorder

ALTERATION IN HEALTH (DIAGNOSIS): Postpartum depression occurs within 6 months of delivery. It is characterized by persistent feelings of sadness and intense mood swings. It occurs in 10% to 15% of new mothers and usually does not resolve without intervention. It is similar to nonpostpartum mood disorders.

MEDICATIONS: Antidepressants

NURSING CARE

- Monitor client-infant interactions; encourage bonding activities.
- Monitor the client's mood and affect.
- Encourage verbalization of feelings; validate and address person conflicts; reinforce personal power and autonomy.
- Reinforce compliance with medication regimen.
- Provide referral, and schedule appointment with an appropriate community resource.
- Monitor the client for indications of postpartum psychosis. Prioritize care to ensure the safety of the client and her infant.

CLIENT EDUCATION

- Advise the client to get plenty of rest; nap when the infant sleeps.
- Remind the client to make time for herself.
- Tell the client to seek counseling, and use resources provided by referred community agencies.

Ⓝ *NCLEX® Connection: Health Promotion and Maintenance, Ante/Intra/Postpartum and Newborn Care*

NCLEX® Connections

When reviewing the following chapters, keep in mind the relevant topics and tasks of the NCLEX outline, in particular:

Client Needs: Health Promotion and Maintenance

ANTE/INTRA/POSTPARTUM AND NEWBORN CARE: Assist client with performing/learning newborn care.

TECHNIQUES OF PHYSICAL ASSESSMENT: Perform comprehensive health assessment.

Client Needs: Basic Care and Comfort

NON-PHARMACOLOGICAL COMFORT INTERVENTIONS: Apply knowledge of pathophysiology to non-pharmacological comfort/palliative care interventions.

NUTRITION AND ORAL HYDRATION: Manage the client's nutritional intake.

Client Needs: Reduction of Risk Potential

CHANGES/ABNORMALITIES IN VITAL SIGNS: Apply knowledge of client pathophysiology when measuring vital signs.

LABORATORY VALUES: Monitor client laboratory values.

SYSTEM SPECIFIC ASSESSMENTS: Assess the client for signs of hypoglycemia or hyperglycemia.

CHAPTER 23 # Newborn Assessment

Understanding physiologic responses of a newborn to birth and physical assessment findings are imperative for providing nursing care following the birth of a newborn. Key areas to know about include Apgar scoring, physical examination of the newborn, New Ballard Scale (gestational age assessment), normal newborn vital signs and measurements, classifications of a newborn by gestational age and weight, diagnostic and therapeutic procedures, and complications of a newborn.

PHYSIOLOGIC RESPONSE OF NEWBORN TO BIRTH

- Adjustments to extrauterine life occur as a newborn's respiratory and circulatory systems are required to rapidly adjust to life outside of the uterus.
- The establishment of respiratory function with the cutting of the umbilical cord is the most critical extrauterine adjustment as air inflates the lungs with the first breath.
- Circulatory changes after birth occur with the expulsion of the placenta and the cutting of the umbilical cord as a newborn begins breathing independently. The three shunts (ductus arteriosus, ductus venosus, and foramen ovale) functionally close during a newborn's transition to extrauterine life with the flow of oxygenated blood in the lungs and readjustment of atrial blood pressure in the heart.

PHYSICAL ASSESSMENT OF NEWBORN FOLLOWING BIRTH

Apgar scoring and a brief physical exam is done immediately following birth to rule out abnormalities. **(23.1)**

EQUIPMENT FOR NEWBORN ASSESSMENT

Bulb syringe: Used for suctioning excess mucus from the mouth and nose.

Stethoscope with a pediatric head: Used to evaluate heart rate, breath sounds, and bowel sounds.

Axillary thermometer: Used to monitor temperature and prevent hypothermia. Rectal temperatures are avoided because they can injure the delicate rectal mucosa; an initial rectal temperature can be obtained to evaluate for anal abnormalities.

Blood pressure cuff 2.5 cm wide: Palpation or electronic method. Blood pressure can be done in all four extremities if evaluating the newborn for cardiac problems.

Scale with protective cover in place: Scale should be at 0; weight should include pounds, ounces, and grams.

Tape measure in centimeters: Measure from crown to heel of foot for length. Measure head circumference at greatest diameter (occipital to frontal). Measure chest circumference beginning at the nipple line, and abdominal circumference above the umbilicus.

Clean gloves: Worn for all physical assessments until discharge.

INITIAL ASSESSMENT

The nurse performs a quick initial assessment to review the newborn's systems and to observe for any abnormalities.

External assessment: Skin color, peeling, birthmarks, foot creases, breast tissue, nasal patency, and meconium staining (can indicate fetal hypoxia)

Chest: Point of maximal impulse location; ease of breathing; auscultation for heart rate and quality of tones; and respirations for crackles, wheezes, and equality of bilateral breath sounds

23.1 Apgar scoring

An Apgar score is assigned based on a quick review of systems that is completed at 1 and 5 min of life. This allows the nurse to rapidly assess extrauterine adaptation and intervene with appropriate nursing actions.
- 0 to 3 indicates severe distress
- 4 to 6 indicates moderate difficulty
- 7 to 10 indicates minimal or no difficulty with adjusting to extrauterine life

APGAR SCORE	0	1	2
HEART RATE	Absent	Slow, less than 100/min	Greater than 100/min
RESPIRATORY RATE	Absent	Slow, weak cry	Good cry
MUSCLE TONE	Flaccid	Some flexion of extremities	Well-flexed
REFLEX IRRITABILITY	None	Grimace	Cry
COLOR	Blue, pale	Pink body, cyanotic hands and feet (acrocyanosis)	Completely pink

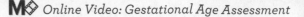

Abdomen: Rounded abdomen and umbilical cord with one vein and two arteries

Neurologic: Muscle tone and reflex reaction (Moro reflex); palpation for the presence and size of fontanels and sutures; assessment of fontanels for fullness or bulge

Other observations: Inspection for gross structural malformations

EXPECTED REFERENCE RANGES

Weight: 2,500 to 4,000 g (5.5 to 8.8 lb)

Length: 45 to 55 cm (18 to 22 in)

Head circumference: 32 to 36.8 cm (12.6 to 14.5 in)

Chest circumference: 30 to 33 cm (12 to 13 in)

GESTATIONAL AGE ASSESSMENT

A gestational age assessment is performed on newborns within the first 48 hr following birth. Neonatal morbidity and mortality are related to gestational age and birth weight. The gestational age assessment involves taking measurements of the newborn and the use of the New Ballard Scale. This scale provides an estimation of gestational age and a baseline to assess growth and development.

New Ballard Scale

A newborn maturity rating scale that assesses neuromuscular and physical maturity
- Each individual assessment parameter displays at least six ranges of development along a continuum.
- Each range of development within an assessment is assigned a number value from –1 to 5. The totals are added to give a maturity rating in weeks gestation (e.g., a score of 35 indicates 38 weeks of gestation).

NEUROMUSCULAR MATURITY
- Posture ranging from fully extended to fully flexed (0 to 4).
- Square window formation with the neonate's wrist (–1 to 4).
- Arm recoil, where the neonate's arm is passively extended and spontaneously returns to flexion (0 to 4).
- Popliteal angle, which is the degree of the angle to which the newborn's knees can extend (–1 to 5).
- Scarf sign, which is crossing the neonate's arm over the chest (–1 to 4).
- Heel to ear, which is how far the neonate's heels reach to her ears (–1 to 4).

PHYSICAL MATURITY
- Skin texture, ranging from sticky and transparent, to leathery, cracked, and wrinkled (–1 to 5).
- Lanugo presence and amount, ranging from none, sparse, abundant, thinning, bald, or mostly bald (–1 to 4).
- Plantar surface creases, ranging from less than 40 mm to creases over the entire sole (–1 to 4).
- Breast tissue amount, ranging from imperceptible, to full areola with a 5 to 10 mm bud (–1 to 4).

- Eyes and ears for amount of eye opening and ear cartilage present (–1 to 4).
- Genitalia development, ranging from flat smooth scrotum to pendulous testes with deep rugae for males (–1 to 4), and prominent clitoris with flat labia to the labia majora covering the labia minora and clitoris for females (–1 to 4).

CLASSIFICATION
Following physical assessment, classification of the newborn by gestational age and birth weight is determined.

Appropriate for gestational age (AGA): Weight is between the 10th and 90th percentile.

Small for gestational age (SGA): Weight is less than the 10th percentile.

Large for gestational age (LGA): Weight is greater than the 90th percentile.

Low birth weight (LBW): Weight of 2,500 g or less at birth.

Intrauterine growth restriction (IUGR): Growth rate does not meet expected norms.

Term: Birth between the beginning of week 37 and prior to the end of 42 weeks of gestation.

Preterm or premature: Born prior to the completion of 37 weeks of gestation.

Postterm (postdate): Born after the completion of 42 weeks of gestation.

Postmature: Born after the completion of 42 weeks of gestation with evidence of placental insufficiency.

VITAL SIGNS

Vital signs are checked in the following sequence: respirations, heart rate, blood pressure, and temperature. The nurse observes the respiratory rate first before the newborn becomes active or agitated by use of the stethoscope, thermometer, and/or blood pressure cuff.

Respiratory rate varies from 30 to 60 breaths/min with short periods of apnea (less than 15 seconds) occurring most frequently during the rapid eye movement sleep cycle. Periods of apnea lasting longer than 15 seconds should be evaluated. Crackles and wheezing are manifestations of fluid or infection in the lungs. Grunting and nasal flaring are clinical findings of respiratory distress.

Normal heart rate ranges from 110 to 160/min with brief fluctuations above and below this range depending on activity level (crying, sleeping). Apical pulse rate is assessed for 1 full minute, preferably when the newborn is sleeping. The pediatric stethoscope head is placed on the fourth or fifth intercostal space at the left midclavicular line over the apex of the newborn's heart. Heart murmurs are documented and reported.

Blood pressure should be 60 to 80 mm Hg systolic and 40 to 50 mm Hg diastolic.

Normal temperature range is 36.5 to 37.5 °C (97.7 to 99.5 °F) axillary. The newborn is at risk for hypothermia and hyperthermia until thermoregulation (ability to produce heat and maintain normal body temperature) stabilizes. If the newborn becomes chilled (cold stress), oxygen demands can increase and acidosis can occur.

A more extensive physical exam is performed on the neonate within 24 hr of birth. Vital signs are obtained. A head-to-toe assessment is performed. Neurological and behavioral assessments are completed by eliciting reflexes and observing responses. Laboratory data is monitored.

PHYSICAL EXAM FROM HEAD TO TOE

Posture

- Lying in a curled-up position with arms and legs in moderate flexion
- Resistant to extension of extremities

Skin

- Skin color should be pink or acrocyanotic with no jaundice present on the first day. Secondary to increased bilirubin, jaundice can appear on the third day of life, but then decrease spontaneously.
- Skin turgor should be present, showing that the newborn is well hydrated. The skin should spring back immediately when pinched.
- Texture should be dry, soft, and smooth, showing good hydration. Cracks in hands and feet can be present. In full-term newborns, desquamation (peeling) occurs a few days after birth.
- Vernix caseosa (protective, thick, cheesy covering) amounts vary, with more present in creases and skin folds.
- Lanugo (fine downy hair) varies regarding the amount present. It is usually found on the pinnae of ears, forehead, and shoulders.

NORMAL DEVIATIONS

- **Milia** (small raised white spots on the nose, chin, and forehead) can be present. These spots disappear spontaneously without treatment (parents should not squeeze the spots).
- **Mongolian spots** (bluish purple spots of pigmentation) are commonly noted on the shoulders, back, and buttocks. These spots are frequently present on newborns who have dark skin. Be sure the parents are aware of Mongolian spots, and document location and presence. **(23.2)**
- **Telangiectatic nevi** (stork bites) are flat pink or red marks that easily blanch and are found on the back of the neck, nose, upper eyelids, and middle of the forehead. They usually fade by the second year of life. **(23.3)**

- **Nevus flammeus** (port wine stain) is a capillary angioma below the surface of the skin that is purple or red, varies in size and shape, is commonly seen on the face, and does not blanch or disappear.
- **Erythema toxicum** (erythema neonatorum) is a pink rash that appears suddenly anywhere on the body of a term newborn during the first 3 weeks. This is frequently referred to as newborn rash. No treatment is required.

Head

- Head should be 2 to 3 cm larger than chest circumference. If the head circumference is greater than or equal to 4 cm larger than the chest circumference, this can be an indication of **hydrocephalus** (excessive cerebral fluid within the brain cavity surrounding the brain). If the head circumference is less than or equal to 32 cm, this can be an indication of **microcephaly** (abnormally small head).
- Anterior fontanel should be palpated and approximately 5 cm on average and diamond shaped. Posterior fontanel is smaller and triangle-shaped. Fontanels should be soft and flat. Fontanels can bulge when the newborn cries, coughs, or vomits, and are flat when the newborn is quiet. Bulging fontanels can indicate increased intracranial pressure, infection, or hemorrhage. Depressed fontanels can indicate dehydration.
- Sutures should be palpable, separated, and can be overlapping (molding), a normal occurrence resulting from head compression during labor.

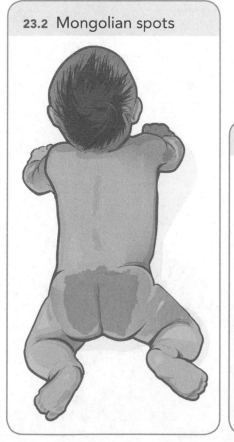

23.2 Mongolian spots

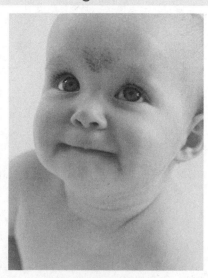

23.3 Telangiectatic nevi

- **Caput succedaneum** (localized swelling of the soft tissues of the scalp caused by pressure on the head during labor) is an expected finding that can be palpated as a soft edematous mass and can cross over the suture line. Caput succedaneum usually resolves in 3 to 4 days and does not require treatment. **(23.4)**
- **Cephalohematoma** is a collection of blood between the periosteum and the skull bone that it covers. It does not cross the suture line. It results from trauma during birth such as pressure of the fetal head against the maternal pelvis in a prolonged difficult labor or forceps delivery. It appears in the first 1 to 2 days after birth and resolves in 2 to 3 weeks. **(23.5)**

Eyes

- Assess eyes for symmetry in size and shape.
- Each eye and the space between the eyes should equal one-third the distance from the inner to the outer canthus of both eyes to rule out chromosomal abnormalities, such as Down syndrome.
- Eyes are usually blue or gray following birth.
- Lacrimal glands are immature, with minimal or no tears.
- Subconjunctival hemorrhages can result from pressure during birth.
- Pupillary and red reflex are present.
- Eyeball movement will demonstrate random, jerky movements.

Ears

- When examining the placement of ears, draw an imaginary line through the inner to the outer canthus of the newborn's eye. The eye should be even with the upper tip of the pinna of the newborn's ear. Ears that are low-set can indicate a chromosome abnormality, such as Down syndrome, or a kidney disorder.
- Cartilage should be firm and well formed. Lack of cartilage indicates prematurity.
- The newborn should respond to voices and other sounds.
- Inspect ears for skin tags.

Nose

- The nose should be midline, flat, and broad with lack of a bridge.
- Some mucus should be present, but with no drainage.
- Newborns are obligate nose breathers and do not develop the response of opening the mouth with a nasal obstruction until 3 weeks after birth. Therefore, a nasal blockage can result in flaring of the nares, cyanosis, or asphyxia.
- Newborns sneeze to clear nasal passages.

Mouth

- Assess for palate closure and strength of sucking.
- Lip movements should be symmetrical.
- Saliva should be scant. Excessive saliva can indicate a tracheoesophageal fistula.
- Epstein's pearls (small white cysts found on the gums and at the junction of the soft and hard palates) are expected findings. They result from the accumulation of epithelial cells and disappear a few weeks after birth.
- Tongue should move freely, be symmetrical in shape, and not protrude. (A protruding tongue can be a sign of Down syndrome.)
- Soft and hard palate should be intact.
- Gums and tongue should be pink. Gray-white patches on the tongue and gums can indicate thrush, a fungal infection caused by Candida albicans, sometimes acquired from the mother's vaginal secretions.

Neck

- Neck should be short, thick, surrounded by skin folds, and exhibit no webbing.
- Neck should move freely from side to side and up and down.
- Absence of head control can indicate prematurity or Down syndrome.

Chest

- Chest should be barrel-shaped.
- Respirations are primarily diaphragmatic.
- Clavicles should be intact.
- Absence of retractions.
- Nipples should be prominent, well formed, and symmetrical.
- Breast nodules can be 3 to 10 mm.

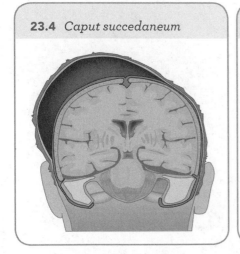

23.4 *Caput succedaneum*

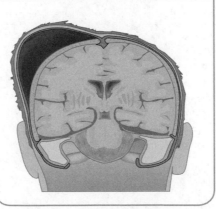

23.5 *Cephalohematoma*

Abdomen

- Umbilical cord should be odorless and exhibit no intestinal structures.
- Abdomen should be round, dome-shaped, and nondistended.
- Bowel sounds should be present 1 to 2 hr following birth.

Anogenital

- Anus should be present, patent, and not covered by a membrane.
- Meconium should be passed within 24 to 48 hr after birth.
- Genitalia of a male newborn should include rugae on the scrotum.
- Testes should be present in the scrotum.
- Male urinary meatus is located at penile tip.
- Genitalia of a female should include labia majora covering the labia minora and clitoris, and are usually edematous.
- Vaginal blood-tinged discharge can occur in female newborns, which is caused by maternal pregnancy hormones. This is an expected finding.
- A hymenal tag should be present.
- Urine should be passed within 24 hr after birth. Uric acid crystals will produce a rust color in the urine the first couple of days of life.

Extremities

- Assess for full range, symmetry of motion, and spontaneous movements.
- Extremities should be flexed.
- Assess for bowed legs and flat feet, which should be present because lateral muscles are more developed than the medial muscles.
- No click should be heard when abducting the hips.
- Gluteal folds should be symmetrical.
- Soles should be well-lined over two-thirds of the feet.
- Nail beds should be pink, and no extra digits are present.

Spine

Spine should be straight, flat, midline and easily flexed.

Reflexes

Sucking and rooting reflex
- EXPECTED FINDING: Elicit by stroking the cheek or edge of mouth. Newborn turns the head toward the side that is touched and starts to suck.
- EXPECTED AGE: Usually disappears after 3 to 4 months but can persist up to 1 year

Palmar grasp
- EXPECTED FINDING: Elicit by placing examiner's finger in palm of newborn's hand. The newborn's fingers curl around examiner's fingers.
- EXPECTED AGE: Lessens by 3 to 4 months

Plantar grasp
- EXPECTED FINDING: Elicit by placing examiner's finger at base of newborn's toes. The newborn responds by curling toes downward.
- EXPECTED AGE: Birth to 8 months

Moro reflex
- EXPECTED FINDING: Elicit by allowing the head and trunk of the newborn in a semisitting position to fall backward to an angle of at least 30°. The newborn will symmetrically extend and then abduct the arms at the elbows and fingers spread to form a "C."
- EXPECTED AGE: Birth to 6 months

Tonic neck reflex (fencer position)
- EXPECTED FINDING: With newborn in supine, neutral position, examiner turns newborn's head quickly to one side. The newborn's arm and leg on that side extend and opposing arm and leg flex.
- EXPECTED AGE: Birth to 3 to 4 months

Babinski reflex
- EXPECTED FINDING: Elicit by stroking outer edge of sole of the foot, moving up toward toes. Toes will fan upward and out. (23.6)
- EXPECTED AGE: Birth to 1 year

Stepping
- EXPECTED FINDING: Elicit by holding the newborn upright with feet touching a flat surface. The newborn responds with stepping movements.
- EXPECTED AGE: Birth to 4 weeks

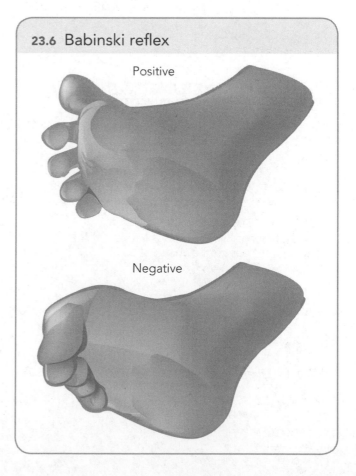

23.6 Babinski reflex

Positive

Negative

Senses

Vision: The newborn should be able to focus on objects 8 to 12 inches away from face. This is approximately the distance from the mother's face when the newborn is breastfeeding. The eyes are sensitive to light, so newborns prefer dim lighting. Pupils are reactive to light, and the blink reflex is easily stimulated. The newborn can track high-contrast objects and prefers bright colors and patterns. Term newborns can see objects as far away as 2.5 feet. Within 2 to 3 months, they can discriminate colors.

Hearing: Hearing is similar to that of an adult once the amniotic fluid drains from the ears. Newborns exhibit selective listening to familiar voices and rhythms of intrauterine life. The newborn turns toward the general direction of a sound.

Touch: Newborns should respond to tactile messages of pain and touch. The mouth is the area most sensitive to touch in the newborn.

Taste: Newborns can taste and prefer sweet to salty, sour, or bitter.

Smell: Newborns have a highly developed sense of smell, prefer sweet smells, and can recognize the mother's smell.

Habitation: This is a protective mechanism whereby the newborn becomes accustomed to environmental stimuli. Response to a constant or repetitive stimulus is decreased. This allows the newborn to select stimuli that promotes continued learning, avoiding overload.

> **!** Provide education to the mother and family about the neonate's appearance, and give reassurance about expected findings that the family can be concerned about (e.g., milia, Epstein's pearls, caput succedaneum).

DIAGNOSTIC AND THERAPEUTIC PROCEDURES FOLLOWING BIRTH

Cord blood is collected at birth. Laboratory tests are conducted to determine ABO blood type and Rh status if the mother's blood type is "O" or she is Rh-negative. A CBC can be done by a capillary stick to evaluate for anemia, polycythemia, infection, or clotting problems. Blood glucose is done to evaluate for hypoglycemia.

EXPECTED LABORATORY VALUES
- **Hgb:** 14 to 24 g/dL
- **Platelets:** 150,000 to 300,000/mm³
- **Hct:** 44% to 64%
- **Glucose:** 40 to 60 mg/dL
- **RBC count:** 4.8 x 10⁶ to 7.1 x 10⁶
- **Bilirubin**
  - 24 hr: 2 to 6mg/dL
  - 48 hr: 6 to 7 mg/dL
  - 3 to 5 days: 4 to 6 mg/dL
- **Leukocytes:** 9,000 to 30,000/mm³

COMPLICATIONS

Airway obstruction related to mucus

NURSING CONSIDERATIONS: Mouth and nose are suctioned with a bulb syringe. Gentle percussion over the chest can help loosen secretions.

Hypothermia

NURSING CONSIDERATIONS
- Monitor axillary temperature. Healthy newborn skin temperature is approximately 36.5 to 37 °C (97.7 to 98.6 °F)
- If temperature is unstable, place the newborn in a radiant warmer, and maintain skin temperature at approximately 36.5 °C (97.7 °F). Ideal method for promoting warmth and maintaining neonate's body temperature for a stable newborn s early skin-to-skin contact with mom. If the infant does not remain skin-to-skin with mom during the first 1 to 2 hr after birth, the nurse places the thoroughly dried infant under the radiant warmer or in a warm incubator until body temperature stabilizes.
- Assess axillary temperature every hour until stable.
- All exams and assessments should be performed under a radiant warmer or during skin-to-skin contact with the mother.

Inadequate oxygen supply

Related to obstructed airway, poorly functioning cardiopulmonary system, or hypothermia

NURSING CONSIDERATIONS
- Monitor respirations and skin color for cyanosis.
- Stabilize the body temperature or clear airway as indicated, administer oxygen, and if needed, prepare for resuscitation.

Application Exercises

1. A nurse is caring for a newborn who was born at 38 weeks of gestation, weighs 3,200 g, and is in the 60th percentile for weight. Based on the weight and gestational age, the nurse should classify this neonate as which of the following?

   A. Low birth weight

   B. Appropriate for gestational age

   C. Small for gestational age

   D. Large for gestational age

2. A nurse is completing a newborn assessment and observes small white nodules on the roof of the newborn's mouth. This finding is a characteristic of which of the following conditions?

   A. Mongolian spots

   B. Milia spots

   C. Erythema toxicum

   D. Epstein's pearls

3. A nurse is assessing the reflexes of a newborn. In checking for the Moro reflex, the nurse should perform which of the following?

   A. Hold the newborn vertically under arms and allow one foot to touch table.

   B. Stimulate the pads of the newborn's hands with stroking or massage.

   C. Stimulate the soles of the newborn's feet on the outer lateral surface of each foot.

   D. Hold the newborn in a semi-sitting position, then allow the newborn's head and trunk to fall backward.

4. A nurse is completing an assessment. Which of the following data indicate the newborn is adapting to extrauterine life? (Select all that apply.)

   A. Expiratory grunting

   B. Inspiratory nasal flaring

   C. Apnea for 10-second periods

   D. Obligatory nose breathing

   E. Crackles and wheezing

5. A nurse is teaching a newly licensed nurse how to bathe a newborn and observes a bluish marking across the newborn's lower back. The nurse should include which of the following information in the teaching?

   A. "This is frequently seen in newborns who have dark skin."

   B. "This is a finding indicating hyperbilirubinemia."

   C. "This is a forceps mark from an operative delivery."

   D. "This is related to prolonged birth or trauma during delivery."

PRACTICE Active Learning Scenario

A nurse in the nursery is admitting a newborn 2 hr following birth. What nursing actions should the nurse use to evaluate newborn physical development? Use the ATI Active Learning Template: Growth and Development to complete this item.

PHYSICAL DEVELOPMENT
- Describe at least three tools for assessment.
- Describe four reflex responses present at birth and how they are elicited.
- Describe newborn heart rate and how it is assessed.

Application Exercises Key

1. A. A newborn who has a low birth weight would weigh less than 2,500 g.

   B. **CORRECT:** This newborn is classified as appropriate for gestational age because the weight is between the 10th and 90th percentile.

   C. A newborn who is small for gestational age would weigh less than the 10th percentile.

   D. A newborn who is large for gestational age would weigh greater than the 90th percentile.

   Ⓝ *NCLEX® Connection: Health Promotion and Maintenance, Health Screening*

2. A. Mongolian spots are dark areas observed in dark-skinned newborns.

   B. Milia are small white bumps that occur on the nose due to clogged sebaceous glands.

   C. Erythema toxicum is a transient maculopapular rash seen in newborns.

   D. **CORRECT:** Epstein's pearls are small white nodules that appear on the roof of a newborn's mouth.

   Ⓝ *NCLEX® Connection: Health Promotion and Maintenance, Health Screening*

3. A. Holding the newborn vertically under the arms and allowing one foot to touch the table elicits the stepping reflex.

   B. Stimulating the pads of the newborn's hands elicits the grasp reflex.

   C. Stimulating the outer lateral portion of the newborn's soles elicits the Babinski reflex.

   D. **CORRECT:** The Moro reflex is elicited by holding the newborn in a semi-sitting position and then allowing the head and trunk to fall backward.

   Ⓝ *NCLEX® Connection: Health Promotion and Maintenance, Health Screening*

4. A. Expiratory grunting is a manifestation of respiratory distress.

   B. Nasal flaring is a manifestation of respiratory distress.

   C. **CORRECT:** Periods of apnea lasting less than 15 seconds are an expected finding.

   D. **CORRECT:** Newborns are obligatory nose breathers.

   E. Crackles and wheezing are manifestations of fluid or infection in the lungs.

   Ⓝ *NCLEX® Connection: Health Promotion and Maintenance, Health Screening*

5. A. **CORRECT:** Mongolian spots are commonly found over the lumbosacral area of newborns who have dark skin and are of African American, Asian, or Native American origin.

   B. Hyperbilirubinemia would present as jaundice.

   C. Forceps marks would most likely present as a cephalohematoma.

   D. Birth trauma would present as ecchymosis.

   Ⓝ *NCLEX® Connection: Health Promotion and Maintenance, Health Screening*

PRACTICE Answer

Using the ATI Active Learning Template: Growth and Development

PHYSICAL DEVELOPMENT

Assessment tools
- Brief initial systems assessment
- Gestational age assessment: Physical measurements and New Ballard Scale
- Vital signs
- Head-to-toe physical assessment

Reflexes
- Sucking and rooting: Turns head to side that is touched and begins to suck when cheek or edge of mouth is stroked.
- Palmar grasp: Grasps object when placed in palm.
- Plantar grasp: Toes curl downward when sole of the foot is touched.
- Moro reflex: Arms and legs symmetrically extend and then abduct while fingers spread to form a "C" when infant's head and trunk are allowed to fall backward to an angle of at least 30°.
- Tonic neck (fencer position): Extends arm and leg on same side when head is turned to that side, and flexes arm and leg of opposite side.
- Babinski: Toes fan upward and out when outer edge of sole of foot is stroked, moving up toward toes.
- Stepping: Makes stepping movements when held upright with feet touching flat surface.

Heart rate
- 100 to 160/min with brief fluctuations above and below, depending on activity level.
- When newborn is sleeping, place pediatric stethoscope head on fourth or fifth intercostal space at the left midclavicular line over apex of the heart. Listen for 1 full minute.
- Note any murmurs.

Ⓝ *NCLEX® Connection: Health Promotion and Maintenance, Health Screening*

CHAPTER 24 *Nursing Care of Newborns*

Newborn care consists of stabilization and/ or resuscitation. This can include establishing a patent airway, maintaining adequate oxygenation, and thermoregulation for the maintenance of body temperature. A physical assessment (physical examination, measurements, and monitoring laboratory studies) is done every 8 hr or as needed.

Nursing interventions and family teaching (umbilical cord care, prophylactic measures, newborn screening, newborn feedings and bathing, and fostering baby-friendly activities) are integrated into a newborn's plan of care.

ASSESSMENT

PHYSICAL ASSESSMENT

- Vital signs should be checked on admission/birth and every 30 min x 2, every 1 hr x 2, and then every 8 hr.
- Weight should be checked daily at the same time, using the same scale.
- Inspect the umbilical cord. Observe for any bleeding from the cord, and ensure that the cord is clamped securely to prevent hemorrhage.
- In the first 6 to 8 hr of life as body systems stabilize and pass through periods of adjustment, observe for periods of reactivity.
  - **First period of reactivity:** The newborn is alert, exhibits exploring activity, makes sucking sounds, and has a rapid heart rate and respiratory rate. Heart rate can be as high as 160 to 180/min, but will stabilize at a baseline of 100 to 120/min during a period that lasts 30 min after birth.
  - **Period of relative inactivity:** The newborn will become quiet and begin to rest and sleep. The heart rate and respirations will decrease, and this period will last from 60 to 100 min after birth.
  - **Second period of reactivity:** The newborn reawakens, becomes responsive again, and often gags and chokes on mucus that has accumulated in his mouth. This period usually occurs 2 to 8 hr after birth and can last 10 min to several hours.
- Using the facility's preferred pain assessment tool, conduct a pain assessment on the newborn every 8 to 12 hr and following painful procedures. Q EBP

LABORATORY TESTS

Hgb and Hct, if prescribed

Blood glucose for hypoglycemia, per facility policy or as prescribed

Metabolic screening
- Newborn genetic screening is mandated in all states. A capillary heel stick should be done 24 hr following birth. For results to be accurate, the newborn must have received formula or breast milk for at least 24 hr. If the newborn is discharged before 24 hr of age, the test should be repeated in 1 to 2 weeks.
- All states require testing for phenylketonuria (PKU). PKU is a defect in protein metabolism in which the accumulation of the amino acid phenylalanine can result in mental retardation. (Treatment in the first 2 months of life can prevent mental retardation.)

Other genetic testing that can be done includes for galactosemia, cystic fibrosis, maple syrup urine disease, hypothyroidism, and sickle cell disease.

Serum bilirubin on all newborns prior to discharge

Collecting blood samples
- Heel stick blood samples are obtained by the nurse, who dons clean gloves.
- Warm the newborn's heel first to increase circulation.
- Cleanse the area with an appropriate antiseptic, and allow for drying.
- A spring-activated lancet is used so that the skin incision is made quickly and painlessly.
- The outer aspect of the heel should be used, and the lancet should go no deeper than 2.4 mm to prevent necrotizing osteochondritis resulting from penetration of bone with the lancet.
- Follow facility protocol for specimen collection, equipment to be used, and labeling of specimens.
- Apply pressure with dry gauze (do not use alcohol because it will cause bleeding to continue) until bleeding stops, and cover with an adhesive bandage.
- Cuddle and comfort the newborn when the procedure is completed to reassure the newborn and promote feelings of safety.

DIAGNOSTIC PROCEDURES

Newborn hearing screening is required in most states. Newborns are screened so that hearing impairments can be detected and treated early. Q EBP

PATIENT-CENTERED CARE

NURSING CARE

Stabilize and/or give resuscitation to the newborn.

Respiratory complications

Monitor for clinical findings of respiratory complications.
- **Bradypnea:** respirations less than or equal to 30/min
- **Tachypnea:** respirations greater than or equal to 60/min
- **Abnormal breath sounds:** expiratory grunting, crackles, and wheezes
- **Respiratory distress:** nasal flaring, retractions, grunting, gasping, and labored breathing

INTERVENTIONS FOR STABILIZATION AND RESUSCITATION OF AIRWAY
- The newborn is able to clear most secretions in air passages by the cough reflex. Routine suctioning of the mouth, then the nasal passages with a bulb syringe, is done to remove excess mucus in the respiratory tract.
- Newborns delivered by cesarean birth are more susceptible to fluid remaining in the lungs than newborns who were delivered vaginally.
- If bulb suctioning is unsuccessful, mechanical suction and/or back blows and chest thrusts can be used, as well as the institution of emergency procedures.
- The bulb syringe should be kept with the newborn, and the newborn's family should be instructed on its use. Family members should be asked to perform a demonstration to show that they understand bulb syringe techniques.
  - Compress bulb before insertion into one side of the mouth.
  - Avoid center of the mouth to prevent stimulating gag reflex.
  - Aspirate mouth first, one nostril, then second nostril.

Identification

Identification (using two identifiers) is applied to the newborn immediately after birth by the nurse. It is an important safety measure to prevent the newborn from being given to the wrong parents, switched, or abducted. Qs
- The newborn, mother, and mother's partner are identified by plastic identification wristbands with permanent locks that must be cut to be removed. Identification bands should include the newborn's name, sex, date, and time of birth, and mother's health record number. The newborn should have one band placed on the ankle and one on the wrist. In addition, the newborn's footprints and mother's thumb prints are taken. The above information is also included with the footprint sheet.
- Each time the newborn is given to the parents, the identification band should be verified against the mother's identification band.
- All facility staff who assist in caring for the newborn are required to wear photo identification badges.

- The newborn is not to be given to anyone who does not have a photo identification badge that distinguishes that person as a staff member of the facility maternal-newborn unit.
- Many facilities have locked maternal-newborn units that require staff to permit entrance or exit. Some facilities have a sensor device on the ID band or umbilical cord clamp that sounds an alarm if the newborn is removed from the facility.

Thermoregulation

Thermoregulation provides a neutral thermal environment that helps a newborn maintain a normal core temperature with minimal oxygen consumption and caloric expenditure. A newborn has a relatively large surface-to-weight ratio, reduced metabolism per unit area, blood vessels close to the surface, and small amounts of insulation.
- The newborn keeps warm by metabolizing brown fat, which is unique to newborns, but only within a very narrow temperature range. Becoming chilled (cold stress) can increase the newborn's oxygen demands and rapidly use up brown fat reserves. Therefore, monitoring temperature regulation is important.
- Monitor for hypothermia in the newborn.
  - Axillary temperature of less than 36.5° C (97.7° F)
  - Cyanosis
  - Increased respiratory rate

INTERVENTIONS TO MAINTAIN THERMOREGULATION
- Core temperature varies within newborns, but it should be kept at approximately 36.5 to 37° C (97.7 to 98.6° F. Heat loss occurs by four mechanisms.
  - **Conduction:** Loss of body heat resulting from direct contact with a cooler surface. Preheat a radiant warmer, warm a stethoscope and other instruments, and pad a scale before weighing the newborn. The newborn should be placed directly on the mother's chest and covered with a warm blanket.
  - **Convection:** Flow of heat from the body surface to cooler environmental air. Place the bassinet out of the direct line of a fan or air conditioning vent, swaddle the newborn in a blanket, and keep the head covered. Any procedure done with the newborn uncovered should be performed under a radiant heat source. Keep ambient temperature of the nursery or mother's room at 22 to 26° C (72 to 78° F).
  - **Evaporation:** Loss of heat as surface liquid is converted to vapor. Gently rub the newborn dry with a warm sterile blanket (adhering to standard precautions) immediately after delivery. If thermoregulation is unstable, postpone the initial bath until the newborn's skin temperature is 36.5° C (97.7° F). When bathing, expose only one body part at a time, washing and drying thoroughly.
  - **Radiation:** Loss of heat from the body surface to a cooler solid surface that is close to, but not in direct contact. Keep the newborn and examining tables away from windows and air conditioners.
- Temperature stabilizes at 37° C (98.6° F) within 4 hr after birth if chilling is prevented.

Bathing

- Bathing can begin once the newborn's temperature has stabilized to at least 36.5° C (97.7° F). A complete sponge bath should be given within the first 1 to 2 hr after birth under a radiant heat source to prevent heat loss. If necessary, the first bath will be postponed until thermoregulation stabilizes.
- Gloves should be worn until the newborn's first bath to avoid exposure to body secretions.

Feeding

Feedings can be started immediately following birth.
- Breastfeeding is initiated as soon as possible after birth as part of baby-friendly initiatives.
- Formula feeding usually is started at about 2 to 4 hr of age. A few sips of sterile water can be given to assess sucking and swallowing reflexes and ensure that there are no anomalies, such as a tracheoesophageal fistula, prior to initiating formula.
  ○ The newborn is fed on demand, which is normally every 3 to 4 hr for bottle-fed newborns and more frequently for breastfed newborns.
  ○ Monitor and document feedings per facility protocol.

Sleep

- Sleep-wake states are variations of consciousness in the newborn consisting of six states along a continuum comprised of deep sleep, light sleep, drowsy, quiet alert, active alert, and crying.
- Newborns sleep approximately 16 to 19 hr/day with periods of wakefulness gradually increasing. Newborns are positioned supine, "safe sleep," to decrease the incidence of sudden infant death syndrome (SIDS). **Qs**
  ○ No bumper pads, loose linens, or toys should be placed in the bassinet.
  ○ Mothers should sleep in close proximity but not in a shared space. Higher incidence rates are noted for SIDS and suffocation with bed sharing/co-sleeping.
  ○ Educate parents about the need for immunizations as a measure to prevent SIDS.

Elimination

- Monitor elimination habits.
  ○ Newborns should void once within 24 hr of birth. They should void 6 to 8 times per 24 hr after day 4.
  ○ Meconium should be passed within the first 24 hr to 48 hr after birth. The newborn will then continue to pass stool 3 to 4 times a day depending on whether he is being breast- or bottle-fed.
  ○ The stools of newborns who are breastfed can appear yellow and seedy. They should have at least 3 stools per day for the first month. These stools are lighter in color and looser than the stools of newborns who are formula-fed.

- Monitor and document output.
  ○ Keep the perineal area clean and dry. The ammonia in urine is irritating to the skin and can cause diaper rash.
  ○ After each diaper change, cleanse the perineal area with clear water or water with a mild soap. Diaper wipes with alcohol should be avoided. Pat dry, and apply triple antibiotic ointment, petroleum jelly, or zinc oxide, depending on facility protocol.

Infection control

Infection control is essential in preventing cross-contamination from newborn to newborn and between newborns and staff. Newborns are at risk for infection during the first few months of life because of immature immune systems.
- Provide individual bassinets equipped with a thermometer, diapers, T-shirts, and bathing supplies.
- All personnel who care for a newborn should scrub with antimicrobial soap from elbows to finger tips before entering the nursery. In between care of the newborn, the nurse should follow facility hygiene protocols. Cover gowns or special uniforms are used to avoid direct contact with clothes.

Family education

Provide family education and promote family-newborn attachment. **QEBP**
- Provide family education while performing all nursing care. Encourage family involvement, allowing the mother and family to perform newborn care with direct supervision and support by the nurse.
- Encourage mothers and family to hold the newborn so that they can experience eye-to-eye contact and interaction.
- Foster sibling interaction in newborn care.

Umbilical cord care

Goal of cord care is to prevent or decrease risk for infection and hemorrhage.

NURSING CONSIDERATIONS
- Cord clamp stays in place for 24 to 48 hr.
- The Association of Women's Health, Obstetric and Neonatal Nurses (2013) recommendations for cord care include cleaning the cord with water (using cleanser sparingly if needed to remove debris) during the initial bath of the newborn.
- Assess stump and base of cord for erythema, edema, and drainage with each diaper change.
- The newborn's diaper should be folded down and away from the umbilical stump.
- Bathing infant by submerging in water should not occur until the cord has fallen off.
- Most cords fall off within the 10 to 14 days.

Erythromycin

- Prophylactic eye care is the mandatory instillation of antibiotic ointment into the eyes to prevent ophthalmia neonatorum.
- Infections can be transmitted during descent through the birth canal. Ophthalmia neonatorum is caused by Neisseria gonorrhoeae or Chlamydia trachomatis and can cause blindness.

NURSING CONSIDERATIONS
- Use a single-dose unit to avoid cross-contamination.
- Apply a 1 to 2 cm ribbon of ointment to the lower conjunctival sac of each eye, starting from the inner canthus and moving outward.
- A possible side effect is chemical conjunctivitis, causing redness, swelling, drainage, and temporarily blurred vision for 24 to 48 hr. Reassure the parents that this will resolve on its own.
- Application can be delayed for 1 hr after birth to facilitate baby-friendly activities during the first period of newborn reactivity.

Vitamin K (phytonadione)

Administered to prevent hemorrhagic disorders. Vitamin K is not produced in the gastrointestinal tract of the newborn until around day 7. Vitamin K is produced in the colon by bacteria that forms once formula or breast milk is introduced into the gut of the newborn.

NURSING CONSIDERATIONS: Administer 0.5 to 1 mg intramuscularly into the vastus lateralis (where muscle development is adequate) within 1 hr after birth.

Hepatitis B immunization

Provides protection against hepatitis B

NURSING CONSIDERATIONS
- Recommended to be administered to all newborns.
- Informed consent must be obtained.
- For newborns born to healthy women, recommended dosage schedule is at birth, 1 month, and 6 months.
- For mothers infected with hepatitis B, hepatitis B immunoglobulin and the hepatitis B vaccine is given within 12 hr of birth. The hepatitis B vaccine is given alone at 1 month, 2 months, and 12 months.

> ! It is important **NOT** to give the vitamin K and the hepatitis B injections in the same thigh. Sites should be alternated.

Cold stress

Ineffective thermoregulation can lead to hypoxia, acidosis, and hypoglycemia. Newborns who have respiratory distress are at a higher risk for hypothermia.

NURSING ACTIONS
- Monitor for manifestations of cold stress (cyanotic trunk, depressed respirations).
- The newborn should be warmed slowly over a period of 2 to 4 hr. Correct hypoxia by administering oxygen. Correct acidosis and hypoglycemia. Q̨EBP

Hypoglycemia

Frequently occurs in the first few hours of life secondary to the use of energy to establish respirations and maintain body heat.
- Newborns of mothers who have diabetes mellitus, are small or large for gestational age, are less than 37 weeks of gestation, or are greater than 42 weeks of gestation, are at risk for hypoglycemia and should have blood glucose monitored within the first 2 hr of life.
- Follow facility protocols regarding frequency of assessing blood glucose levels.

NURSING ACTIONS
- Monitor for jitteriness; twitching; a weak, high-pitched cry; irregular respiratory effort; cyanosis; lethargy; eye rolling; seizures; and a blood glucose level less than 40 mg/dL by heel stick.
- Have the mother breastfeed immediately or give donor breast milk or formula to elevate blood glucose levels. Brain damage can result if brain cells are depleted of glucose.

Hemorrhage

Due to improper cord care or placement of clamp

NURSING ACTIONS
- Ensure that the clamp is tight. If seepage of blood is noted, a second clamp should be applied.
- Notify the provider if bleeding continues.

Application Exercises

1. A nurse is preparing to administer prophylactic eye ointment to a newborn to prevent ophthalmia neonatorum. Which of the following medications should the nurse anticipate administering?

   A. Ofloxacin

   B. Nystatin

   C. Erythromycin

   D. Ceftriaxone

2. A newborn was not dried completely after birth. Which of the following mechanisms should the nurse understand causes heat loss?

   A. Conduction

   B. Convection

   C. Evaporation

   D. Radiation

3. A nurse is caring for a newborn immediately following birth. Which of the following nursing interventions is the highest priority?

   A. Initiating breastfeeding

   B. Performing the initial bath

   C. Giving a vitamin K injection

   D. Covering the newborn's head with a cap

4. A nurse is preparing to administer a vitamin K (phytonadione)injection to a newborn. Which of the following responses should the nurse make to the newborn's mother regarding why this medication is given?

   A. "It assists with blood clotting."

   B. "It promotes maturation of the bowel."

   C. "It is a preventative vaccine."

   D. "It provides immunity."

5. A nurse is taking a newborn to a mother following a circumcision. Which of the following actions should the nurse take for security purposes?

   A. Ask the mother to state her full name.

   B. Look at the name on the newborn's bassinet.

   C. Match the mother's identification band with the newborn's band.

   D. Compare name on the bassinet and room number.

PRACTICE Active Learning Scenario

A nurse is conducting a class for parents on care of the newborn. What should the nurse include in this class? Use the ATI Active Learning Template: Basic Concept to complete this item.

UNDERLYING PRINCIPLES: Describe three mechanisms that promote airway clearance.

NURSING INTERVENTIONS: Describe appropriate bulb syringe technique.

1. A. Ofloxacin is an antibiotic, but it is not used for ophthalmia neonatorum.

   B. Nystatin is used to treat *Candida albicans*, an oral yeast infection.

   C. **CORRECT:** One medication of choice for ophthalmia neonatorum is erythromycin ophthalmic ointment 0.5%. This antibiotic provides prophylaxis against *Neisseria gonorrhoeae* and *Chlamydia trachomatis*.

   D. Ceftriaxone is an antibiotic, but it is not used for ophthalmia neonatorum.

   ⓝ *NCLEX® Connection: Pharmacological and Parenteral Therapies, Medication Administration*

2. A. Conduction is the loss of heat from the body surface area to cooler surfaces that the newborn can be in contact with.

   B. Convection is the flow of heat from the body surface area to cooler air.

   C. **CORRECT:** Evaporation is the loss of heat that occurs when a liquid is converted to a vapor. In a newborn, heat loss by evaporation occurs as a result of vaporization of the moisture from the skin.

   D. Radiation is the loss of heat to a cooler surface that is not in direct contact with the newborn.

   ⓝ *NCLEX® Connection: Health Promotion and Maintenance, Aging Process*

3. A. Initiating breastfeeding is important following birth, but it is not the priority action.

   B. Initial baths are not given until the newborn's temperature is stable. It is not the priority action.

   C. Vitamin K can be given immediately after birth, but it is not the priority action.

   D. **CORRECT:** The greatest risk to the newborn is cold stress. Therefore the highest priority intervention is to prevent heat loss. Covering the newborn's head with a cap prevents cold stress due to excessive evaporative heat loss.

   ⓝ *NCLEX® Connection: Management of Care, Establishing Priorities*

4. A. **CORRECT:** Vitamin K is deficient in a newborn because the colon is sterile. Until bacteria are present to stimulate vitamin K production, the newborn is at risk for hemorrhagic disease.

   B. Vitamin K does not assist the bowel to mature.

   C. Vitamin K is not part of the vaccines that are administered.

   D. Vitamin K does not provide immunity.

   ⓝ *NCLEX® Connection: Pharmacological and Parenteral Therapies, Medication Administration*

5. A. Asking the mother to state her full name is not appropriate verification because two identifiers should be used.

   B. Looking at the name on the bassinet is not appropriate verification because two identifiers should be used.

   C. **CORRECT:** Each time the newborn is taken to the mother, the mother's identification band should be verified against the newborn's identification band.

   D. Comparing the name on the bassinet with the room number is not appropriate verification because it does not include two identifiers involving the mother and newborn.

   ⓝ *NCLEX® Connection: Safety and Infection Control, Accident/Error/Injury Prevention*

PRACTICE Answer

Using the ATI Active Learning Template: Basic Concept

UNDERLYING PRINCIPLES: Mechanisms that promote airway clearance
- Infant's cough reflex
- Mechanical suctioning, back blows/chest thrusts
- Use of the bulb syringe for suctioning

NURSING INTERVENTIONS: Bulb syringe technique
- Depress the bulb.
- Insert syringe into side of mouth, avoiding center of the mouth.
- Suction mouth first, then one nostril, then second nostril.

ⓝ *NCLEX® Connection: Safety and Infection Control, Home Safety*

UNIT 4   NEWBORN NURSING CARE
SECTION: LOW-RISK NEWBORN

CHAPTER 25 *Newborn Nutrition*

Acquiring an understanding of the nutritional needs of newborns (breastfeeding, human pasteurized milk/donor milk, formula/bottle-feeding) is essential. This includes nutrition considerations, complications, and interventions.

NUTRITIONAL NEEDS FOR THE NEWBORN

Desirable growth and development of the newborn is enhanced by good nutrition. Feeding the newborn provides an opportunity for parents to meet the newborn's nutritional needs as well as an opportunity for them to bond with the newborn. Whether the mother chooses to breastfeed, use donor milk, or formula (bottle) feed, nurses should provide education and support.

- Normal newborn weight loss immediately after birth and subsequent weight gain should be as follows.
  - **Loss of 5% to 10% after birth (regain 10 to 14 days after birth)**
  - **Gain of 110 to 200 g/week for first 3 months**
- Healthy newborns need a fluid intake of 100 to 140 mL/kg/24 hr. Newborns do not need to be given water because they receive sufficient water from breast milk or formula.
- Adequate caloric intake is essential to provide energy for growth, digestion, metabolic needs, and activity. For the first 3 months, the newborn requires 110 kcal/kg/day. From 3 to 6 months, the requirement decreases to 100 kcal/kg/day. Both breast milk and formula provide 20 kcal/oz.
- Carbohydrates should make up 40% to 50% of the newborn's total caloric intake. The most abundant carbohydrate in breast milk or formula is lactose.
- At least 15% of calories must come from fat (triglycerides). The fat in breast milk is easier to digest than the fat in cow's milk.
- For adequate growth and development, a newborn must receive 2.25 to 4 g/kg/day of protein.
- Breast milk contains the vitamins necessary to provide adequate newborn nutrition. According to the American Academy of Pediatrics, all infants who are breastfed or partially breastfed should receive 400 IU of vitamin D daily beginning in the first few days of life. Infant formula has vitamins added, but vitamin D supplements also are recommended. Mothers who are breastfeeding and are vegetarians who exclude meat, fish, and dairy products should provide vitamin B_{12} supplementation to their newborns. Q EBP

- The mineral content of commercial newborn formula and breast milk is adequate with the exception of iron and fluoride.
  - Iron is low in all forms of milk, but it is absorbed better from breast milk. Newborns who only breastfeed for the first 6 months maintain adequate hemoglobin levels and do not need additional iron supplementation. After 6 months of age, all newborns need to be fed iron-fortified cereal and other foods rich in iron. Newborns who are formula-fed should receive iron-fortified newborn formula until 12 months of age. Mothers who breastfeed their newborns are encouraged to do so for the newborn's first 12 months of life.
  - Fluoride levels in breast milk and formulas are low. A fluoride supplement should be given to newborns not receiving fluoridated water after 6 months of age.
- Solids are not introduced until 6 months of age. If introduced too early, food allergies can develop.

BREASTFEEDING

Breastfeeding is the optimal source of nutrition for newborns. Breastfeeding is recommended exclusively for the first 6 months of age by the American Academy of Pediatrics. Newborns should be breastfed every 2 to 3 hr. Parents should awaken the newborn to feed at least every 3 hr during the day and at least every 4 hr during the night until the newborn is feeding well and gaining weight adequately. Breastfeeding should occur 8 to 12 times within a 24-hr window. Then, a feed-on-demand schedule can be followed.

- For the first few days after birth, the baby receives colostrum (early milk). Colostrum is secreted from the mother's breasts during postpartum days 1 to 3. It contains immunoglobulin A (IgA), which provides passive immunity to the newborn.
- Nursing interventions can help a new mother be successful in breastfeeding. This includes the provision of adequate calories and fluids to support breastfeeding. The practice of rooming-in (allowing mothers and newborns to remain together) should be encouraged as part of baby-friendly initiatives. Lactation consultants can improve the mother's efforts and success in breastfeeding. Q TC

ADVANTAGES OF BREASTFEEDING

Parents should be presented with factual information about the nutritional and immunological needs of their newborn. The nurse should present information about both breastfeeding and bottle feeding in a nonjudgmental manner. The optimal time to provide newborn nutritional information is during pregnancy, so that the parents make a decision prior to hospital admission.

BENEFITS OF BREASTFEEDING
- Reduces the risk of infection by providing IgA antibodies, lysozymes, leukocytes, macrophages, and lactoferrin that prevents infections.
- Promotes rapid brain growth due to large amounts of lactose.

- Provides protein and nitrogen for neurological cell building and improves the newborn's ability to regulate calcium and phosphorus levels.
- Contains electrolytes and minerals.
- Breast milk is easy for the newborn to digest.
- Breastfeeding is convenient and inexpensive.
- Reduces incidence of sudden infant death syndrome (SIDS), allergies, and childhood obesity.
- Promotes maternal–infant bonding and attachment.

Benefits specific to the infant: Decreased risk for gastrointestinal infections, celiac disease, asthma, lower respiratory tract infections, otitis media, sudden infant death syndrome (SIDS), obesity in adolescence and adulthood, diabetes mellitus types 1 and 2, and acute lymphocytic and myeloid leukemia

Benefits specific to the mother: Decreased postpartum bleeding and more rapid uterine involution, decreased risk for ovarian and breast cancer, diabetes mellitus type 2, hypertension, hypercholesterolemia, cardiovascular disease, and rheumatoid arthritis

Benefits specific to families and society: Convenient, less expensive than formula, reduces annual health care costs, and reduces environmental burden related to disposal of formula packaging and equipment

NURSING INTERVENTIONS

Successful breastfeeding

- Place the newborn skin-to-skin on the mother's chest immediately after birth. Initiate breastfeeding as soon as possible or within the first 30 min following birth.
- Explain breastfeeding techniques to the mother. Have the mother wash her hands, get comfortable, and have caffeine-free, nonalcoholic fluids to drink during breastfeeding.
- Explain the let-down reflex (stimulation of maternal nipple releases oxytocin that causes the let-down of milk).
- Reassure the mother that uterine cramps are normal during breastfeeding, resulting from oxytocin, which also promote uterine involution.
- Express a few drops of colostrum or milk and spread it over the nipple to lubricate the nipple and entice the newborn.
- Show the mother the proper latch-on position. Have her support the breast in one hand with the thumb on top and four fingers underneath. With the newborn's mouth in front of the nipple, the newborn can be stimulated to open his mouth by tickling his lower lip with the tip of the nipple. The mother pulls the newborn to the nipple with his mouth covering part of the areola as well as the nipple.
- Explain to the mother that when her newborn is latched on correctly, his nose, cheeks, and chin will be touching her breast. Hunger cues include hand to mouth or hand to hand movements, sucking motions, and rooting reflex.
- Demonstrate the four basic breastfeeding positions: football hold (under the arm), cradle (most common) or modified cradle (across the lap), and side-lying. **(25.1)**

- Encourage the mother to breastfeed at least 15 to 20 min per breast to ensure that her newborn receives adequate fat and protein, which is richest in the breast milk as it empties the breast. Newborns need to be breastfed at least 8 to 12 times in a 24 hr. period.
- Avoid educating mothers regarding the duration of newborn feedings. Mothers should be instructed to evaluate when the newborn has completed the feeding, including slowing of newborn suckling, a softened breast, or sleeping. Both breasts should be offered to ensure that each breast receives equal stimulation and emptying.
- Explain to the mother that newborns will nurse on demand after a pattern is established.
- Show the mother how to insert a finger in the side of the newborn's mouth to break the suction from the nipple prior to removing the newborn from the breast to prevent nipple trauma.
- Show the mother how to burp the newborn when she alternates breasts. The newborn should be burped either over the shoulder or in an upright position with his chin supported. The mother should gently pat the newborn on his back to elicit a burp.
- Tell the mother to begin the newborn's next feeding with the breast she stopped feeding him with in the previous feeding.
- Tell the mother how to tell if her newborn is receiving adequate feeding (gaining weight, voiding 6 to 8 diapers per day, and contentedness between feedings).
- Explain to the mother that the newborn can have loose, pale, and/or yellow stools during breastfeeding, and that this is normal.
- Tell the mother to avoid nipple confusion in the newborn by not offering supplemental formula, pacifier, or soothers until breastfeeding has been established typically 2 to 3 weeks. Supplementation can be provided using a small feeding or syringe feeding, if needed. When supplementation is deemed necessary, giving the baby expressed breast milk is best.
- Tell the mother to always place her newborn on his back after feedings.
- Promote rooming-in efforts.
- Offer referral to breastfeeding support groups.
- Contact a lactation consultant to offer additional recommendations and support, especially to mothers who have concerns about adequate breast milk or mothers who have been unsuccessful with breastfeeding in the past.
- Herbal products, such as fenugreek or blessed thistle, and prescription medications, such as metoclopramide, have been reported to increase breast milk production. There is insufficient data to confirm or deny their effect on lactation. Mothers should check with the provider before taking over-the-counter or prescription medications. Q EBP

Successful storage of breast milk obtained by a breast pump

- Inform the mother that breast milk can still be provided to the newborn during periods of separation by using a breast pump or hand expression.
  - Breast pumps can be manual, electric, or battery-operated and pumped directly into a bottle or freezer bag.
  - One or both breasts can be pumped, and suction is adjustable for comfort.
- Teach the parents that breast milk must be stored according to guidelines for proper containers, labeling, refrigerating, and freezing.
  - Breast milk can be stored at room temperature under very clean conditions for up to 8 hr. It can be refrigerated in sterile bottles for use within 8 days, or can be frozen in sterile containers in the freezer compartment of a refrigerator for up to 6 months. Breast milk can be stored in a deep freezer for 12 months.
  - Thawing the milk in the refrigerator for 24 hr is the best way to preserve the immunoglobulins present in it. It also can be thawed by holding the container under running lukewarm water or placing it in a container of lukewarm water. The bottle should be rotated often, but not shaken when thawing in this manner.
  - Thawing by microwave is contraindicated because it destroys some of the immune factors and lysozymes contained in the milk. Microwave thawing also leads to the development of hot spots in the milk because of uneven heating, which can burn the newborn.
  - Do not refreeze thawed milk.
  - Used portions of breast milk must be discarded.

HUMAN MILK FEEDING/DONOR MILK

If the mother is not able to provide the breast milk, the recommended alternative is pasteurized donor milk from a milk bank (obtain informed consent). However, in many cases, it's not readily accessible, and a commercial infant formula is used.

FORMULA (BOTTLE) FEEDING

Formula feeding can be a successful and adequate source of nutrition if the mother chooses not to breastfeed. The newborn should be fed every 3 to 4 hr. Parents should awaken the newborn to feed at least every 3 hr during the day and at least every 4 hr during the night until the newborn is feeding well and gaining weight adequately. Then, a feed-on-demand schedule can be followed.

NURSING INTERVENTIONS

- Teach the parents how to prepare formula (mix according to instructions), bottles, and nipples. Review the importance of hand washing prior to formula preparation.
- Teach the parents about the different forms of formula (ready-to-feed, concentrated, and powder) and how to prepare each correctly.

- Bottles and accessories can be put in the dishwasher, boiled, or washed by hand in hot soapy water using a good bottle and nipple brush.
- Teach parents to wash the lid of a can of concentrated formula with hot soapy water, and shake before opening it.

25.1 Breastfeeding positions

Football hold

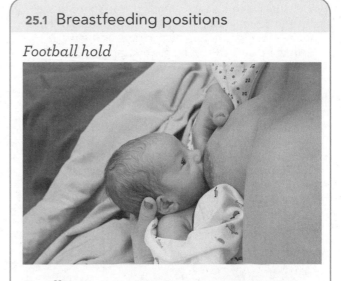

Cradle

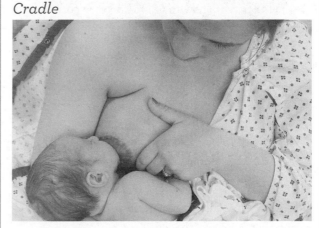

Modified cradle
The mother positions the baby as in the cradle position shown above, but reverses the function of each arm.

Side-lying

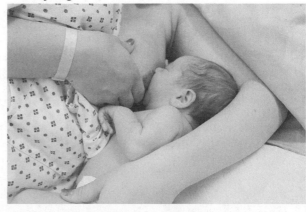

- Instruct parents to use tap water to mix concentrated or powder formula. If the water source is questionable, tap water should be boiled first.
- Instruct parents that prepared formula can be refrigerated for up to 48 hr.
- Teach the parents to check the flow of formula from the bottle to ensure it is not coming out too slow or too fast.
- Advise parents not to use formula past the expiration date located on the container.
- Show the parents how to cradle the newborn in their arms in a semi-upright position. The newborn should not be placed in the supine position during bottle feeding because of the danger of aspiration. Newborns who bottle feed do best when held close and at a 45° angle.
- Instruct the mother how to place the nipple on top of the newborn's tongue.
- Keep the nipple filled with formula to prevent the newborn from swallowing air.
- Always hold the bottle and never prop the bottle for feeding.
- Give newborn opportunities to burp several times during a feeding
- Place the newborn on his back after feedings.
- Tell the parents to discard any unused formula remaining in the bottle when the newborn is finished feeding due to the possibility of bacterial contamination. **Qs**
- Teach the parents how to tell if their newborn is being adequately fed (gaining weight; bowel movements are yellow, soft and formed; and satisfaction between feedings). Breastfed infants usually have 3 or more bowel movements a day; formula-fed infants less frequent. Breastfed and formula-fed infants usually have 6 or more wet diapers a day.

RISK FACTORS FOR IMPAIRED NEWBORN NUTRITION

Risk factors for failure to thrive (newborn) can be related to ineffective feeding patterns of the newborn or inadequate breastfeeding by the mother.

NEWBORN FACTORS
- Inadequate breastfeeding
- Illness/infection
- Malabsorption
- Other conditions that increase energy needs

MATERNAL FACTORS
- Inadequate or slow milk production
- Inadequate emptying of the breast
- Inappropriate timing of feeding
- Inadequate breast tissue
- Pain with feeding
- Maternal hemorrhage
- Illness/infection

MONITORING NEWBORN FOR ADEQUATE GROWTH

- Monitor the newborn for adequate growth and weight gain.
  - Weights are done daily in the newborn nursery. Every newborn should be seen and examined at the doctor's office within 72 hr (2 to 3 days) after discharge from the hospital. Growth is assessed by placing the newborn's weight on a growth chart. Adequate growth should be within the 10th to 90th percentile. Poor weight gain would be below 10%, and too much weight gain would be above 90%.
  - The newborn's length and head circumference are also routinely monitored.
- Assess the mother's ability to feed her newborn, whether by breast or bottle.
- Calculate the newborn's 24-hr I&O, if indicated, to ensure adequate nutrition.

ASSESSMENT OF NEWBORN NUTRITION

Assessment of newborn nutrition begins during pregnancy and continues after birth by reviewing the parents' attitudes and choices about their newborn's feeding. Breastfeeding is the preferred method. However, if the mother chooses not to breastfeed, she must not be made to feel guilty.

NEWBORN
- Maturity level
- History of labor and delivery
- Birth trauma
- Maternal risk factors
- Congenital defects
- Physical stability
- State of alertness
- Presence of bowel sounds

MOTHER
- Previous experience with breastfeeding
- Knowledge about breastfeeding
- Cultural factors
- Feelings about breastfeeding
- Physical features of breasts
- Physical/psychological readiness
- Support of family and significant others

INTERVENING FOR NEWBORN NUTRITION

Provide the mother with education about feeding-readiness cues exhibited by newborns and encourage the mother to begin feeding her newborn upon cues rather than waiting until the newborn is crying. Cues include the following.
- Hand-to-mouth or hand-to-hand movements
- Sucking motions
- Rooting
- Mouthing

COMPLICATIONS FOR NEWBORN NUTRITION

There can be special considerations when a newborn has difficulty receiving adequate nutrition. Nursing interventions can often help these newborns receive adequate nutrition.

NEWBORNS WHO ARE SLEEPY
- Unwrap the newborn.
- Change the newborn's diaper.
- Hold the newborn upright, and turn him from side to side.
- Talk to the newborn.
- Massage the newborn's back, and rub his hands and feet.
- Apply a cool cloth to the newborn's face.

NEWBORNS WHO ARE FUSSY
- Swaddle the newborn.
- Hold the newborn close, move, and rock him gently.
- Reduce the newborn's environmental stimuli.
- Place the newborn skin-to-skin.

Failure to thrive

Failure to thrive is slow weight gain. A newborn usually falls below the 5th percentile on the growth chart.

NEWBORNS WHO ARE BREASTFEEDING
- Evaluate positioning and latch-on during breastfeeding. **(25.1)**
- Massage the breast during feeding. ○EBP

- Determine feeding patterns and length of feedings.
- If the newborn is spitting up, the newborn can have an allergy to dairy products. Determine the maternal intake of dairy products. The mother can need to eliminate dairy from her diet. Instruct her to consume other food sources high in calcium or calcium supplements.

NEWBORNS WHO ARE FORMULA FEEDING
- Evaluate how much and how often the newborn is feeding.
- If the newborn is spitting up or vomiting, he can have an allergy or intolerance to cow's milk-based formula and can require a soy-based formula.

PRACTICE Active Learning Scenario

A nurse is teaching about the use of a breast pump and storing breast milk with a group of new mothers. What information should the nurse include in the teaching? Use the ATI Active Learning Template: Basic Concept to complete this item.

RELATED CONTENT

List the types of breast pumps.

Describe use of the pump.

NURSING INTERVENTIONS

Describe storage and freezing of milk.

Describe procedures for thawing milk.

Application Exercises

1. A nurse is giving instructions to a mother about how to breastfeed her newborn. Which of the following actions by the mother indicates understanding of the teaching?

   A. The mother places a few drops of water on her nipple before feeding.

   B. The mother gently removes her nipple from the infant's mouth to break the suction.

   C. When she is ready to breastfeed, the mother gently strokes the newborn's neck with her finger.

   D. When latched on, the infant's nose, cheek, and chin are touching the breast.

2. A nurse is teaching a group of new parents about proper techniques for bottle feeding. Which of the following instructions should the nurse provide?

   A. Burp the newborn at the end of the feeding.

   B. Hold the newborn close in a supine position.

   C. Keep the nipple full of formula throughout the feeding.

   D. Refrigerate any unused formula.

3. A nurse is caring for a newborn. Which of the following actions by the newborn indicates readiness to feed?

   A. Spits up clear mucus

   B. Attempts to place his hand in his mouth

   C. Turns his head toward sounds

   D. Lies quietly with his eyes open

4. A nurse is reviewing formula preparation with parents who plan to bottle-feed their newborn. Which of the following information should the nurse include in the teaching? (Select all that apply.)

   A. Use a disinfectant wipe to clean the lid of the formula can.

   B. Store prepared formula in the refrigerator for up to 72 hr.

   C. Place used bottles in the dishwasher.

   D. Check the nipple for appropriate flow of formula.

   E. Use tap water to dilute concentrated formula.

5. A nurse is reviewing breastfeeding positions with the mother of a newborn. Which of the following positions should the nurse discuss?

   A. Over-the-shoulder

   B. Supine

   C. Chin-supported

   D. Cradle

Application Exercises Key

1. A. The infant is enticed to suck when the mother spreads colostrum on the nipple.

    B. The mother should insert a finger in the side of the newborn's mouth to break the suction before removing her nipple.

    C. The mother should stroke the newborn's lips with her nipple to promote sucking.

    D. **CORRECT:** Effective latching-on includes the infant's nose, cheek and chin touching the mother's breast.

    (N) *NCLEX® Connection: Health Promotion and Maintenance, Ante/Intra/Postpartum and Newborn Care*

2. A. The newborn should be burped after each ½ oz of formula.

    B. The newborn should be cradled in a semi-upright position.

    C. **CORRECT:** The nipple should always be kept full of formula to prevent the newborn from sucking in air during the feeding.

    D. Any unused formula should be discarded due to the possibility of bacterial contamination.

    (N) *NCLEX® Connection: Health Promotion and Maintenance, Ante/Intra/Postpartum and Newborn Care*

3. A. Spitting up, coughing, or gagging on mucus is an attempt by the newborn to clear his airway.

    B. **CORRECT:** Readiness-to-feed cues include the newborn making hand-to-mouth and hand-to-hand movements, sucking motions, rooting, and mouthing.

    C. The infant turns his head toward sounds in the environment as a sensory response indicating normal central nervous system functioning.

    D. Lying quietly with eyes open is an alerting behavior, indicating normal newborn reactivity.

    (N) *NCLEX® Connection: Health Promotion and Maintenance, Ante/Intra/Postpartum and Newborn Care*

4. A. Chemicals from the disinfectant wipe can remain on the lid during opening and mix with the formula.

    B. Once formula is prepared, it can be refrigerated for up to 48 hr.

    C. **CORRECT:** Bottles can be placed in a dishwasher or washed by hand in hot soapy water using a good bottle brush.

    D. **CORRECT:** The flow of formula from the nipple should be checked to determine that it is not too fast or too slow.

    E. **CORRECT:** Tap water is used to mix concentrated or powder formula. If the water is from a questionable source, it should be boiled first.

    (N) *NCLEX® Connection: Health Promotion and Maintenance, Ante/Intra/Postpartum and Newborn Care*

5. A. An over-the-shoulder position can be used when burping the newborn.

    B. The supine position is appropriate for the sleeping newborn.

    C. Holding the newborn upright with the chin supported is a position that can be used when burping the newborn.

    D. **CORRECT:** The cradle position for breastfeeding includes the mother laying the newborn across her forearm with her hand supporting the lower back and buttocks.

    (N) *NCLEX® Connection: Health Promotion and Maintenance, Ante/Intra/Postpartum and Newborn Care*

PRACTICE Answer

Using the ATI Active Learning Template: Basic Concept

RELATED CONTENT

Types of breast pumps
- Manual
- Electric
- Battery-operated

Use of the pump: Pumping of one or both breasts using adjustable suction for comfort to obtain breast milk for storage in a bottle or freezer bag

NURSING INTERVENTIONS

Storage
- Store at room temperature under very clean conditions for up to 8 hr.
- Refrigerate in sterile bottles for use within 8 days.
- Freeze in sterile containers in the freezer of a refrigerator for up to 6 months.
- Store in a deep freezer for up to 12 months.

Thawing
- Thaw milk in the refrigerator for 24 hr to preserve immunoglobulins.
- Hold container under running lukewarm water or place in a pan of lukewarm water; bottle should be rotated, but not shaken.
- Do not thaw in a microwave.

(N) *NCLEX® Connection: Health Promotion and Maintenance, Ante/Intra/Postpartum and Newborn Care*

CHAPTER 26 *Nursing Care and Discharge Teaching*

Discharge teaching and newborn care include bathing, umbilical cord care, circumcision, car seat safety, environmental safety, newborn behaviors, feeding, elimination and clinical findings of illness to report to the provider.

Prior to discharge, a nurse should provide anticipatory guidance to prepare new parents to care for their newborn at home. Mothers and newborns are normally discharged 48 hr following a vaginal delivery or 72 hr following a cesarean birth. Serious complications can result if improper discharge instructions are given to the parents prior to taking the newborn home.

A nurse should inquire about the family's current experience and knowledge regarding newborn care, anticipate the learning needs of the parents, and assess their readiness for learning to provide education about newborn care.

Parents should be made aware of general guidelines about newborn behavior and care. These guidelines include causes of crying in the newborn, quieting techniques, sleeping patterns, hunger cues, and feeding, bathing, and clothing the newborn.

Parents need to be aware of the importance of well-newborn checkups, immunization schedules, and when to call the provider for signs of illness.

Providing a safe protective environment at home should be stressed to new parents and should include instruction about proper car seat usage, which is a very important part of the discharge instruction process. Qs

ASSESSMENT OF FAMILY READINESS FOR HOME CARE OF THE NEWBORN

- Previous newborn experience and knowledge
- Parent-newborn attachment
- Adjustment to the parental role
- Social support
- Educational needs
- Sibling rivalry issues
- Readiness of the parents to have their home and lifestyle altered to accommodate their newborn
- Parents' ability to verbalize and demonstrate newborn care following teaching

INTERVENTIONS FOR HOME CARE OF THE NEWBORN

Through verbal discussion, pamphlets, and demonstration, the nurse provides education to the client and family regarding newborn behavior, quieting techniques, newborn care, signs of newborn well-being and illness, and issues of newborn safety. Qpcc

CRYING

Inform the parents that newborns cry when they are hungry, overstimulated, wet, cold, hot, tired, bored, or need to be burped. Assure the mother that, in time, she will learn what her newborn's cry means. Instruct the mother not to feed her newborn every time he cries. Overfeeding can lead to stomach aches and diarrhea. After checking the newborn, it is okay to let her cry for short periods of time.

QUIETING TECHNIQUES

- Swaddling
- Close skin contact
- Nonnutritive sucking with pacifier
- Rhythmic noises to simulate utero sounds
- Movement (a car ride, vibrating chair, infant swing, rocking newborn)
- Placing the newborn on his stomach across a holder's lap while gently bouncing legs
- En face position for eye contact (when parents and newborns faces are about 30 cm (12 in) apart and on the same plane
- Stimulation

SLEEP-WAKE CYCLE

- Reinforce to the parents that placing the newborn in the supine position for sleeping greatly decreases the risk of sudden infant death syndrome.
- Newborns sleep approximately 16 to 19 hr/day with periods of wakefulness gradually increasing.
- Many parents believe that adding solid food to the newborn's diet will help with sleep patterns. During the first 6 months of life, the American Academy of Pediatrics recommends only breastfeeding. Most newborns will sleep through the night without a feeding by 4 to 5 months of age. The provider will instruct the parents when to add solid food to the newborn's diet.

- Keep the newborn's environment quiet and dark at night.
- Place the newborn in a crib or bassinet to sleep. The newborn should never sleep in the parents' bed due to the risk of suffocation.
- Most newborns get their days and nights mixed up. Provide basic suggestions for helping the parents develop a predictable routine. Bring the newborn out into the center of the action in the afternoon, and keep him there for the rest of the evening. Bathe him right before bedtime so that he feels soothed. Give him his last feeding around 2300, and then place him into a crib or bassinet.
- When awake, the newborn can be placed on his abdomen to promote muscle development for crawling. The infant should be supervised.
- For nighttime feedings and diaper changes, keep a small night-light on to avoid having to turn on bright lights. Speak softly, and handle the newborn gently so that he goes back to sleep easily.

ORAL AND NASAL SUCTIONING

Review correct technique with the parents.

POSITIONING AND HOLDING OF THE NEWBORN (HEAD SUPPORT)

Teach the parents that the newborn has minimal head control. The head should be supported when the newborn is lifted because the head is larger and heavier than the rest of the body.

FOUR BASIC WAYS TO HOLD THE NEWBORN
- **Cradle hold:** Cradle the newborn's head in the bend of the elbow. This permits eye-to-eye contact and is a good position for feeding.
- **Upright position:** Hold the newborn upright, and face him toward the holder while supporting his head, upper back, and buttocks.
- **Football hold:** Support half of the newborn's body in the holder's forearm with the newborn's head and neck resting in the palm of the hand. This is a good position for breastfeeding and when shampooing the newborn's hair.
- **Colic hold:** Place the newborn face-down along the holder's forearm with the hand firmly between the newborn's legs. The newborn's cheek should be by the holder's elbow on the outside. The newborn should be able to see the ground, and the holder's arm should be close to the body, using it to brace and steady the newborn. This is a good position for quieting a fussy newborn.

SWADDLING

Parents should be shown how to swaddle their newborn. Swaddling the newborn snugly in a receiving blanket helps the newborn to feel more secure. Swaddling brings the newborn's extremities in closer to his trunk, which is similar to the intrauterine position. Q EBP

BATHING

- After the initial bath, the newborn's face, diaper area, and skin folds are cleansed daily. Complete bathing is performed two to three times per week using a mild soap that does not contain hexachlorophene.
- Bathing by immersion is not done until the newborn's umbilical cord has fallen off and the circumcision has healed, if applicable. Wash the area around the cord, taking care not to get the cord wet. Move from the cleanest to dirtiest part of the newborn's body, beginning with his eyes, face, and head; proceed to the chest, arms, and legs; and wash the groin area last.
- Teach the parents proper newborn bathing techniques by a demonstration. Have the parents return the demonstration.
- Bathing should take place at the convenience of the parents, but not immediately after feeding to prevent spitting up and vomiting.
- Organize all equipment so that the newborn is not left unattended. Never leave the newborn alone in the tub or sink.
- Make sure the hot water heater is set at 49° C (120.2° F) or less. The room should be warm, and the bath water should be 36.6° to 37.2° C (98° to 99° F). Test the water for comfort on inner wrist prior to bathing the newborn.
- Avoid drafts or chilling of the newborn. Expose only the body part being bathed, and dry the newborn thoroughly to prevent chilling and heat loss.
- The newborn's eyes should be cleaned using a clean portion of the wash cloth. Clear water should be used to clean each eye, moving from the inner to the outer canthus.
- Each area of the newborn's body should be washed, rinsed, and dried, with no soap left on the skin.
- Wrap the newborn in a towel, and swaddle him in a football hold to shampoo his head. Rinse shampoo from the newborn's head, and dry to avoid chilling.
- In male newborns, to cleanse an uncircumcised penis, wash with soap and water and rinse the penis. The foreskin should not be forced back or constriction can result.
- In female newborns, wash the vulva by wiping from front to back to prevent contamination of the vagina or urethra from rectal bacteria.
- Applying a fragrance-free, hypoallergenic, moisturizing emollient immediately after bathing can help prevent dry skin.

FEEDING/ELIMINATION

- Mothers who are breastfeeding should be seen by the lactation consultant.
- Every newborn should be seen and examined at the doctor's office within 72 hr (2 to 3 days) after discharge from the hospital
- The newborn is offered the breast immediately after birth and frequently thereafter. Newborns need to be breastfed at least 8 to 12 times in a 24-hr period. Newborns who are breastfed will average 15 to 20 min per breast and 30 to 40 min for the total feeding. Feedings should be 8 to 12 times in a 24-hr period. Feeding for a newborn who is breastfeeding should be on demand or every 2 to 3 hr. Newborns who are formula-fed should also be fed on demand or every 3 to 4 hr. Parents should awaken the newborn to feed at least every 3 hr during the day and at least every 4 hr at night. Once the newborn is feeding well and gaining weight adequately, going to demand feeding is appropriate.
- Inform parents that adhering to specific timing of feedings is to be avoided. Parents should be instructed to recognize when the newborn has completed the feeding. No other fluids are offered to the newborn unless indicated by the provider.
- The mother's milk supply is equal to the demand of the newborn. Eventually, the newborn will empty a breast within 5 to 10 min, but can need to continue to suck to meet comfort needs.
- Frequent feedings (every 2 hr can be indicated), and manual expression of milk to initiate flow can be needed.
- Most newborns spit up a small amount after feedings. Keep the newborn upright and quiet for a few minutes after feedings.
- Breastfed newborns should have three or more bowel movements per day; formula (bottle) fed newborns are less frequent. Breastfed newborns should have six or more wet diapers per day; formula-fed infants have a similar number of voids.

DIAPERING

To avoid diaper rash, the newborn's diaper area should be kept clean and dry. Diapers should be changed frequently, and the perineal area cleaned with warm water or wipes and dried thoroughly to prevent skin breakdown.

CORD CARE

- Before discharge, the cord clamp is removed.
- Prevent cord infection by keeping the cord dry, and keep the top of the diaper folded underneath it.
- Sponge baths are given until the cord falls off, which occurs around 10 to 14 days after birth. Tub bathing and submersion can follow.
- Cord infection (a complication of improper cord care) can result if the cord is not kept clean and dry.
  - Monitor for manifestations of a cord that is moist and red, has a foul odor, or has purulent drainage.
  - Notify the provider immediately if findings of cord infection are present.

CIRCUMCISION CARE

Circumcision is the surgical removal of the foreskin of the penis.

- Circumcision is a personal choice made by the newborn's family for reasons of health and hygiene, religious conviction (Jewish male on eighth day after birth), tradition, culture, or social norms. Parents should make a well-informed decision in consultation with the provider.
- Circumcision should not be done immediately following birth because the newborn's level of vitamin K is at a low point, and the newborn would be at risk for hemorrhage.

HEALTH BENEFITS OF CIRCUMCISION
- Easier hygiene
- Decreased risk of urinary tract infections
- Decreased risk of STIs, including HIV
- Prevention of penile problems, such as phimosis
- Decreased risk of penile cancer and cervical cancer in female partners. Qᴘᴄᴄ

26.1 Circumcision Plastibell

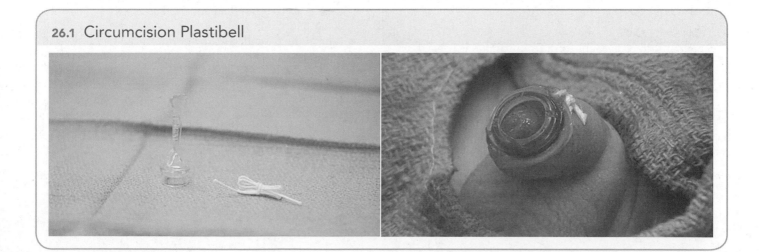

CONTRAINDICATIONS FOR CIRCUMCISION
- Newborns born with hypospadias (abnormal positioning of urethra on ventral under-surface of the penis) and epispadias (urethral canal terminates on dorsum of penis) because the prepuce skin can be needed for surgical repair of the defect
- Familiar history of bleeding disorders
- Newborns who are circumcised and whose parents decline vitamin K can be more likely to experience bleeding at the circumcision site, especially if they are breastfed

Diagnostic and therapeutic procedures and management

ANESTHESIA: Anesthesia is required for circumcision. Types of anesthesia include a ring block, dorsal-penile nerve block, topical anesthetic (eutectic mixture of local anesthetics), and concentrated oral sucrose. Nonpharmacologic methods, such as swaddling and nonnutritive sucking can be used to enhance pain management.

EQUIPMENT FOR PERFORMING CIRCUMCISION: Gomco (Yellen) or Mogen clamp, or Plastibell device
- The provider applies the Gomco (Yellen) or Mogen clamp to the penis, loosens the foreskin, and inserts the cone under the foreskin to provide a cutting surface for removal of the foreskin and to protect the penis. The wound is covered with sterile petroleum gauze to prevent infection and control bleeding.
- The provider slides the Plastibell device between the foreskin and the glans of the penis. The provider ties a suture tightly around the foreskin at the coronal edge of the glans. This applies pressure as the excess foreskin is removed from the penis. After 5 to 7 days, the Plastibell drops off, leaving a clean, healed excision. No petroleum is used for circumcision with the Plastibell. **(26.1)**

Preprocedure

NURSING ASSESSMENT
The newborn should be assessed for the following.
- A history of bleeding tendencies in the family (hemophilia and clotting disorders)
- Hypospadias or epispadias
- Ambiguous genitalia (when the newborn has genitalia that can include both male and female characteristics).
- Illness or infection.

NURSING ACTIONS
- Signed informed consent form from parents is needed.
- Gather and prepare supplies.
- Administer medication to newborn as prescribed.
- Assist with procedure.
  - Place the newborn on the restraining board, and provide a radiant heat source to prevent cold stress. Do not leave the newborn unattended. Have bulb syringe readily available.
  - Comfort the newborn as needed.
  - Document time and type of circumcision, excessive bleeding, and newborn voiding following procedure.

Postprocedure

NURSING ASSESSMENT
The newborn should be assessed for the following.
- Bleeding every 15 to 30 min for the first hour and then hourly for the next 4 to 6 hr
- The first voiding

NURSING ACTIONS
- Remove the newborn from the restraining board, and swaddle to provide comfort.
- Monitor for bleeding and voiding per facility protocol. Apply gauze lightly to penis if bleeding or oozing is observed.
- Fan-fold diapers to prevent pressure on the circumcised area.
- Liquid acetaminophen 10 to 15 mg/kg can be administered orally after the procedure and repeated every 4 to 6 hr as prescribed for a maximum of 30 to 45 mg/kg/day.

PARENT TEACHING
- Signed informed consent from parents is needed.
- Explain to the parents that the newborn will not be able to be bottle feed for up to 2-3 hr prior to the procedure to prevent vomiting and aspiration based on the preferences of the provider. Newborns who are breastfed can nurse up until the procedure.
- Explain that the newborn is restrained on a special board during the procedure.
- Teach the parents to keep the area clean. Change the newborn's diaper at least every 4 hr, and clean the penis with warm water with each diaper change. With clamp procedures, apply petroleum jelly with each diaper change for at least 24 hr after the circumcision to keep the diaper from adhering to the penis.
- Avoid wrapping the penis in tight gauze, which can impair circulation to the glans.
- A tub bath should not be given until the circumcision is healed. Until then, warm water should be trickled gently over the penis.
- Notify the provider if there is any redness, discharge, swelling, strong odor, tenderness, decrease in urination, or excessive crying from the newborn.
- Tell the parents that a film of yellowish mucus can form over the glans by day two, and it is important not to wash it off.
- Teach the parents to avoid using premoistened towelettes to clean the penis because they contain alcohol.
- Inform the parents that the newborn can be fussy or can sleep for several hours after the circumcision. Provide comfort measures for 24 to 48 hr, to include acetaminophen as prescribed.
- Inform the parents that the circumcision will heal completely within a couple of weeks.

Complications and nursing management

Hemorrhage
- Monitor the newborn for bleeding.
- Provide gentle pressure on the penis using a small gauze square. Gelfoam powder or sponge can be applied to stop bleeding. If bleeding persists, notify the provider that a blood vessel can need to be ligated. Have a nurse continue to hold pressure until the provider arrives while another nurse prepares the circumcision tray and suture material.

Cold stress/hypoglycemia
- Monitor the newborn for excessive loss of heat resulting in increased respirations and lowered body temperature.
- Swaddle and feed the newborn as soon as the procedure is over.

Other complications
- Report any frank bleeding, foul-smelling drainage, or lack of voiding to the provider.
- Provide discharge instructions to the parents about manifestations of infection, comfort measures, medications, and when to notify the provider.

CLOTHING

Instruct the parents about how to properly clothe their newborn.
- The best clothing is soft and made of cotton.
- Clothes should be washed separately with mild detergent and hot water.
- Dress lightly for indoors and on hot days. Too many layers of clothing or blankets can make the newborn too hot.
- On cold days, cover the newborn's head when outdoors.
- A general rule is to dress the newborn as the parents would dress themselves.

HOME SAFETY

- Never leave the newborn unattended with pets or other small children.
- Keep small objects (coins) out of the reach of newborns due to choking hazard.
- Never leave the newborn alone on a bed, couch, or table. Newborns move enough to reach the edge and fall off.
- Never place the newborn on his stomach to sleep during the first few months of life. The back-lying position is the position of choice. The newborn can be placed on his abdomen when awake and being supervised.
- Never provide a newborn with a soft surface to sleep on (pillows or water bed). The newborn's mattress should be firm. Never put pillows, toys, bumper pads, or loose blankets in a crib. Crib linens should be tight-fitting.
- Do not tie anything around the newborn's neck.
- Monitor the safety of the newborn's crib. The space between the mattress and sides of the crib should be less than 2 fingerbreadths. The slats on the crib should be no more than 5.7 cm (2.25 in) apart.

- The newborn's crib or playpen should be away from window blinds and drapery cords. Newborns can become strangled in them.
- The bassinet or crib should be placed on an inner wall, not next to a window, to prevent cold stress by radiation.
- If an infant carrier is placed on a high place, such as a table, an adult should always be within arm's reach.
- Smoke detectors should be on every floor of a home and should be checked monthly to ensure that they are working. Batteries should be changed twice a year. (Change batteries when daylight savings time occurs or on a child's birthday.)
- Eliminate potential fire hazards. Keep a crib and playpen away from heaters, radiators, and heat vents. Linens could catch fire if they come into contact with heat sources.
- Control the temperature and humidity of the newborn's environment by providing adequate ventilation.
- Avoid exposing the newborn to cigarette smoke in a home or elsewhere. Secondhand exposure increases the newborn's risk of developing respiratory illnesses.
- All visitors should wash their hands before touching the newborn. Any individual who has an infection should be kept away from the newborn.
- Carefully handle the newborn. Do not toss the newborn up in the air or swing him by her extremities.
- Provide community resources to clients who can need additional and ongoing assessment and instruction on newborn care (adolescent parents).

CAR SEAT SAFETY

Use an approved rear-facing car seat in the back seat, preferably in the middle (away from air bags and side impact), to transport the newborn. Keep infants in rear-facing car seats until age 2 or until the child reaches the maximum height and weight for the seat. **Qs**

NEWBORN WELLNESS CHECKUPS

- Every newborn should be seen and examined at the doctor's office within 72 hr (2 to 3 days) after discharge. The American Academy of Pediatrics recommends wellness checks at 2 to 5 days, 1 month, 2 months, 4 months, 6 months, 9 months, 12 months, 15 months, 18 months, 2 years, 2.5 years, 3 years, 4 years, and every year thereafter.
- Review the schedule for immunizations with the parents. Stress the importance of receiving these immunizations on a schedule for the newborn to be protected against diphtheria, tetanus, pertussis, hepatitis B, *Haemophilus influenzae*, polio, measles, mumps, rubella, influenza, rotavirus, pneumococcal, and varicella.

MANIFESTATIONS OF ILLNESS TO REPORT

Instruct parents regarding the signs of illness and to report them immediately.
- A temperature greater than 38° C (100.4° F) or less than 36.6° C (97.9° F)
- Poor feeding or little interest in food
- Forceful vomiting or frequent vomiting
- Decreased urination
- Diarrhea or decreased bowel movements
- Labored breathing with flared nostrils or an absence of breathing for greater than 15 seconds
- Jaundice
- Cyanosis
- Lethargy
- Inconsolable crying
- Difficulty waking
- Bleeding or purulent drainage around umbilical cord or circumcision
- Drainage developing in eyes.

CARDIOPULMONARY RESUSCITATION

Encourage parents to seek CPR training.

COMPLICATIONS RELATED TO NEWBORN HOME CARE

Complications stemming from improper understanding of discharge instructions can include the following.
- An infected cord or circumcision from improper care or tub bathing too soon.
- Falls; suffocation; strangulation; burns resulting in injuries, fractures, aspiration; or even death due to improper safety precautions.
- Respiratory infections due to passive smoke or inhaled powders.
- Improper or no use of a car seat resulting in injuries or death.
- Serious infections due to lack of noncompliance with immunization schedule.

Application Exercises

1. A nurse is reviewing care of the umbilical cord with the parent of a newborn. Which of the following instructions should the nurse include in the teaching?

   A. Cover the cord with a small gauze square.

   B. Trickle clean water over the cord with each diaper change.

   C. Apply hydrogen peroxide to the cord twice a day.

   D. Keep the diaper folded below the cord.

2. A nurse is reviewing contraindications for circumcision with a newly hired nurse. Which of the following conditions are contraindications? (Select all that apply.)

   A. Hypospadias

   B. Hydrocele

   C. Family history of hemophilia

   D. Hyperbilirubinemia

   E. Epispadias

3. A nurse is providing discharge teaching to the parents of a newborn regarding circumcision care. Which of the following statements made by a parent indicates an understanding of the teaching?

   A. "His circumcision will heal within a couple of days."

   B. "I should remove the yellow mucus that will form."

   C. "I will clean his penis with each diaper change."

   D. "I will give him a tub bath within a couple of days."

4. A nurse is caring for a newborn immediately following a circumcision using a Gomco procedure. Which of the following actions should the nurse implement?

   A. Apply Gelfoam powder to the site.

   B. Place the newborn in the prone position.

   C. Apply petroleum gauze to the site.

   D. Avoid changing the diaper until the first voiding.

5. A nurse is reviewing car seat safety with the parents of a newborn. Which of the following instructions should the nurse include in the teaching regarding car seat position?

   A. Front seat, rear-facing

   B. Front seat, forward-facing

   C. Back seat, rear-facing

   D. Back seat, forward-facing

PRACTICE Active Learning Scenario

A nurse is leading a discussion with a group of parents on bathing a newborn. What information should the nurse include in the teaching? Use the ATI Active Learning Template: Basic Concept to complete this item.

NURSING INTERVENTIONS

- Describe two interventions that relate to general skin care.
- Describe two interventions that relate to promoting infant safety.
- Describe two interventions that relate to the correct order of giving a bath.
- Describe two interventions that prevent complications in the newborn.

Application Exercises Key

1. A. Covering the cord with a gauze square prevents the cord from drying and encourages infection.

   B. Water should not be applied to the cord.

   C. The cord should be kept clean and dry. Hydrogen peroxide is not applied to the cord site.

   D. **CORRECT:** Folding the diaper below the cord prevents urine from the diaper penetrating the cord site.

   Ⓝ NCLEX® Connection: Health Promotion and Maintenance, Ante/Intra/Postpartum and Newborn Care

2. A. **CORRECT:** Hypospadias involves a defect in the location of the urethral opening and is a contraindication to circumcision.

   B. Hydrocele, a collection of fluid in the scrotal sac, is not a contraindication to circumcision.

   C. **CORRECT:** A family history of hemophilia is a contraindication for circumcision.

   D. Hyperbilirubinemia is not a contraindication for circumcision.

   E. **CORRECT:** Epispadias involves a defect in the location of the urethral opening and is a contraindication to circumcision.

   Ⓝ NCLEX® Connection: Reduction of Risk Potential, Therapeutic Procedures

3. A. The circumcision will heal within a couple of weeks.

   B. The yellow mucus should remain in place as part of the healing process.

   C. **CORRECT:** The penis should be cleaned with warm water with each diaper change.

   D. A tub bath should not be given until the circumcision is healed.

   Ⓝ NCLEX® Connection: Health Promotion and Maintenance, Ante/Intra/Postpartum and Newborn Care

4. A. Gelfoam powder is used to control bleeding when there is a risk for hemorrhage

   B. Newborns should not be placed in the prone position.

   C. **CORRECT:** Petroleum gauze is applied to the site for 24 hr to prevent the skin edges from sticking to the diaper.

   D. Diapers are changed more frequently to inspect the site.

   Ⓝ NCLEX® Connection: Reduction of Risk Potential, Therapeutic Procedures

5. A. This is not an appropriate position for the car seat.

   B. This is not an appropriate position for the car seat.

   C. **CORRECT:** The newborn should be restrained in a car seat in a rear-facing position in the back seat until 2 years of age.

   D. This is not an appropriate position for the car seat.

   Ⓝ NCLEX® Connection: Safety and Infection Control, Accident/Error/Injury Prevention

PRACTICE Answer

Using ATI Active Learning Template: Basic Concept

NURSING INTERVENTIONS

Skin Care
- The eyes are cleaned using a clean portion of the wash cloth.
- The newborn should be washed, rinsed, and dried with no soap left on the skin.
- Use a mild soap that does not contain hexachlorophene.

Infant Safety
- Do not leave the newborn unattended during the bath.
- Hot water heater should be set at 49° C (120.2° F) or less.
- The room should be warm, and the bath water should be at 36.6° to 37.2° C (98° to 99° F).
- Bath water should be tested on the inner wrist prior to use.

Order of Giving the Bath
- Move from the cleanest to the dirtiest areas of the newborn's body, which includes starting with the eyes, face, and head; proceeding to the chest, arms, and legs; and washing the groin area last.
- The eyes are cleaned by moving from the inner to the outer canthus.

Preventing Complications
- Bathing by immersion is not done until the umbilical cord falls off and the circumcision is healed.
- Do not bathe the newborn immediately after feeding to prevent spitting up and vomiting.
- After cleansing the uncircumcised newborn male, the foreskin should not be forced back.
- In female newborns, wash the vulva by wiping from front to back.

Ⓝ NCLEX® Connection: Health Promotion and Maintenance, Ante/Intra/Postpartum and Newborn Care

CHAPTER 27 *Assessment and Management of Newborn Complications*

Assessment and management of newborn complications includes assessment, risk factors, and collaborative care. It is essential for a nurse to immediately identify complications and implement appropriate interventions. Ongoing emotional support to a client and significant other is also imperative to the plan of care.

Complications include neonatal substance withdrawal, hypoglycemia, respiratory distress syndrome (RDS)/asphyxia/meconium aspiration, preterm newborn, small for gestational age (SGA) newborn, large for gestational age (LGA)/macrosomic newborn, postmature newborn, newborn infection/sepsis (sepsis neonatorum), birth trauma or injury, hyperbilirubinemia, and congenital anomalies.

Neonatal substance withdrawal

Maternal substance use during pregnancy consists of any use of alcohol or drugs. Intrauterine drug exposure can cause anomalies, neurobehavioral changes, and evidence of withdrawal in the neonate. These changes depend on the specific drug or combination of drugs used, dosage, route of administration, metabolism and excretion by the mother and fetus, timing of drug exposure, and length of drug exposure.

- Substance withdrawal in the newborn occurs when the mother uses drugs that have addictive properties during pregnancy. This includes illegal drugs, alcohol, tobacco, and prescription medications.
- Fetal alcohol syndrome (FAS) results from the chronic or periodic intake of alcohol during pregnancy. Alcohol is considered teratogenic, so the daily intake of alcohol increases the risk of FAS. Newborns who have FAS are at risk for specific congenital physical defects and long-term complications.

LONG-TERM COMPLICATIONS

- Feeding problems
- Central nervous system dysfunction (cognitive impairment, cerebral palsy)
- Attention deficit disorder
- Language abnormalities
- Microcephaly
- Delayed growth and development
- Poor maternal–newborn bonding

ASSESSMENT

RISK FACTORS

- Maternal use of substances prior to knowing she is pregnant
- Maternal substance use during pregnancy

EXPECTED FINDINGS

Monitor the neonate for abstinence syndrome (withdrawal) and increased wakefulness using the neonatal abstinence scoring system that assesses for and scores the following.

- **CNS:** High-pitched, shrill cry; incessant crying; irritability; tremors; hyperactivity with an increased Moro reflex; increased deep-tendon reflexes; increased muscle tone; disturbed sleep pattern; hypertonicity; convulsions
- **Metabolic, vasomotor, and respiratory findings:** Nasal congestion with flaring, frequent yawning, skin mottling, retractions, apnea, tachypnea greater than 60/min, sweating, temperature greater than 37.2° C (99° F)
- **Gastrointestinal:** Poor feeding; regurgitation (projectile vomiting); diarrhea; excessive, uncoordinated, constant sucking

OPIATE WITHDRAWAL: Manifestations of neonatal abstinence syndrome

HEROIN WITHDRAWAL
- Low birth weight
- Small for gestational age (SGA)
- Manifestations of neonatal abstinence syndrome
- Increased risk of sudden infant death syndrome (SIDS)

METHADONE WITHDRAWAL
Manifestations of neonatal abstinence syndrome:
Increased incidence of seizures, sleep pattern disturbances, higher birth weights (compared to with heroin exposure)

MARIJUANA WITHDRAWAL
- Preterm birth, meconium staining
- Long-term effects, such as deficits in attention, cognition, memory, and motor skills

AMPHETAMINE WITHDRAWAL: Preterm or SGA, drowsiness, jitteriness, sleep pattern disturbances, respiratory distress, frequent infections, poor weight gain, emotional disturbances, and delayed growth and development

ALCOHOL WITHDRAWAL: Jitteriness, irritability, increased tone and reflex responses, and seizures

FETAL ALCOHOL SYNDROME
- Facial anomalies: small eyes, flat midface, smooth philtrum, thin upper lip, eyes with a wide spaced appearance, epicanthal folds, strabismus, ptosis, poor suck, small teeth, and cleft lip or palate
- Deafness
- Abnormal palmar creases and irregular hair
- Many vital organ anomalies, such as heart defects, including atrial and ventricular septal defects, tetralogy of Fallot, and patent ductus arteriosus
- Developmental delays and neurologic abnormalities
- Prenatal and postnatal growth delays
- Sleep disturbances

TOBACCO: Prematurity, low birth weight, increased risk for SIDS, increased risk for bronchitis, pneumonia, and developmental delays

LABORATORY TESTS

Blood tests should be done to differentiate between neonatal drug withdrawal and central nervous system disorders.
- CBC
- Blood glucose
- Electrolyte imbalance
- Thyroid-stimulating hormone, thyroxine, triiodothyronine
- Drug screen of urine or meconium to reveal the substance used by the mother
- Hair analysis

DIAGNOSTIC PROCEDURES

Chest x-ray for FAS to rule out congenital heart defects

PATIENT-CENTERED CARE

NURSING CARE

Nursing care for maternal substance use and neonatal effects or withdrawal include the following in addition to normal newborn care.
- Perform ongoing assessment of the newborn using the neonatal abstinence scoring system assessment, as prescribed.
- Elicit and assess the newborn's reflexes.
- Monitor the newborn's ability to feed and digest intake. Offer small frequent feedings.
- Swaddle the newborn with legs flexed.
- Offer non-nutritive sucking.
- Monitor the newborn's fluids and electrolytes with skin turgor, mucous membranes, fontanels, daily weights, and I&O.
- Reduce environmental stimuli (decrease lights, lower noise level).

MEDICATIONS

Based on withdrawal symptoms.

Morphine sulfate
CLASSIFICATION: Opioid

Phenobarbital
CLASSIFICATION: Anticonvulsant

INTENDED EFFECT: Decrease CNS irritability and control seizures for newborns who have alcohol or opioid withdrawal.

NURSING CONSIDERATIONS
- Assess IV site frequently (phenobarbital).
- Check for any medication incompatibilities.
- Decrease environmental stimuli.
- Cluster cares to minimize stimulation.
- Swaddle the newborn to reduce self-stimulation and protect the skin from abrasions.
- Monitor and maintain fluids and electrolytes.
- Administer frequent, small feedings of high-calorie formula; can require gavage feedings.
- Elevate the newborn's head during and following feedings, and burp the newborn to reduce vomiting and aspiration. Qs
- Try various nipples to compensate for a poor suck reflex.
- Have suction available to reduce the risk for aspiration.
- For newborns who are withdrawing from cocaine, avoid eye contact and use vertical rocking and a pacifier.
- Prevent infection.
- Initiate a consult with child protective services.
- Consult lactation services to evaluate whether breastfeeding is desired or contraindicated to avoid passing narcotics in breast milk. Methadone is not contraindicated during breastfeeding.

CLIENT EDUCATION

- Refer the mother to a drug and/or alcohol treatment center.
- Discuss the importance of SIDS prevention activities due to the increased rate in newborns of mothers who used methadone.

Hypoglycemia

The newborn's source of glucose stops when the umbilical cord is clamped. A healthy term newborn's blood glucose level can drop to 30 mg/dL the first 1 to 2 hr following birth. If newborns have other physiological stress, they can experience hypoglycemia due to inadequate gluconeogenesis or increased use of glycogen stores.
- Hypoglycemia is a serum glucose level less than 40 mg/dL. Routine assessment of all newborns, especially newborns who are LGA and SGA, should include monitoring for hypoglycemia.
- Hypoglycemia differs for a newborn who is preterm or term. Hypoglycemia in the first 3 days of life in the term newborn is defined as a blood glucose level less than 40 mg/dL.
- Untreated hypoglycemia can result in seizures, brain damage, or death.

ASSESSMENT

RISK FACTORS

- Maternal diabetes mellitus
- Preterm infant
- LGA or SGA
- Stress at birth, such as cold stress and asphyxia

EXPECTED FINDINGS

PHYSICAL ASSESSMENT FINDINGS
- Poor feeding
- Jitteriness/tremors
- Hypothermia
- Diaphoresis
- Weak cry
- Lethargy
- Flaccid muscle tone
- Seizures/coma
- Irregular respirations
- Cyanosis
- Apnea

LABORATORY TESTS

Blood glucose levels less than 45 mg/dL should be followed up with a serum glucose level.

PATIENT-CENTERED CARE

NURSING CARE

- Obtain blood by heel stick for glucose monitoring.
- An asymptomatic at-risk newborn who has a blood glucose level 25 mg/dL in the first 4 hr, or less than 35 mg/dL from 4 hr to 24 hr of age, should be offered oral feedings to increase levels to greater than 45 mg/dL.
- Initiate IV dextrose for a symptomatic newborn.
- Provide frequent oral and/or gavage feedings or continuous parenteral nutrition early after birth to treat hypoglycemia.
- Monitor the neonate's blood glucose level closely per facility protocol.
- Monitor IV if the neonate is unable to feed orally.
- Maintain skin-to-skin contact to treat hypothermia.

Respiratory distress syndrome, asphyxia, and meconium aspiration

- RDS occurs as a result of surfactant deficiency in the lungs and is characterized by poor gas exchange and ventilatory failure.
- Surfactant is a phospholipid that assists in alveoli expansion. Surfactant keeps alveoli from collapsing and allows gas exchange to occur.
- Atelectasis (collapsing of a portion of lung) increases the work of breathing. As a result, respiratory acidosis and hypoxemia can develop.
- Birth weight alone is not an indicator of fetal lung maturity.

- Complications from RDS are related to oxygen therapy and mechanical ventilation.
  - Pneumothorax
  - Pneumomediastinum
  - Retinopathy of prematurity
  - Bronchopulmonary dysplasia
  - Infection
  - Intraventricular hemorrhage

ASSESSMENT

RISK FACTORS

- Preterm gestation
- Perinatal asphyxia (meconium staining, cord prolapse, nuchal cord)
- Maternal diabetes mellitus
- Premature rupture of membranes
- Maternal use of barbiturates or narcotics close to birth
- Maternal hypotension
- Cesarean birth without labor
- Hydrops fetalis (massive edema of the fetus caused by hyperbilirubinemia)
- Maternal bleeding during the third trimester
- Hypovolemia
- Genetics: male gender, Caucasian descent

EXPECTED FINDINGS

PHYSICAL ASSESSMENT FINDINGS
- Tachypnea (respiratory rate greater than 60/min)
- Nasal flaring
- Expiratory grunting
- Retractions
- Labored breathing with prolonged expiration
- Fine crackles on auscultation
- Cyanosis
- Unresponsiveness, flaccidity, and apnea with decreased breath sounds (manifestations of worsened RDS)

LABORATORY TESTS

- ABGs
- Complete blood count with differential
- Culture and sensitivity of the blood, urine, and cerebrospinal fluid
- Blood glucose

DIAGNOSTIC PROCEDURES

Chest x-ray

PATIENT-CENTERED CARE

NURSING CARE

- Suction the newborn's mouth, trachea, and nose as needed.
- Maintain thermoregulation.
- Provide mouth and skin care.
- Correct respiratory acidosis with ventilatory support.

- Correct metabolic acidosis by administering sodium bicarbonate.
- Maintain adequate oxygenation, prevent lactic acidosis, and avoid the toxic effects of oxygen.
- Monitor pulse oximetry.
- Provide parenteral nutrition as prescribed.
- Monitor laboratory results, I&O, and weight to evaluate hydration status.
- Decrease stimuli.

MEDICATIONS

Beractant, calfactant, lucinactant

CLASSIFICATION: Lung surfactant

INTENDED EFFECT: Restores surfactant and improves respiratory compliance for newborns who are premature and have RDS

NURSING CONSIDERATIONS
- Perform a respiratory assessment including ABGs, respiratory rhythm, and rate and skin color before and after administration of agent.
- Provide suction to the newborn prior to administration of the medication.
- Assess endotracheal tube placement.
- Avoid suctioning of the endotracheal tube for 1 hr after administration of the medication.

> Factors that can accelerate lung maturation in the fetus while in utero include increased gestational age, intrauterine stress, exogenous steroid use, and ruptured membranes.

Preterm newborn

- A preterm newborn's birth occurs after 20 weeks of gestation and before completion of 37 weeks of gestation.
- A late preterm newborn's birth occurs from 34 to 36 weeks of gestation.
- An early term newborn's birth occurs from 37 to 38⁶/₇ weeks of gestation.
- Preterm newborns are at risk for a variety of complications due to immature organ systems. The degree of complications depends on gestational age. There is a decreased risk for complications the closer the newborn is to 40 weeks of gestation.
  - Goals include meeting the newborn's growth and development needs, and anticipating and managing associated complications such as RDS and sepsis.
  - The main priority in treating newborns who are preterm is supporting the cardiac and respiratory systems as needed. Most newborns who are preterm are cared for in a neonatal intensive care unit (NICU). Meticulous care and observation in the NICU is necessary until the newborn can receive oral feedings, maintain body temperature, and weighs approximately 2 kg (4.4 lb).

COMPLICATIONS

Respiratory distress syndrome: Decreased surfactant in the alveoli occurs, regardless of a newborn's birth weight

Bronchopulmonary dysplasia: Causes the lungs to become stiff and noncompliant, requiring a newborn to receive mechanical ventilation and oxygen. It is sometimes difficult to remove the newborn from ventilation and oxygen after initial placement.

Aspiration: A result of a newborn who is premature not having an intact gag reflex or the ability to effectively suck or swallow

Apnea of prematurity: A result of immature neurological and chemical mechanisms

Intraventricular hemorrhage: Bleeding in or around the ventricles of the brain

Retinopathy of prematurity: Disease caused by abnormal growth of retinal blood vessels and is a complication associated with oxygen administration to the newborn; can cause mild to severe eye and vision problems

Patent ductus arteriosus: Occurs when the ductus arteriosus reopens after birth due to neonatal hypoxia

Necrotizing enterocolitis: An inflammatory disease of the gastrointestinal mucosa due to ischemia. It results in necrosis and perforation of the bowel. (Short-gut syndrome can be the result secondary to removal of most or part of the small intestine due to necrosis.)

Additional complications: Infection, hyperbilirubinemia, anemia, hypoglycemia, and delayed growth and development

ASSESSMENT

RISK FACTORS

- Maternal gestational hypertension
- Multiple pregnancies that are closely spaced
- Adolescent pregnancy
- Lack of prenatal care
- Maternal substance use, smoking
- Previous history of preterm delivery
- Abnormalities of the uterus
- Cervical incompetence
- Placenta previa
- Preterm labor
- Preterm premature rupture of membranes

EXPECTED FINDINGS

PHYSICAL ASSESSMENT FINDINGS
- Ballard assessment showing a physical and neurological assessment totaling less than 37 weeks of gestation
- Periodic breathing consisting of 5- to 10-second respiratory pauses, followed by 10- to 15-second compensatory rapid respirations

- Manifestations of increased respiratory effort and/or respiratory distress including nasal flaring or retractions of the chest wall during inspirations, expiratory grunting, and tachypnea
- Apnea: a pause in respirations 20 seconds or greater
- Low birth weight
- Minimal subcutaneous fat deposits
- Head that is large in comparison with his body, and small fontanels
- Wrinkled features with abundance of lanugo covering back, forearms, forehead, and sides of face, and few or no creases on soles of feet
- Skull and rib cage that feel soft
- Eyes closed if the newborn is born at 22 to 24 weeks of gestation
- Weak grasp reflex
- Inability to coordinate suck and swallow; weak or absent gag, suck, and cough reflex; weak swallow
- Hypotonic muscles, decreased level of activity, and a weak cry for more than 24 hr
- Lethargy, tachycardia, and poor weight gain

LABORATORY TESTS

- CBC showing decreased Hgb and Hct as a result of slow production of RBCs
- Urinalysis and specific gravity
- Increased PT and aPTT time with an increased tendency to bleed
- Serum glucose
- Calcium
- Bilirubin
- ABGs

DIAGNOSTIC PROCEDURES

- Chest x-ray
- Head ultrasounds
- Echocardiography
- Eye exams

PATIENT-CENTERED CARE

NURSING CARE

- Perform rapid initial assessment.
- Perform resuscitative measures if needed.
- Monitor the newborn's vital signs.
- Assess the newborn's ability to consume and digest nutrients. Before feeding by breast or nipple, the newborn must have an intact gag reflex and be able to suck and swallow to prevent aspiration.
- Monitor I&O and daily weight.
- Monitor the newborn for bleeding from puncture sites and the gastrointestinal tract.

- Ensure and maintain thermoregulation in a newborn who is preterm by using a radiant heat warmer
  - Manifestations of hypothermia: Apnea, cyanosis, hypoglycemia, feeding intolerance, lethargy, irritability, bradycardia.
- Administer respiratory support measures, such as surfactant and/or oxygen administration.
- Administer parental or enteral nutrition and fluids as prescribed (most preterm newborns who are less than 34 weeks of gestation will receive fluids either by IV and/or gavage feedings). Provide for nonnutritive sucking, such as using a pacifier while gavage feeding.
- Minimize the newborn's stimulation. Cluster nursing care. Touch the newborn very smoothly and lightly. Keep lighting dim and noise levels reduced.
- Position the newborn in neutral flexion with his extremities close to his body to conserve body heat. Prone and side-lying positions are preferred to supine with body containment using blanket rolls and swaddling, but only in the nursery under monitored supervision.
- Perform a skin assessment tool daily to minimize risk of skin breakdown.
- Encourage skin to skin contact (Kangaroo care) whenever possible to reduce preterm infant stress.
- Protect the newborn against infection by enforcing hand hygiene and gowning procedures.
  - Equipment should not be shared with other newborns.
  - **Evidence of infection:** Temperature instability, lethargy, irritability, cyanosis, bradycardia or tachycardia, apnea or tachypnea, feeding intolerance, glucose instability
- Observe the newborn for findings of dehydration or overhydration (resulting from IV nutrition and fluid administration).
  - **Dehydration**
    - Urine output less than 1 mL/kg/hr
    - Urine-specific gravity greater than 1.015
    - Weight loss
    - Dry mucous membranes
    - Absent skin turgor
    - Depressed fontanel
  - **Overhydration**
    - Urine output greater than 3 mL/kg/hr
    - Urine-specific gravity less than 1.001
    - Edema
    - Increased weight gain
    - Crackles in lungs
    - Intake greater than output

CLIENT EDUCATION

Keep parents informed about and engaged in the care of their preterm newborn.

Small for gestational age newborn

- SGA describes a newborn whose birth weight is at or below the 10th percentile and who has intrauterine growth restriction.
- Common complications of newborns who are SGA are perinatal asphyxia, meconium aspiration, hypoglycemia, polycythemia, and instability of body temperature.

ASSESSMENT

RISK FACTORS

- Congenital or chromosomal anomalies
- Maternal infections, disease, or malnutrition
- Gestational hypertension and/or diabetes
- Maternal smoking, drug, or alcohol use
- Multiple gestations
- Placental factors (small placenta, placenta previa, decreased placental perfusion)
- Fetal congenital infections such as rubella or toxoplasmosis

EXPECTED FINDINGS

PHYSICAL ASSESSMENT FINDINGS
- Weight below 10th percentile
- Normal skull, but reduced body dimensions
- Hair is sparse on scalp
- Wide skull sutures from inadequate bone growth
- Dry, loose skin
- Decreased subcutaneous fat
- Decreased muscle mass, particularly over the cheeks and buttocks
- Thin, dry, yellow, and dull umbilical cord rather than gray, glistening, and moist
- Drawn abdomen rather than well-rounded
- Respiratory distress and hypoxia
- Wide-eyed and alert, which is attributed to prolonged fetal hypoxia
- Hypotonia
- Evidence of meconium aspiration
- Hypoglycemia
- Acrocyanosis

LABORATORY TESTS

- Blood glucose for hypoglycemia
- CBC will show polycythemia resulting from fetal hypoxia and intrauterine stress.
- ABGs may be prescribed due to chronic hypoxia in utero due to placental insufficiency.

DIAGNOSTIC PROCEDURES

Chest x-ray to rule out meconium aspiration syndrome

PATIENT-CENTERED CARE

NURSING CARE

- Support respiratory efforts, and suction the newborn as necessary to maintain an open airway. Qs
- Provide a neutral thermal environment for the newborn (isolette or radiant heat warmer) to prevent cold stress.
- Initiate early feedings. (A newborn who is SGA will require feedings that are more frequent.)
- Administer parenteral nutrition if necessary.
- Maintain adequate hydration.
- Conserve the newborn's energy level.
- Prevent skin breakdown.
- Protect the newborn from infection.

CLIENT EDUCATION

Provide support to the newborn's parents and extended family, and encourage them to participate in caring for the newborn. Anticipate home care needs.

Large for gestational age (macrosomic) newborn

- LGA occurs in neonates who weigh above the 90th percentile or more than 4,000 g (8 lb, 13 oz).
- Neonates who are LGA can be preterm, postmature, or full-term.
- Newborns who are macrosomic are at risk for birth injuries (shoulder dystocia, clavicle fracture or a cesarean birth, asphyxia, hypoglycemia, polycythemia and Erb-Duchenne paralysis due to birth trauma).
- Uncontrolled hyperglycemia during pregnancy (leading risk factor for LGA) can lead to congenital defects with the most common being congenital heart defects, tracheoesophageal fistula, and CNS anomalies.

ASSESSMENT

RISK FACTORS

- Newborns who are postmature
- Maternal diabetes mellitus during pregnancy (high glucose levels stimulate continued insulin production by the fetus)
- Fetal cardiovascular disorder of transposition of the great vessels
- Genetic factors
- Maternal obesity
- A mother who is multiparous

EXPECTED FINDINGS

PHYSICAL ASSESSMENT FINDINGS
- Weight above 90th percentile (4,000 g)
- Large head
- Plump and full-faced (cushingoid appearance) from increased subcutaneous fat
- Manifestations of hypoxia including tachypnea, retractions, cyanosis, nasal flaring, and grunting
- Birth trauma (e.g., fractures, shoulder dystocia, intracranial hemorrhage, and CNS injury)
- Sluggishness, hypotonic muscles, and hypoactivity
- Tremors from hypocalcemia
- Hypoglycemia
- Respiratory distress from immature lungs or meconium aspiration

Findings of increased intracranial pressure: dilated pupils, vomiting, bulging fontanels, high-pitched cry

LABORATORY TESTS

- Blood glucose levels to monitor closely for hypoglycemia
- ABGs may be prescribed due to chronic hypoxia in utero secondary to placental insufficiency.
- CBC shows polycythemia (Hct greater than 65%) from in utero hypoxia.
- Hyperbilirubinemia resulting from polycythemia as excessive RBCs break down after birth.
- Hypocalcemia can result in response to a long and difficult birth.

DIAGNOSTIC PROCEDURES

Chest x-ray to rule out meconium aspiration syndrome

PATIENT-CENTERED CARE

NURSING CARE

Prior to delivery

- Prepare the client for a possible vacuum-assisted or cesarean birth.
- Prepare to place the client in McRoberts position (lithotomy position with legs flexed to chest to maximize pelvic outlet).
- Prepare to apply suprapubic pressure to aid in the delivery of the anterior shoulder, which is located inferior to the maternal symphysis pubis.
- Assess the newborn for birth trauma, such as a broken clavicle or Erb-Duchenne paralysis.

For a newborn who is LGA following delivery

- Obtain early and frequent heel sticks (blood glucose testing).
- Initiate early feedings or IV therapy to maintain glucose levels within the expected reference range.
- Provide thermoregulation with an isolette.
- Identify and treat any birth injuries.

Postmature infant

- A newborn who is postmature is born after the completion of 42 weeks of gestation. Postmaturity of the infant can be associated with either of the following.
  - **Dysmaturity from placental degeneration and uteroplacental insufficiency** (placenta functions effectively for approximately 40 weeks) resulting in chronic fetal hypoxia and fetal distress in utero. The fetal response is polycythemia, meconium aspiration, and/or neonatal respiratory problems. Perinatal mortality is higher when a postmature placenta fails to meet increased oxygen demands of the fetus during labor.
  - **Continued growth of the fetus in utero** because the placenta continues to function effectively and the newborn becomes LGA at birth. This leads to a difficult delivery, cephalopelvic disproportion, as well as high insulin reserves and insufficient glucose reserves at birth. The neonatal response can be birth trauma, perinatal asphyxia, a clavicle fracture, seizures, hypoglycemia, and/or temperature instability (cold stress).
- A newborn who is postmature can be either SGA or LGA depending on how well the placenta functions during the last weeks of pregnancy.
- Newborns who are postmature have an increased risk for aspirating the meconium passed by the fetus in utero.
- Persistent pulmonary hypertension (persistent fetal circulation) is a complication that can result from meconium aspiration. There is an interference in the transition from fetal to neonatal circulation, and the ductus arteriosus (connecting the main pulmonary artery and the aorta) and foramen ovale (shunt between the right and left atria) remain open, and fetal pathways of blood flow continue.

ASSESSMENT

RISK FACTORS

In most cases, the cause of a pregnancy that extends beyond 40 weeks of gestation is unknown, but there is a higher incidence in first pregnancies and in women who have had a previous postmature pregnancy.

EXPECTED FINDINGS

PHYSICAL ASSESSMENT FINDINGS
- Wasted appearance, thin with loose skin, having lost some of the subcutaneous fat
- Peeling, cracked, and dry skin; leathery from decreased protection of vernix and amniotic fluid
- Long, thin body
- Meconium staining of fingernails and umbilical cord
- Hair and nails can be long
- Alertness similar to a 2-week-old newborn
- Difficulty establishing respirations secondary to meconium aspiration
- Hypoglycemia due to insufficient stores of glycogen
- Clinical findings of cold stress
- Neurological manifestations that become apparent with the development of fine motor skills
- Macrosomia

LABORATORY TESTS

- Blood glucose levels to monitor for hypoglycemia
- ABGs secondary to chronic hypoxia in utero due to placental insufficiency
- CBC can show polycythemia from decreased oxygenation in utero
- Hct elevated from polycythemia and dehydration

DIAGNOSTIC PROCEDURES

- Cesarean birth
- Chest x-ray to rule out meconium aspiration syndrome

PATIENT-CENTERED CARE

NURSING CARE

- Monitor vital signs.
- Administer and monitor IV fluids.
- Moisturize the skin with a petrolatum-based ointment
- Use mechanical ventilation if necessary.
- Administer oxygen as prescribed.
- Prepare and/or assist with exchange transfusion if hematocrit is high.
- Provide thermoregulation in an isolette to avoid cold stress.
- Provide early feedings to avoid hypoglycemia.
- Identify and treat any birth injuries.

Newborn infection, sepsis (sepsis neonatorum)

- Infection can be contracted by the newborn before, during, or after delivery. Newborns are more susceptible to micro-organisms due to their limited immunity and inability to localize infection. The infection can spread rapidly into the bloodstream.
- Newborn sepsis is the presence of micro-organisms or their toxins in the blood or tissues of the newborn during the first month after birth. Manifestations of sepsis are subtle and can resemble other diseases; the nurse often notices them during routine care of the newborn.
- Organisms frequently responsible for newborn infections include *Staphylococcus aureus*, *Staphylococcus epidermidis*, *Escherichia coli*, *Haemophilus influenzae*, and streptococcus ß-hemolytic, Group B.
- Prevention of infection and newborn sepsis starts perinatally with maternal screening for infections, prophylactic interventions, and the use of sterile and aseptic techniques during delivery. Prophylactic antibiotic treatment of the eyes of all newborns and appropriate umbilical cord care also help to prevent newborn infection and sepsis.

ASSESSMENT

RISK FACTORS

- Premature rupture of membranes
- Prolonged labor
- Toxoplasmosis, rubella, cytomegalovirus, and herpes (TORCH)
- Chorioamnionitis
- Preterm birth
- Low birth weight
- Maternal substance use
- Maternal urinary tract infection
- Meconium aspiration
- HIV transmitted from the mother to the newborn perinatally through the placenta and postnatally through the breast milk

EXPECTED FINDINGS

PHYSICAL ASSESSMENT FINDINGS

- Temperature instability
- Suspicious drainage (eyes, umbilical stump)
- Poor feeding pattern, such as weak suck or decreased intake
- Vomiting and diarrhea
- Hypoglycemia, hyperglycemia
- Abdominal distention
- Apnea, retractions, grunting, nasal flaring
- Decreased oxygen saturation
- Color changes, such as pallor, jaundice, and petechiae
- Tachycardia or bradycardia
- Tachypnea
- Low blood pressure
- Irritability and seizure activity
- Poor muscle tone and lethargy

LABORATORY TESTS

- CBC with differential, C-reactive protein
- Blood, urine, and cerebrospinal fluid cultures and sensitivities
- Chemical profile shows a fluid and electrolyte imbalance.

PATIENT-CENTERED CARE

NURSING CARE

- Assess infection risks. (Review maternal health record.)
- Monitor for clinical findings of opportunistic infection.
- Monitor vital signs continuously.
- Monitor I&O and daily weight.
- Monitor fluid and electrolyte status.
- Monitor the newborn's visitors for infection.
- Obtain specimens (blood, urine, stool) to assist in identifying the causative organism.
- Initiate and maintain IV therapy as prescribed to administer electrolyte replacements, fluids, and medications
- Isolation precautions as indicated.

- Administer medications as prescribed (antibiotics, antivirals, or antifungals).
- Initiate and maintain respiratory support as needed.
- Assess IV site for evidence of infection.
- Provide newborn care to maintain temperature.
- Clean and sterilize all equipment to be used.

CLIENT EDUCATION

DISCHARGE INSTRUCTIONS
- Provide the family with education about infection control.
  - Instruct them how to use clean bottles and nipples for each feeding.
  - Discard any unused formula.
  - Supervise hand hygiene
- Promote adequate rest for newborn, and decrease physical stimulation.
- Provide emotional support to the family.

Birth trauma or injury

Birth injury occurs during childbirth resulting in physical injury to a newborn. Most injuries are minor and resolve rapidly. Other injuries can require some intervention. A few are serious enough to be fatal.

TYPES OF BIRTH INJURIES
- **Skull:** Linear fracture, depressed fracture
- **Scalp:** Caput succedaneum, hemorrhage
- **Intracranial:** Epidural or subdural hematoma, contusions
- **Spinal cord:** Spinal cord transaction or injury, vertebral artery injury
- **Plexus:** Brachial plexus injury, Klumpke's palsy
- **Cranial and peripheral nerve:** Radial nerve palsy, diaphragmatic paralysis

ASSESSMENT

RISK FACTORS

- Maternal age: younger than 16 or older than 35
- Fetal macrosomia
- Abnormal or difficult presentations
- Prolonged labor
- Precipitous labor
- Oligohydramnios
- Cephalopelvic disproportion
- Multifetal gestation
- Congenital abnormalities
- Internal FHR monitoring
- Forceps or vacuum extraction
- External version
- Cesarean birth

EXPECTED FINDINGS

PHYSICAL ASSESSMENT FINDINGS
- Irritability, seizures within the first 72 hr, and decreased level of consciousness are manifestations of a subarachnoid hemorrhage.
- Facial flattening and unresponsiveness to grimace that accompanies crying or stimulation, as well as eyes remaining open, are findings to assess for facial paralysis.
- A weak or hoarse cry is characteristic of laryngeal nerve palsy from excessive traction on the neck.
- Flaccid muscle tone can signal joint dislocations and separation during birth.
- Flaccid muscle tone of the extremities suggests nerve-plexus injuries or long bone fractures.
- Limited motion of an arm, crepitus over a clavicle, and absence of the Moro reflex on the affected side are manifestations of clavicular fractures.
- A flaccid arm with the elbow extended and the hand rotated inward, absence of the Moro reflex on the affected side, sensory loss over the lateral aspect of the arm, and intact grasp reflex are manifestations of Erb-Duchenne paralysis (brachial paralysis).
- Localized discoloration, ecchymosis, petechiae, and edema over the presenting part are seen with soft-tissue injuries.

DIAGNOSTIC PROCEDURES

Birth injuries are normally diagnosed by a CT scan, x-ray of suspected area of fracture, or neurological exam to determine paralysis of nerves.

PATIENT-CENTERED CARE

NURSING CARE

- Review maternal history for factors that can predispose the newborn to injuries.
- Review Apgar scoring that might indicate a possibility of birth injury.
- Perform frequent head-to-toe physical assessments.
- Obtain vital signs and temperature.
- Promote parent-newborn interaction as much as possible.
- Administer treatment to the newborn based on the injury and according to the provider's prescriptions.

CLIENT EDUCATION

DISCHARGE INSTRUCTIONS
- Educate the newborn's parents and family regarding the injury and the management of the injury.
- Promote parent-newborn bonding.

Hyperbilirubinemia

Hyperbilirubinemia is an elevation of serum bilirubin levels resulting in jaundice. Jaundice normally appears on the head (especially the sclera and mucous membranes), and then progresses down the thorax, abdomen, and extremities.

Jaundice can be physiologic or pathologic.
- **Physiologic jaundice** is considered benign (resulting from normal newborn physiology of increased bilirubin production due to the shortened lifespan and breakdown of fetal RBCs and liver immaturity). The newborn who has physiological jaundice exhibits an increase in unconjugated bilirubin levels 72 to 120 hr after birth, with a rapid decline to 3 mg/dL 5 to 10 days after birth.
- **Pathologic jaundice** is a result of an underlying disease. Pathologic jaundice appears before 24 hr of age or is persistent after day 14. In the term newborn, bilirubin levels increase more than 0.5 mg/dL/hr, peaks at greater than 12.9 mg/dL, or is associated with anemia and hepatosplenomegaly. Pathologic jaundice is usually caused by a blood group incompatibility or an infection, but can be the result of RBC disorders.

Acute bilirubin encephalopathy is when the bilirubin is deposited in the brain. This occurs once all of the binding sites for the bilirubin are used within the body, resulting in necrosis of neurons. Bilirubin levels higher than 25 mg/dL that place the newborn at risk. This can result in permanent damage including dystonia and athetosis, upward gaze, hearing loss, and cognitive impairments.

Kernicterus is an irreversible, chronic result of bilirubin toxicity. The newborn demonstrates many of the same manifestations of bilirubin encephalopathy with hypotonia, severe cognitive impairments, and spastic quadriplegia.

ASSESSMENT

RISK FACTORS

- Increased RBC production or breakdown
- Rh or ABO incompatibility
- Decreased liver function
- Maternal ingestion of diazepam, salicylates, or sulfonamides close to birth
- Maternal diabetes
- Oxytocin during labor
- Neonatal hyperthyroidism
- Ecchymosis or hemangioma
- Prematurity

EXPECTED FINDINGS

PHYSICAL ASSESSMENT FINDINGS
- Yellowish tint to skin, sclera, and mucous membranes.
- To verify jaundice, press the newborn's skin on the cheek or abdomen lightly with one finger. Then, release pressure, and observe the newborn's skin color for yellowish tint as the skin is blanched.
- Note the time of jaundice onset.

- Assess the underlying cause by reviewing the maternal prenatal, family, and newborn history.
- Hypoxia, hypothermia, hypoglycemia, and metabolic acidosis can occur as a result of hyperbilirubinemia and can increase the risk of brain damage.

LABORATORY TESTS

- An elevated serum bilirubin level can occur (direct and indirect bilirubin). Monitor the newborn's bilirubin levels every 4 hr until the level returns to normal. Qs
- Assess maternal and newborn blood type to determine whether there is ABO incompatibility. This occurs if the newborn has blood type A or B, and the mother is type O.
- Review Hgb and Hct.
- A direct Coombs' test reveals the presence of antibody-coated (sensitized) Rh-positive RBCs in the newborn.
- Check electrolyte levels for dehydration from phototherapy.

DIAGNOSTIC PROCEDURES

Transcutaneous bilirubin level is a noninvasive method to measure a newborn's bilirubin level.

PATIENT-CENTERED CARE

NURSING CARE

- Observe the skin and mucous membranes for jaundice.
- Monitor vital signs.
- Set up phototherapy if prescribed.
  - Maintain an eye mask over the newborn's eyes for protection of corneas and retinas.
  - Keep the newborn undressed. For a male newborn, a surgical mask should be placed (like a bikini) over the genitalia to prevent possible testicular damage from heat and light waves. Be sure to remove the metal strip from the mask to prevent burning.
  - Avoid applying lotions or ointments to the skin because they absorb heat and can cause burns.
  - Remove the newborn from phototherapy every 4 hr, and unmask the newborn's eyes, checking for inflammation or injury.
  - Reposition the newborn every 2 hr to expose all of the body surfaces to the phototherapy lights and prevent pressure sores.
  - Check the lamp energy with a photometer per facility protocol.
  - Turn off the phototherapy lights before drawing blood for testing.
- Observe the newborn for effects of phototherapy.
  - Bronze discoloration: not a serious complication
  - Maculopapular skin rash: not a serious complication
  - Development of pressure areas
  - Dehydration: poor skin turgor, dry mucous membranes, decreased urinary output
  - Elevated temperature
- Encourage the parents to hold and interact with the newborn when phototherapy lights are off.

- Monitor elimination and daily weights, watching for evidence of dehydration.
- Check the newborn's axillary temperature every 4 hr during phototherapy because temperature can become elevated.
- Feed the newborn early and frequently, every 3 to 4 hr. This will promote bilirubin excretion in the stools.
- Encourage continued breastfeeding of the newborn. Supplementation with formula may be prescribed.
- Maintain adequate fluid intake to prevent dehydration.
- Reassure the parents that most newborns experience some degree of jaundice.
- Explain hyperbilirubinemia, its causes, diagnostic tests, and treatment to parents.
- Explain that the newborn's stool contains some bile that will be loose and green.
- Administer an exchange transfusion for newborns who are at risk for kernicterus.

THERAPEUTIC PROCEDURES

Phototherapy: The newborn's bilirubin should start to decrease within 4 to 6 hr after starting treatment.

CLIENT EDUCATION

DISCHARGE INSTRUCTIONS
- Educate the parents regarding the newborn's plan of care.
- Advise parents that infants who have low to moderate risk of hyperbilirubinemia should receive follow up care within two days. Infants at higher risk should be seen within 24 hr.

Congenital anomalies

Newborns can be born with congenital anomalies involving all systems. Anomalies are often diagnosed prenatally. A nurse should provide emotional support to the parents whose newborn is facing procedures or surgeries to correct the defects.

When congenital anomalies are present at birth, they can involve any of the body systems. Major anomalies causing serious problems include the following.
- **Congenital heart disease:** Atrial septal defects, ventricular septal defects, coarctation of the aorta, tetralogy of Fallot, transposition of the great vessels, stenosis, atresia of valves
- **Neurological defects:** Neural tube defects, hydrocephalus, anencephaly, encephalocele, meningocele, myelomeningocele
- **Gastrointestinal problems:** Cleft lip/palate, diaphragmatic hernia, imperforate anus, tracheoesophageal fistula/esophageal atresia, duodenal atresia, omphalocele, gastroschisis, umbilical hernia, intestinal obstruction
- **Musculoskeletal deformities:** Clubfoot, polydactyly, developmental dysplasia of the hip
- **Genitourinary deformities:** Hypospadias, epispadias, exstrophy of the bladder
- **Metabolic disorders:** Phenylketonuria, galactosemia, hypothyroidism
- **Chromosomal abnormalities**

Congenital anomalies are generally identified soon after birth by Apgar scoring and a brief assessment indicating the need for further investigation. Once identified, congenital anomalies are treated in a pediatric setting.
- **Cleft lip/palate:** Failure of the lip or hard or soft palate to fuse
- **Tracheoesophageal atresia:** Failure of the esophagus to connect to the stomach
- **Duodenal atresia:** Common in newborns who have Down syndrome; when the first part of the small bowel has not developed properly and is not open, and stomach contents are unable to pass. Surgical intervention is required.
- **Phenylketonuria (PKU):** Inability to metabolize the amino acid phenylalanine
- **Galactosemia:** Inability to metabolize galactose into glucose
- **Hypothyroidism:** Slow metabolism caused by maternal iodine deficiency or maternal antithyroid medications during pregnancy
- **Neurologic anomalies (spina bifida):** A neural tube defect in which the vertebral arch fails to close
- **Hydrocephalus:** Excessive spinal fluid accumulation in the ventricles of the brain
- **Patent ductus arteriosus:** A noncyanotic heart defect in which the ductus arteriosus connecting the pulmonary artery and the aorta fails to close after birth
- **Tetralogy of Fallot:** Cyanotic heart defect characterized by a ventricular septal defect, the aorta positioned over the ventricular septal defect, stenosis of the pulmonary valve, and hypertrophy of the right ventricle
- **Down syndrome:** Trisomy 21, which is the most common trisomic abnormality with 47 chromosomes in each cell

ASSESSMENT

RISK FACTORS

GENETIC AND/OR ENVIRONMENTAL FACTORS
- Maternal age greater than 40 years
- Chromosome abnormalities, such as Down syndrome
- Viral infections, such as rubella
- Excessive body heat exposure during the first trimester (neural tube defects)
- Medications and substance use during pregnancy
- Maternal obesity
- Radiation exposure
- Maternal metabolic disorders (phenylketonuria, diabetes mellitus)
- Poor maternal nutrition such as folic acid deficiency (neural tube defects)
- Newborns who are preterm
- Newborns who are SGA
- Oligohydramnios or polyhydramnios

EXPECTED FINDINGS

Monitor the newborn for evidence of congenital anomalies.

Cleft lip/palate: Opening in the lip or palate

Tracheoesophageal atresia: Excessive mucous secretions and drooling, periodic cyanotic episodes and choking, abdominal distention after birth, immediate regurgitation after birth

Duodenal atresia: Abdominal distention, bilious vomiting, failure to pass meconium in the first 24 hr

PKU: Can result in cognitive impairment if untreated; not evident at birth, but will be identified with neonatal screening

Galactosemia: Can result in failure to thrive, cataracts, jaundice, cirrhosis of the liver, sepsis, and cognitive impairment if untreated; this will not be evident at birth, but will be identified with neonatal screening

Hypothyroidism: Can result in hypothermia, poor feeding, lethargy, jaundice, and cretinism if untreated

Neurologic anomalies (spina bifida): Protrusion of the meninges and/or spinal cord

Hydrocephalus: Enlarged head and bulging fontanels; sun-setting sign is common in which the whites of the eyes are visible above the iris

Patent ductus arteriosus: Murmurs, abnormal heart rate or rhythm, breathlessness, and fatigue while feeding

Tetralogy of Fallot: Respiratory difficulties, cyanosis, tachycardia, tachypnea, and diaphoresis

Down syndrome: Oblique palpebral fissures or upward slant of eyes, epicanthal folds, flat facial profile with a depressed nasal bridge and a small nose, protruding tongue, small low-set ears, short broad hands with a fifth finger that has one flexion crease instead of two, a deep crease across the center of the palm (frequently referred to as a simian crease), hyperflexibility, hypotonic muscles

NURSING ASSESSMENT

- Newborn's ability to take in adequate nourishment
- Newborn's ability to eliminate waste products
- Vital signs and axillary temperature
- Newborn-parental bonding, observing the parent's response to the diagnosis of a congenital defect, and encouraging the parents to verbalize concerns ☰PCC

DIAGNOSTIC AND THERAPEUTIC PROCEDURES

- Prenatal screening for congenital anomalies can be done by ultrasound and multiple-marker screening (triple and quad screen).
- Confirmation of a diagnosis depends on the anomaly.
- Prenatal diagnosis or confirmation of congenital anomalies is often made by amniocentesis, chorionic villi sampling, or ultrasound.

- Routine testing of newborns for metabolic disorders (inborn errors of metabolism)
  - A Guthrie test for PKU is done to show elevations of phenylalanine in the blood and urine. It is not reliable until the newborn has ingested sufficient amounts of protein.
  - Monitor blood and urine levels of galactose (galactosemia).
  - Measure thyroxine (hypothyroidism).
  - Cytologic studies (karyotyping of chromosomes), such as a buccal smear, uses cells scraped from the mucosa from inside the newborn's mouth.

PATIENT-CENTERED CARE

NURSING CARE

Nursing interventions for congenital anomalies are dependent upon the type and extent of the anomaly.
- Establish and maintain adequate respiratory status.
- Establish and maintain extrauterine circulation.
- Establish and maintain adequate thermoregulation.
- Administer medications as prescribed, such as thyroid replacement for hypothyroidism.
- Educate the parents regarding preoperative and postoperative treatment procedures.
- Encourage the parents to hold, touch, and talk to the newborn.
- Ensure that parents provide consistent care to the newborn.
- Provide parents with information about parent groups or support systems.

Neurologic anomalies (spina bifida)

- Protect the membrane with a sterile covering and plastic to prevent drying.
- Observe for leakage of cerebrospinal fluid.
- Handle the newborn gently by positioning him prone to prevent trauma.
- Prevent infection by keeping the area free from contamination by urine and feces.
- Measure the circumference of the newborn's head to identify hydrocephalus.
- Assess the newborn for increased intracranial pressure.

Hydrocephalus

- Frequently reposition the newborn's head to prevent sores.
- Measure the newborn's head circumference daily.
- Assess for manifestations of increased intracranial pressure, such as vomiting and a shrill cry.

Patent ductus arteriosus

Educate the parents about surgical treatment.

Tetralogy of Fallot

- Conserve the newborn's energy to reduce the workload on the heart.
- Administer gavage feedings, or give oral feedings with a specialized nipple.
- Elevate the newborn's head and shoulders to improve respirations and reduce the cardiac workload.
- Prevent infection.
- Place the newborn in a knee-chest position during respiratory distress.

Cleft lip/palate

- Encourage expression of parental concerns, grief, and fears.
- Monitor the newborn's weight daily while hospitalized.
- Monitor for manifestations of dehydration.
- Encourage parental attachment.
- Suction nose and mouth gently with bulb syringe as needed to clear airway.
- Position infant facilitate drainage of sections.
- Educate parents on feeding requirements of infants.

NUTRITION

Provide adequate nutrition.

Cleft lip/palate: Determine the most effective nipple for feeding. Can use specialized bottles, cups, or syringes to feed the infant. Infants who have cleft lip can achieve breastfeeding with changes in positioning. Feed the newborn in the upright position to decrease aspiration risk. Feed the newborn slowly, and burp him frequently so that he does not swallow air. Cleanse his mouth with water after feedings.

Tracheoesophageal atresia: Withhold feedings until esophageal patency is determined. Elevate the head of the newborn's crib to prevent gastric juice reflux. Supervise the first feeding to observe for this anomaly.

Duodenal atresia: Withhold feedings until surgical repair is done and the newborn has begun to pass stools. Administer IV fluids as prescribed. Monitor for jaundice.

PKU: Specialized synthetic formula in which phenylalanine is removed or reduced. The mother should restrict meat, dairy products, diet drinks (artificial sweeteners), and protein during pregnancy. Aspartame must be avoided.

Galactosemia: Give the newborn a soy-based formula because galactose is present in milk. Eliminate lactose and galactose in the newborn's diet. Breastfeeding is also contraindicated.

PRACTICE Active Learning Scenario

A nurse educator is reviewing hyperbilirubinemia with a newly hired nurse. What should the nurse educator include in this review? Use the ATI Active Learning Template: System Disorder to complete this item.

ALTERATION IN HEALTH (DIAGNOSIS): Describe the difference between physiologic and pathologic jaundice, acute bilirubin encephalopathy, and kernicterus.

DIAGNOSTIC PROCEDURES: Describe the procedure that can be used to verify the presence of jaundice.

NURSING CARE: Describe care of the infant receiving phototherapy.

Application Exercises

1. A nurse is caring for a client who is at 42 weeks gestation and in labor. The client asks the nurse what should she expect because her baby is postmature. Which of the following statements should the nurse make?

   A. "Your baby will have excess body fat."

   B. "Your baby will have flat areola without breast buds."

   C. "Your baby's heels will easily move to his ears."

   D. "Your baby's skin will have a leathery appearance."

2. A nurse is caring for an infant who has a high bilirubin level and is receiving phototherapy. Which of the following is the priority finding in the newborn?

   A. Conjunctivitis

   B. Bronze skin discoloration

   C. Sunken fontanels

   D. Maculopapular skin rash

3. A nurse is called to the birthing room to assist with the assessment of a newborn who was born at 32 weeks of gestation. The newborn's birth weight is 1,100 g. Which of the following are expected findings in this newborn? (Select all that apply.)

   A. Lanugo

   B. Long nails

   C. Weak grasp reflex

   D. Translucent skin

   E. Plump face

4. A nurse is caring for a newborn who is preterm and has respiratory distress syndrome. Which of the following should the nurse monitor to evaluate the newborn's condition following administration of synthetic surfactant?

   A. Oxygen saturation

   B. Body temperature

   C. Serum bilirubin

   D. Heart rate

5. A nurse is teaching a newly licensed nurse about neonatal abstinence syndrome. Which of the following statements by the newly licensed nurse indicate understanding of the teaching?

   A. "The newborn will have decreased muscle tone."

   B. "The newborn will have a continuous high-pitched cry."

   C. "The newborn will sleeps for 2 to 3 hours after a feeding."

   D. "The newborn will have mild tremors when disturbed."

Application Exercises Key

1.   A. Excess body fat is seen in a newborn who is macrosomic.

    B. Flat areolas without breast buds are seen in a newborn who is preterm.

    C. Heels that are movable fully to the ears are seen in newborn who is preterm.

    D. **CORRECT:** Leathery, cracked, and wrinkled skin is seen in a newborn who is postmature due to placental insufficiency.

    Ⓝ *NCLEX® Connection: Health Promotion and Maintenance, Ante/Intra/Postpartum and Newborn Care*

2.   A. Conjunctivitis is an important finding, but it is not the priority.

    B. Bronze skin discoloration is an important finding, but it is not the priority.

    C. **CORRECT:** Using the safety and risk reduction framework, sunken fontanels is the priority finding. Infants receiving phototherapy are at risk for dehydration from loose stools due to increased bilirubin excretion.

    D. Maculopapular skin rash is an important finding, but it is not the priority.

    Ⓝ *NCLEX® Connection: Physiological Adaptation, Alterations in Body Systems*

3.   A. **CORRECT:** Characteristics of a preterm newborn include the presence of abundant lanugo.

    B. Long nails are a finding in a newborn who is postmature.

    C. **CORRECT:** A weak grasp reflex is characteristic of a preterm newborn.

    D. **CORRECT:** Skin that is thin, smooth, shiny, and translucent is a finding in a preterm newborn.

    E. A plump face would be observed in a newborn who is macrosomic.

    Ⓝ *NCLEX® Connection: Health Promotion and Maintenance, Health Screening*

4.   A. **CORRECT:** Surfactant stabilizes the alveoli and helps increase oxygen saturation.

    B. Surfactant administration has no direct effect on body temperature.

    C. Surfactant administration has no direct effect on bilirubin levels.

    D. Surfactant administration has no direct effect on heart rate.

    Ⓝ *NCLEX® Connection: Pharmacological and Parenteral Therapies, Expected Actions/Outcomes*

5.   A. Increased muscle tone is seen in a newborn who has neonatal abstinence syndrome.

    B. **CORRECT:** A continuous high-pitched cry is often an indication of CNS disturbances in a newborn who has neonatal abstinence syndrome.

    C. A newborn who has neonatal abstinence syndrome can have sleep pattern disturbances and would have difficulty sleeping for 2 to 3 hr after feeding.

    D. A newborn who has neonatal abstinence syndrome often has moderate to severe tremors when undisturbed. Most newborns exhibit mild tremors when disturbed.

    Ⓝ *NCLEX® Connection: Physiological Adaptation, Illness Management*

PRACTICE Answer

Using the ATI Active Learning Template: System Disorder

ALTERATION IN HEALTH (DIAGNOSIS)

- Physiologic jaundice is considered benign (resulting from normal newborn physiology of increased bilirubin production due to the shortened lifespan and breakdown of fetal RBCs and liver immaturity). The newborn who has physiological jaundice exhibits an increase in unconjugated bilirubin levels 72 to 120 hr after birth, with a rapid decline to 3 mg/dL 5 to 10 days after birth.
- Pathologic jaundice is a result of an underlying disease. Pathologic jaundice appears before 24 hr of age or is persistent after day 14. In the term newborn, bilirubin levels increase more than 0.5 mg/dL/hr, peaks at greater than 12.9 mg/dL, or is associated with anemia and hepatosplenomegaly. Pathologic jaundice is usually caused by a blood group incompatibility or an infection, but can be the result of RBC disorders.
- Acute bilirubin encephalopathy is when the bilirubin is deposited in the brain. This occurs once all of the binding sites for the bilirubin are used within the body, resulting in necrosis of neurons. Bilirubin levels greater than 25 mg/dL place the newborn at risk for permanent damage, including dystonia, athetosis, upward gaze, hearing loss, and cognitive impairments.
- Kernicterus is an irreversible, chronic result of bilirubin toxicity. The newborn demonstrates many of the same manifestations of bilirubin encephalopathy with hypotonia, severe cognitive impairments, and spastic quadriplegia.

Ⓝ *NCLEX® Connection: Physiological Adaptation, Alterations in Body Systems*

DIAGNOSTIC PROCEDURES: Press the newborn's skin on the cheek or abdomen lightly with one finger. Then release pressure, and observe for a yellowish tint to the skin as the skin is blanched.

NURSING CARE

Maintain an eye mask over the newborn's eyes.

Keep the newborn undressed. Place a mask (like a bikini) over the genitalia of a male newborn.

Remove the newborn from phototherapy every 4 hr, and unmask the eyes.

Reposition the newborn every 2 hr to expose all body surfaces to the phototherapy lights and prevent pressure sores.

Check the lamp energy with a photometer following facility protocol.

Turn off the phototherapy lights before drawing blood for testing.

References

Berman, A., Snyder, S., & Frandsen, G. (2016). *Kozier & Erb's fundamentals of nursing: Concepts, process, and practice* (10th ed.). Upper Saddle River, NJ: Prentice-Hall.

Burchum, J. R., & Rosenthal, L. D. (2016). *Lehne's pharmacology for nursing care* (9th ed.). St. Louis: Elsevier.

Dudek, S. G. (2014). *Nutrition essentials for nursing practice* (7th ed.). Philadelphia: Lippincott Williams & Wilkins.

Grodner, M., Escott-Stump, S., & Dorner, S. (2016). *Nutritional foundations and clinical applications of nutrition: A nursing approach* (6th ed.). St. Louis, MO: Mosby.

Halter, M. J. (2014). *Varcarolis' foundations of psychiatric mental health nursing: A clinical approach* (7th ed.). St. Louis, MO: Saunders.

Hockenberry, M. J., & Wilson, D. (2015) *Wong's nursing care of infants and children* (10th ed.). St. Louis, MO: Mosby.

Lowdermilk, D. L., Perry, S. E., Cashion, M. C., & Aldean, K. R. (2016). *Maternity & women's health care* (11th ed.). St. Louis, MO: Elsevier.

Pagana, K. D. & Pagana, T. J. (2014). *Mosby's manual of diagnostic and laboratory tests* (5th ed.). St. Louis, MO: Elsevier.

Pillitteri, A. (2014). *Maternal and child health nursing: Care of the childbearing and childrearing family* (7th ed.). Philadelphia: Lippincott Williams & Wilkins

Potter, P. A., Perry, A. G., Stockert, P., & Hall, A. (2013). *Fundamentals of nursing* (8th ed.). St. Louis, MO: Mosby.

Skidmore-Roth, L. (2016). *Mosby's 2016 nursing drug reference* (29th ed.). St. Louis, MO: Elsevier.

Taketomo, C. K., Hodding, J. H., & Kraus D. M. (2014). *Lexi-Comp's pediatric & neonatal dosage handbook: A comprehensive resource for all clinicians treating pediatric and neonatal patients (pediatric dosage handbook)* (21st ed.). Hudson, Ohio: Lexi-Comp.

STUDENT NAME _____

CONCEPT_____ REVIEW MODULE CHAPTER_____

Related Content

(E.G., DELEGATION,
LEVELS OF PREVENTION,
ADVANCE DIRECTIVES)

Underlying Principles

Nursing Interventions

WHO? WHEN? WHY? HOW?

STUDENT NAME _____

PROCEDURE NAME _____ REVIEW MODULE CHAPTER_____

Description of Procedure

Indications

Interpretation of Findings

Potential Complications

CONSIDERATIONS

Nursing Interventions (pre, intra, post)

Client Education

Nursing Interventions

Growth and Development

STUDENT NAME _____

DEVELOPMENTAL STAGE _____   REVIEW MODULE CHAPTER_____

EXPECTED GROWTH AND DEVELOPMENT

Physical Development	Cognitive Development	Psychosocial Development	Age-Appropriate Activities

Health Promotion

Immunizations	Health Screening	Nutrition	Injury Prevention

ACTIVE LEARNING TEMPLATE: *Medication*

STUDENT NAME _____

MEDICATION _____ REVIEW MODULE CHAPTER_____

CATEGORY CLASS_____

PURPOSE OF MEDICATION

Expected Pharmacological Action

Therapeutic Use

Complications

Medication Administration

Contraindications/Precautions

Nursing Interventions

Interactions

Client Education

Evaluation of Medication Effectiveness

STUDENT NAME _____

SKILL NAME_____ REVIEW MODULE CHAPTER_____

Description of Skill

Indications

CONSIDERATIONS

Nursing Interventions (pre, intra, post)

Outcomes/Evaluation

Client Education

Potential Complications

Nursing Interventions

System Disorder

STUDENT NAME _____

DISORDER/DISEASE PROCESS _____ REVIEW MODULE CHAPTER_____

Alterations in Health (Diagnosis)

Pathophysiology Related to Client Problem

Health Promotion and Disease Prevention

ASSESSMENT

Risk Factors

Expected Findings

Laboratory Tests

Diagnostic Procedures

SAFETY CONSIDERATIONS

PATIENT-CENTERED CARE

Nursing Care

Medications

Client Education

Therapeutic Procedures

Interprofessional Care

Complications

STUDENT NAME _____

PROCEDURE NAME _____ REVIEW MODULE CHAPTER_____

Description of Procedure

Indications

CONSIDERATIONS

Nursing Interventions (pre, intra, post)

Outcomes/Evaluation

Client Education

Potential Complications

Nursing Interventions